Blood and Circulatory Disorders

SOURCEBOOK

Fourth Edition

Health Reference Series

Fourth Edition

Blood and Circulatory Disorders

SOURCEBOOK

*Basic Consumer Health Information about Blood and
Circulatory System Disorders, Such as Anemia, Leukemia,
Lymphoma, Rh Disease, Hemophilia, Thrombophilia, Other
Bleeding and Clotting Deficiencies, and Artery, Vascular, and
Venous Diseases, Including Facts about Blood Types, Blood
Donation, Bone Marrow and Stem Cell Transplants, Tests and
Medications, and Tips for Maintaining Circulatory Health*

*Along with a Glossary of Related Terms and a List of
Resources for Additional Help and Information*

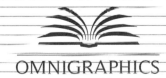

OMNIGRAPHICS

615 Griswold, Ste. 901, Detroit, MI 48226

Bibliographic Note
Because this page cannot legibly accommodate all the copyright notices, the Bibliographic Note portion of the Preface constitutes an extension of the copyright notice.

* * *

Health Reference Series
Keith Jones, *Managing Editor*
***

OMNIGRAPHICS
A PART OF RELEVANT INFORMATION
***

Copyright © 2016 Omnigraphics
ISBN 978-0-7808-1476-9
E-ISBN 978-0-7808-1475-2

Library of Congress Cataloging-in-Publication Data

Names: Omnigraphics, Inc.

Title: Blood and circulatory disorders sourcebook: basic consumer health information about blood and circulatory system disorders, such as anemia, leukemia, lymphoma, Rh disease, hemophilia, thrombophilia, other bleeding and clotting deficiencies, and artery, vascular, and venous diseases, including facts about blood types, blood donation, bone marrow and stem cell transplants, tests and medications, and tips for maintaining circulatory health; along with a glossary of related terms and a list of resources for additional help and information.

Description: Fourth edition. | Detroit, MI: Omnigraphics, [2016] | Series: Health reference series | Includes bibliographical references and index.

Identifiers: LCCN 2016024898 (print) | LCCN 2016025720 (ebook) | ISBN 9780780814769 (hardcover: alk. paper) | ISBN 9780780814752 (ebook) | ISBN 9780780814752 (eBook)

Subjects: LCSH: Blood--Diseases--Popular works. | Blood-vessels--Diseases--Popular works.

Classification: LCC RC636 .B556 2016 (print) | LCC RC636 (ebook) | DDC 616.1/3--dc23

LC record available at https://lccn.loc.gov/2016024898

Table of Contents

Part III: Blood Disorders

Part IV: Bleeding and Clotting Disorders

Part V: Circulatory Disorders

Part VI: Additional Help and Information

Preface

About This Book

Blood plays many important roles in the human body. It carries oxygen and nutrients to the body's cells, helps fight infection, and works to heal wounds. When a disorder inhibits its ability to meet the body's needs or prevents blood from flowing or coagulating properly, a myriad of problems can result. According to the Centers for Disease Control and Prevention (CDC), millions of people across the United States of all ages, race, sex, and socioeconomic status are affected by blood disorders such as anemia, sickle cell disease, and haemophilia.

Blood and Circulatory Disorders Sourcebook, Fourth Edition, offers facts about blood function and composition, the maintenance of a healthy circulatory system, and the types of concerns that arise when processes go awry. It discusses the diagnosis and treatment of many common blood cell disorders, bleeding disorders, and circulatory disorders, including anemia, hemochromatosis, leukemia, lymphoma, hemophilia, hypercoagulation, thrombophilia, atherosclerosis, blood pressure irregularities, coronary artery and heart disease, and peripheral vascular disease. Blood donation, cord blood banking, blood transfusions, and bone marrow and stem cell transplants are also discussed. The book concludes with a glossary of related terms and a list of resources for further help and information.

How to Use This Book

This book is divided into parts and chapters. Parts focus on broad areas of interest. Chapters are devoted to single topics within a part.

Part I: Understanding Blood and the Circulatory System explains the composition and types of blood and how it functions in the body. It also describes blood donation and cord blood banking procedures. The part concludes with information on maintaining a healthy circulatory system and how aging affects the heart and blood vessels.

Part II: Diagnosing and Treating Blood and Circulatory Disorders provides information about medical tests commonly used to identify and monitor blood and circulatory disorders. It offers facts about many of the medications often used in the treatment of these disorders and discusses such procedures as blood transfusion and bone marrow transplants.

Part III: Blood Disorders describes ailments that affect the composition of the blood itself. These include anemia and other hemoglobin disorders, cancers of the blood, plasma cell disorders, and white blood cell disorders. Information about the causes of these disorders is provided, and treatment strategies are discussed.

Part IV: Bleeding and Clotting Disorders provides information about bleeding disorders resulting from insufficient clotting, such as hemophilia and von Willebrand disease, and those resulting from excess clotting, including deep vein thrombosis and pulmonary embolism. Methods of diagnosis and treatment options are included.

Part V: Circulatory Disorders describes disorders affecting the veins, arteries, and heart. It includes information about aneurysms, stroke, blood pressure irregularities, atherosclerosis, carotid artery disease, coronary artery disease, heart disease, peripheral vascular disease, and venous disorders such as arteriovenous malformation and varicose veins. Information about causes and diagnosis, as well as treatment options, is provided.

Part VI: Additional Help and Information includes a glossary of terms related to blood and circulatory disorders and a directory of resources offering additional help and support.

Bibliographic Note

This volume contains documents and excerpts from publications issued by the following U.S. government agencies: Agency for

Healthcare Research and Quality (AHRQ); Centers for Disease Control and Prevention (CDC); Centers for Medicare and Medicaid Services (CMS); *Eunice Kennedy Shriver* National Institute of Child Health and Human Development (NICHD); Genetic and Rare Diseases Information Center (GARD); Health Resources and Services Administration (HRSA); National Cancer Institute (NCI); National Center for Complementary and Integrative Health (NCCIH); National Heart Lung and Blood Institute (NHLBI); National Institute of Arthritis and Musculoskeletal and Skin Diseases (NIAMS); National Institute of Diabetes and Digestive and Kidney Diseases (NIDDK); National Institute of General Medical Sciences (NIGMS); National Institute of Neurological Disorders and Stroke (NINDS); National Institute on Aging (NIA); National Institute of Allergy and Infectious Diseases (NIAID); National Institutes of Health (NIH); and U.S. Food and Drug Administration (FDA).

In addition, this volume contains copyrighted documents from the following organization: The Nemours Foundation

It may also contain original material produced by Omnigraphics and reviewed by medical consultants.

About the Health Reference Series

The *Health Reference Series* is designed to provide basic medical information for patients, families, caregivers, and the general public. Each volume takes a particular topic and provides comprehensive coverage. This is especially important for people who may be dealing with a newly diagnosed disease or a chronic disorder in themselves or in a family member. People looking for preventive guidance, information about disease warning signs, medical statistics, and risk factors for health problems will also find answers to their questions in the *Health Reference Series*. The *Series*, however, is not intended to serve as a tool for diagnosing illness, in prescribing treatments, or as a substitute for the physician/patient relationship. All people concerned about medical symptoms or the possibility of disease are encouraged to seek professional care from an appropriate health care provider.

A Note about Spelling and Style

Health Reference Series editors use *Stedman's Medical Dictionary* as an authority for questions related to the spelling of medical terms and the *Chicago Manual of Style* for questions related to grammatical structures, punctuation, and other editorial concerns. Consistent adherence is not always possible, however, because the individual volumes within the *Series* include many documents from a wide variety of different producers, and the editor's primary goal is to present material from each source as accurately as is possible. This sometimes means that information in different chapters or sections may follow other guidelines and alternate spelling authorities.

Medical Review

Omnigraphics contracts with a team of qualified, senior medical professionals who serve as medical consultants for the *Health Reference Series*. As necessary, medical consultants review reprinted and originally written material for currency and accuracy. Citations including the phrase, "Reviewed (month, year)" indicate material reviewed by this team. Medical consultation services are provided to the *Health Reference Series* editors by:

Dr. Vijayalakshmi, MBBS, DGO, MD
Dr. Senthil Selvan, MBBS, DCH, MD
Dr. K. Sivanandham, MBBS, DCH, MS (Research), PhD

Our Advisory Board

We would like to thank the following board members for providing initial guidance on the development of this series:

- Dr. Lynda Baker, Associate Professor of Library and Information Science, Wayne State University, Detroit, MI

- Nancy Bulgarelli, William Beaumont Hospital Library, Royal Oak, MI

- Karen Imarisio, Bloomfield Township Public Library, Bloomfield Township, MI

- Karen Morgan, Mardigian Library, University of Michigan-Dearborn, Dearborn, MI

- Rosemary Orlando, St. Clair Shores Public Library, St. Clair Shores, MI

Health Reference Series *Update Policy*

The inaugural book in the *Health Reference Series* was the first edition of *Cancer Sourcebook* published in 1989. Since then, the *Series* has been enthusiastically received by librarians and in the medical community. In order to maintain the standard of providing high-quality health information for the layperson the editorial staff at Omnigraphics felt it was necessary to implement a policy of updating volumes when warranted.

Medical researchers have been making tremendous strides, and it is the purpose of the *Health Reference Series* to stay current with the most recent advances. Each decision to update a volume is made on an individual basis. Some of the considerations include how much new information is available and the feedback we receive from people who use the books. If there is a topic you would like to see added to the update list, or an area of medical concern you feel has not been adequately addressed, please write to:

Managing Editor
Health Reference Series
Omnigraphics
615 Griswold, Ste. 901
Detroit, MI 48226

Part One

Understanding Blood and the Circulatory System

Chapter 1

Blood Function and Composition

Anatomy

Blood is one of the connective tissues. As a connective tissue, it consists of cells and cell fragments (formed elements) suspended in an intercellular matrix (plasma). Blood is the only liquid tissue in the body that measures about 5 liters in the adult human and accounts for 8 percent of the body weight.

The body consists of metabolically active cells that need a continuous supply of nutrients and oxygen. Metabolic waste products need to be removed from the cells to maintain a stable cellular environment. Blood is the primary transport medium that is responsible for meeting these cellular demands.

Blood cells are formed in the bone marrow, the soft, spongy center of bones. New (immature) blood cells are called blasts. Some blasts stay in the marrow to mature. Some travel to other parts of the body to mature.

The activities of the blood may be categorized as transportation, regulation, and protection.

These functional categories overlap and interact as the blood carries out its role in providing suitable conditions for cellular functions.

This chapter includes text excerpted from "Anatomy," National Cancer Institute (NCI), April 7, 2004. Reviewed July 2016.

The transport functions include:

- Carrying oxygen and nutrients to the cells.

- Transporting carbon dioxide and nitrogenous wastes from the tissues to the lungs and kidneys where these wastes can be removed from the body.

- Carrying hormones from the endocrine glands to the target tissues.

The regulation functions include:

- Helping regulate body temperature by removing heat from active areas, such as skeletal muscles, and transporting it to other regions or to the skin where it can be dissipated.

- Playing a significant role in fluid and electrolyte balance because the salts and plasma proteins contribute to the osmotic pressure.

- Functioning in pH regulation through the action of buffers in the blood.

The protection functions include:

- Preventing fluid loss through hemorrhage when blood vessels are damaged due to its clotting mechanisms.

- Helping (phagocytic white blood cells) to protect the body against microorganisms that cause disease by engulfing and destroying the agent.

- Protecting (antibodies in the plasma) against disease by their reactions with offending agents.

Composition of the Blood

When a sample of blood is spun in a centrifuge, the cells and cell fragments are separated from the liquid intercellular matrix. Because the formed elements are heavier than the liquid matrix, they are packed in the bottom of the tube by the centrifugal force. The light yellow colored liquid on the top is the plasma, which accounts for about 55 percent of the blood volume. The percentage of the total blood volume that is occupied by red blood cells is called the hematocrit, or packed cell volume (PCV). The white blood cells and platelets form a thin white layer, called the "buffy coat," between plasma and red blood cells.

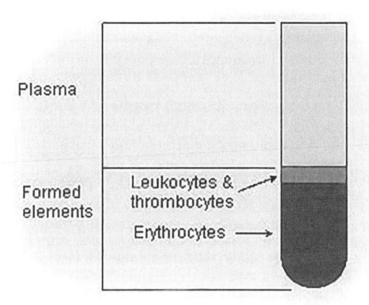

Figure 1.1. *Blood Components*

Plasma

The watery fluid portion of blood (90 percent water) in which the corpuscular elements are suspended. It transports nutrients as well as wastes throughout the body. Various compounds, including proteins, electrolytes, carbohydrates, minerals, and fats, are dissolved in it.

Formed Elements

The formed elements are cells and cell fragments suspended in the plasma. The three classes of formed elements are the erythrocytes (red blood cells), leukocytes (white blood cells), and the thrombocytes (platelets).

Erythrocytes (Red Blood Cells)

Erythrocytes, or red blood cells, are the most numerous of the formed elements. Erythrocytes are tiny biconcave disks, thin in the middle and thicker around the periphery. The shape provides a combination of flexibility for moving through tiny capillaries with a maximum surface area for the diffusion of gases. The primary function of erythrocytes is to transport oxygen and, to a lesser extent, carbon dioxide.

Leukocytes (White Blood Cells)

Leukocytes, or white blood cells, are generally larger than erythrocytes, but they are fewer in number. Even though they are considered to be blood cells, leukocytes do most of their work in the tissues. They use the blood as a transport medium. Some are phagocytic, others produce antibodies; some secrete histamine and heparin, and others neutralize histamine. Leukocytes are able to move through the capillary walls into the tissue spaces, a process called diapedesis. In the tissue spaces they provide a defense against organisms that cause disease and either promote or inhibit inflammatory responses.

There are two main groups of leukocytes in the blood. The cells that develop granules in the cytoplasm are called granulocytes and those that do not have granules are called agranulocytes. Neutrophils, eosinophils, and basophils are granulocytes. Monocytes and lymphocytes are agranulocytes.

Neutrophils, the most numerous leukocytes, are phagocytic and have light-colored granules. Eosinophils have granules and help counteract the effects of histamine. Basophils secrete histomine and heparin and have blue granules. In the tissues, they are called mast cells. Lymphocytes are agranulocytes that have a special role in immune processes. Some attack bacteria directly; others produce antibodies.

Thrombocytes (Platelets)

Thrombocytes, or platelets, are not complete cells, but are small fragments of very large cells called megakaryocytes. Megakaryocytes develop from hemocytoblasts in the red bone marrow. Thrombocytes become sticky and clump together to form platelet plugs that close breaks and tears in blood vessels. They also initiate the formation of blood clots.

Blood Cell Lineage

The production of formed elements, or blood cells, is called hemopoiesis. Before birth, hemopoiesis occurs primarily in the liver and spleen, but some cells develop in the thymus, lymph nodes, and red bone marrow. After birth, most production is limited to red bone marrow in specific regions, but some white blood cells are produced in lymphoid tissue.

All types of formed elements develop from a single cell type—stem cell (pleuripotential cells or hemocytoblasts). Seven different cell lines, each controlled by a specific growth factor, develop from the hemocytoblast. When a stem cell divides, one of the "daughters" remains a stem cell and the other becomes a precursor cell, either a lymphoid cell or a myeloid cell. These cells continue to mature into various blood cells.

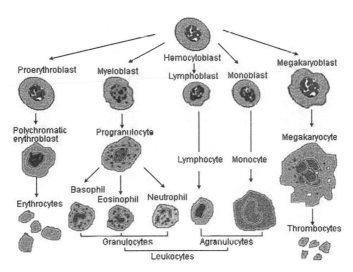

Figure 1.2. *Lineage*

Leukemia can develop at any point in cell differentiation. The illustration above shows the development of the formed elements of the blood.

Chapter 2

Blood Types

About 5 million Americans need blood transfusions every year, for all sorts of reasons. Sometimes, a transfusion is an emergency (like losing blood after an accident). Sometimes it's expected (as with treatment for cancer). Whatever the reason, blood transfusions are one of the most common hospital rules.

While transfusions are common, there's a lot more to them than just taking blood from one person and using it to help someone else. It's very important to keep the blood supply safe. So, each unit of blood goes through many tests to check for infectious diseases and establish the blood type.

Four Blood Groups

It might seem like blood is blood—it all looks pretty much the same to the naked eye. But although all blood contains the same basic components (red cells, white cells, platelets, and plasma), not everyone has the same types of **markers** on the surface of their red blood cells. These markers (also called **antigens**) are proteins and sugars that our bodies use to identify the blood cells as belonging in our own system.

Blood cell markers are microscopic. But they can make the difference between blood being accepted or rejected after a transfusion. So medical experts group blood into types based on the different markers.

This chapter includes text excerpted from "Blood Types," ©1995–2016. The Nemours Foundation/KidsHealth®. Reprinted with permission.

The four main blood groups are:

1. **Type A.** This blood type has a marker known as "A."

2. **Type B.** This blood type has a marker known as "B."

3. **Type AB**. The blood cells in this type have both A and B markers.

4. **Type O.** This blood type has neither A or B markers.

Plus Rh Factor

Some people have an additional marker, called Rh factor, in their blood. Because each of the four main blood groups (A, B, AB, and O) may or may not have Rh factor, scientists further classify blood as either "positive" (meaning it has Rh factor) or "negative" (without Rh factor).

Having any of these markers (or none of them) doesn't make a person's blood any healthier or stronger. It's just a genetic difference, like having green eyes instead of blue or straight hair instead of curly.

Make Eight Blood Types

The different markers that can be found in blood make up eight possible blood types:

1. **O negative.** This blood type doesn't have A or B markers, and it doesn't have Rh factor.

2. **O positive.** This blood type doesn't have A or B markers, but it does have Rh factor. O positive blood is one of the two most common blood types (the other being A positive).

3. **A negative.** This blood type has A marker only.

4. **A positive.** This blood type has A marker and Rh factor, but not B marker. Along with O positive, it's one of the two most common blood types.

5. **B negative.** This blood type has B marker only.

6. **B positive.** This blood type has B marker and Rh factor, but not A marker.

7. **AB negative.** This blood type has A and B markers, but not Rh factor.

8. **AB positive.** This blood type has all three types of markers—A, B, and Rh factor.

Blood banks and hospitals keep careful tabs on blood type to be sure that donated blood matches the blood type of the person receiving the transfusion. Giving someone the wrong blood type can cause serious health problems.

Why Blood Type Matters

The immune system produces proteins known as **antibodies** that act as protectors if foreign cells enter the body. **Depending on which blood type you have, your immune system will produce antibodies to react against other blood types.**

If a patient is given the wrong blood type, the antibodies immediately set out to destroy the invading cells. This aggressive, whole-body response can give someone a fever, chills, and low blood pressure. It can even lead vital body systems—like breathing or kidneys—to fail.

Here's an example of how the blood type-antibody process works: Let's say you have Type A blood. Because your blood contains the A marker, it produces B antibodies. If B markers (found in Type B or AB blood) enter your body, your Type A immune system gets fired up against them. That means you can only get a transfusion from someone with A or O blood, not from someone with B or AB blood.

In the same way, if you have the B marker, your body produces A antibodies. So as a person with Type B blood, you could get a transfusion from someone with B or O blood, but not A or AB.

Things are a little different for people with Type AB or Type O blood. If you have both A and B markers on the surface of your cells (Type AB blood), your body does not need to fight the presence of either. **This means that someone with AB blood can get a transfusion from someone with A, B, AB, or O blood.**

But if you have Type O blood, meaning your red blood cells have neither A or B markers, your body will have both A and B antibodies and will therefore feel the need to defend itself against A, B, and AB blood. **So a person with O blood can only get a transfusion with O blood.**

Type O negative blood can be given to people with any blood type. That's because it has none of the markers that can set off a reaction. People with this blood type are considered "universal donors" and are in great demand at blood banks.

Because Type AB positive blood has all the markers, people with this type can receive any blood type. They're called "universal recipients."

Blood transfusions are one of the most frequent lifesaving procedures hospitals perform. So there's always a need for blood donors. About 15% of blood donors are high school and college students—an impressive number when you consider you have to be 16 or 17 to donate blood.

Chapter 3

Donating and Preserving Blood

Chapter Contents

Section 3.1

Blood Donation Overview

Blood Donation

Blood donation is a voluntary procedure in which one person gives some of their blood to help another person. People need to receive blood donations if they are having surgery, if they lost blood from an injury, or if they have certain illnesses such as hemophilia, sickle cell disease, anemia, or some types of cancer.

Blood Donors

A blood donor is a person who volunteers to give some of their blood through blood donation. Certain requirements must be met in order to become a blood donor. Blood donors must be healthy adults between the ages of 17 and 70 years who weigh at least 110 pounds and have normal blood pressure and body temperature. Donors are eligible to give blood once every 56 days.

Certain restrictions exist to protect both blood donors and blood donation recipients. People who are not able to donate blood include pregnant women, people who have recently had a tattoo or piercing, people who are ill, and those taking specific medications. People who have recently travelled to certain countries may also be disqualified from donating blood.

Blood Donation Process

Blood donations are typically collected at blood drives, blood banks, or at a medical facility. The process usually begins with a donor screening interview, which is conducted in private. During this interview, a health professional asks a series of questions to determine whether a person is able to donate blood. Questions may focus on past and present health conditions and personal behaviors such as drug use or sexually transmitted diseases. These questions are asked every time a person donates blood so that any changes in the donor's health can be identified.

After the initial screening interview, the blood donation process takes about ten minutes. About one pint (480 ml) of blood is collected from each blood donor. This amount is equal to about eight percent of the average adult's total blood volume. The donor's body will replace the volume of donated blood within 24 to 48 hours. The amount of red blood cells in that volume of blood will be replaced by the donor's body in ten to 12 weeks.

Blood donations are tested and screened to ensure the blood is safe to give to another person. These tests usually screen for blood-borne diseases such as hepatitis, HIV, West Nile virus, and other viruses. Blood that tests positive for any of the screened diseases is discarded as medical waste and the donor is notified of the test results so that they may seek treatment if needed. Donated blood is also checked to identify the blood type (A, B, AB, O).

Types of Donated Blood

Most donated blood is processed to separate the whole blood into the different components that make up human blood, such as platelets, plasma, and red blood cells. This is done because most blood donation recipients only need to receive a certain component of blood.

The different types of blood donation are:

- Whole blood that contains red and white blood cells, plasma, platelets, antibodies, and other components. This type of blood donation is called homologous.

- Plasma that is extracted from donated blood with a centrifuge, which is a machine that spins at a high rate of speed to separate the blood into its components. The plasma is then drawn out of the blood, and the red blood cells are returned to the donor. This type of blood donation is called apheresis.

- Platelets are extracted from blood using a different centrifuge process, and both red blood cells and the plasma are returned to the donor. This type of blood donation is called pheresis.

- Autologous donation refers to blood that is donated by a person for their own use. This type of blood donation is rare and is usually done in special cases.

- Directed or designated donation refers to blood that is donated for use by a specific person. This type of blood donation is also rare and done only in special cases.

Risks of Donating Blood

The blood donation process is safe and there are no health risks associated with donating blood. Sterile, prepackaged equipment is used to collect blood donations and new equipment is used for each donor. The blood donor may develop a small bruise on their arm at the site from which blood was drawn. Some blood donors feel light-headed or slightly dizzy after giving blood. For this reason, most blood donors are given water, fruit juice, and a small snack and asked to sit for a few minutes after their blood is collected. For the first few hours after donating blood, it is recommended that blood donors refrain from physical activity and drink plenty of fluids.

References

1. "Donating Blood: Topic Overview," WebMD. March 12, 2014.
2. "Blood Donation," Better Health. March 2013.

Section 3.2

Apheresis

This section includes text excerpted from "NIH Clinical Center Patient Education Materials Apheresis for Transfusion," National Institutes of Health (NIH), December 2015.

Apheresis is a type of procedure in which a machine draws whole blood from a patient, removes one type of cell (such as white blood cells or stem cells), then returns the rest of the blood to the patient.

Various types of machines are used to do apheresis. These machines use sterile, disposable parts to prevent blood-borne infections. The needs of your protocol will determine the type of machine used for your apheresis and how long the procedure will last.

Preparation

Eat Well

You may eat your usual foods, but avoid fatty foods (such as bacon, sausage, and hamburger) the night before and the morning of your procedure. Be sure to eat breakfast before arriving for your apheresis appointment, unless your nurse coordinator has told you otherwise.

Drink Enough Liquid

Drink at least 64 ounces of water, sports drinks, juice, or decaffeinated drinks per day for the 2 days prior to your procedure.

Wear Comfortable Clothing

Wear short sleeves and loose-fitting clothing. If you prefer to wear a hospital gown, the clinic staff can give you one.

Procedure

Before the Procedure

When you arrive in the clinic, a nurse will take your vital signs (temperature, pulse, blood pressure), prick your finger to test your hemoglobin level, and ask you to sign a consent form giving them permission to do apheresis. If you are donating cells for someone other than yourself, you will be asked a series of questions that help to make sure it is both safe for you to have the procedure and safe to give your cells to another person. It is important that you answer all of the questions honestly. Feel free to ask any questions at that time. All of this will take about 1–1½ hours.

Starting the Procedure

A nurse will examine your arms for the best sites to insert a steel needle and an intravenous (IV) catheter (a small, flexible plastic tube that stays inside of your vein). These sites will be cleansed thoroughly, the needle and IV catheter will be inserted, a set of labs will be drawn, and tubing from the apheresis machine will be attached to the needle and the catheter.

Some people's veins are too small for the size of needles used during the procedure. If this is the case for you, your nurse coordinator will arrange for you to have a temporary central venous catheter (central line) placed just before you go to the clinic. You will be asked not to eat or drink anything after midnight, the night prior to your procedure. After your central line has been placed, you will be brought to the clinic and will be allowed to eat your breakfast.

During the Procedure

You will receive a blood-thinning medication (anticoagulant) so that your blood does not clot in the machine. Some people may feel the following minor side effects from this medication: tingling, numbness (around the lips, nose, and mouth), coolness all over, and slight nausea. To help prevent these symptoms, you will be given calcium through the IV catheter in your arm. If you have these symptoms or feel anything unusual, please tell your nurse immediately. The clinic staff will adjust the amount of calcium that you are receiving or pause the procedure until you are comfortable again. A clinic nurse will be with you throughout your procedure.

After the Procedure

When the procedure is over, your nurse will remove the needles and put a bandage over each needle entry site. Please keep these bandages on for 3 to 4 hours.

If you have a central line and are an outpatient, then you will be sent to the day hospital to have it removed. If you are an inpatient, you will return to your room to have it removed. You will be required to stay in bed for a while, to be sure you are not bleeding from the insertion site, before you are allowed to get up or go home.

Before you leave the clinic, the staff will make sure that you feel alright, and they may offer you some snacks and juice. Adjust your daily activity until the following day (about 24 hours):

- Avoid lifting heavy objects

- Avoid strenuous exercis

- Take the elevator, not the stairs

- Drink lots of non-alcoholic/ non-caffeinated beverages

Section 3.3

Cord Blood Banking

This section includes text excerpted from "Cord Blood: What You Need to Know," U.S. Food and Drug Administration (FDA), July 30, 2014.

Approved Uses

Cord blood is approved only for use in "hematopoietic stem cell transplantation" procedures, which are done in patients with disorders affecting the hematopoietic (blood forming) system. Cord blood contains blood-forming stem cells that can be used in the treatment of patients with blood cancers such as leukemias and lymphomas, as well as certain disorders of the blood and immune systems, such as sickle cell disease and Wiskott-Aldrich syndrome.

"Cord blood is useful because it is a source of stem cells that form into blood cells. Cord blood can be used for transplantation in people who need regeneration, that is, 'regrowth,' of these blood-forming cells," Wonnacott says.

For instance, in many cancer patients, the disease is found in the blood cells. Chemotherapy treatment of these patients kills both cancer cells and the healthy blood-forming stem cells. Transplanted stem cells from cord blood can help regrow the healthy blood cells after the chemotherapy.

However, cord blood is not a cure-all.

"Because cord blood contains stem cells, there have been stem cell fraud cases related to cord blood," says Wonnacott. "Consumers may think that stem cells can cure any disease, but science doesn't show this to be the case. Patients should be skeptical if cord blood is being promoted for uses other than blood stem cell regeneration."

About Cord Blood Banking

After cord blood is collected, it is frozen and can be safely stored for many years. "The method of freezing, called 'cryopreservation,' is very important to maintain the integrity of the cells," Wonnacott says. "Cord blood needs to be stored carefully."

You may choose to store your baby's cord blood in a private bank so it can be available if needed in the future by your child or first- or second-degree relatives. Private cord banks typically charge fees for blood collection and storage.

Or you may donate the cord blood to a public bank so that doctors can use for a patient who needs a hematopoietic stem cell transplant.

FDA regulates cord blood in different ways, depending on the source, level of processing and intended use.

Cord blood stored for personal use, for use in first- or second-degree relatives, and that also meets other criteria in U.S. Food and Drug Administration (FDA) regulations, does not require the agency's approval before use. Private cord banks must still comply with other FDA requirements, including establishment registration and listing, current good tissue practice regulations, and donor screening and testing for infectious diseases (except when cord blood is used for the original donor). These FDA requirements ensure safety of these products by minimizing the risk of contamination and transmission of infectious diseases.

Cord blood stored for use by a patient unrelated to the donor meets the legal definitions of both a "drug" and a "biological product." Cord blood in this category must meet additional requirements and be licensed under a biologics license application, or be the subject of an investigational new drug application before use. The FDA requirements help to ensure that these products are safe and effective for their intended use.

Not every cord blood unit will meet requirements for public banking, adds Safa Karandish, M.T., an FDA consumer safety officer. If that happens, some of this donated cord blood may be used for non-clinical research.

Tips for Consumers

If you're considering donating to a cord blood bank, you should look into your options during your pregnancy to have enough time to decide before your baby is born. For public banking, ask whether your delivery hospital participates in a cord blood banking program.

If you have questions about collection procedures and risks, or about the donation process, ask your healthcare provider.

Be skeptical of claims that cord blood is a miracle cure—it is not. Some parents may consider using a private bank as a form of "insurance" against future illness. But remember that, currently, the only approved use of cord blood is for treatment of blood-related illnesses.

Also know that in some cases your stored cord blood may not be suitable for use in the child who donated it. "For instance, you can't cure some diseases or genetic defects with cord blood that contains the same disease or defect," Karandish says.

Parents from minority ethnic groups may especially want to consider donation to a public bank, says Wonnacott, because more donations from these populations will help more minority patients who need a stem cell transplant. (The recipients must be "matched" to donors, so doctors are more likely to find a good match among donors from the recipient's ethnic group.)

"When it comes to public banking, there's a proven need for cord blood," Wonnacott says. "And there's a need especially among minorities to have stem cell transplants available. Cord blood is an excellent source for stem cell transplants."

And these transplants can be life-changing for patients.

Chapter 4

Maintaining a Healthy Circulatory System

Keeping Your Arteries Healthy

The well-being of your arteries depends on a healthy endothelium, the inner lining of your blood vessels.

"Endothelial cells are the prima donnas within the blood vessels. They control almost every activity that occurs in the vessels, and they're fundamentally altered with age," says Dr. Edward Lakatta, M.D., chief of the Laboratory of Cardiovascular Science at the National Institutes of Health. "People who maintain a healthy endothelium as they get older and those who make an effort to do things that promote the repair of injured endothelium can reduce the risk of heart attacks and strokes caused by atherosclerosis or hypertension."

Although scientists still have much to learn about the endothelium and what can be done to keep it healthy, a number of studies suggest that certain modifiable risk factors can have an important impact on the cardiovascular system. For instance, regular moderate exercise, such as running, walking, or swimming can reduce body fat, increase lean muscle mass, decrease blood pressure, increase HDL cholesterol (the "good" cholesterol) levels, and lessen the extent of arterial stiffening. All of these exercise-induced changes can have a positive influence on endothelial cells.

This chapter includes text excerpted from "Blood Vessels and Aging: The Rest of the Journey," National Institute on Aging (NIA), National Institutes of Health (NIH), July 2014.

23

In addition, scientists have long known that tobacco smoke contains numerous toxic compounds, such as carbon monoxide, that promote endothelial cell damage. Smoking also increases blood pressure and heart rate. Free radicals in smoke slash the amount of nitric oxide available in the blood stream. Nitric oxide, as you may recall, is a signaling molecule that helps keep arteries pliable. Because nicotine causes narrowing of blood vessels, less oxygen is transported to the heart. If you smoke, blood platelets become stickier and are more apt to form clots in your arteries.

As mentioned earlier, high blood pressure—hypertension—causes blood vessels to thicken, diminishes production of nitric oxide, promotes blood clotting, and contributes to the development of atherosclerotic plaques in the arteries. Blood pressure is considered high when systolic pressure exceeds 140 mmHg and when diastolic blood pressure is higher than 90mmHg.

Excessive weight increases the risk of high blood pressure and can increase the likelihood that you'll have high blood triglycerides and low HDL cholesterol, Dr. Lakatta says. Being overweight can also increase the probability you'll develop insulin resistance, a precursor of diabetes.

Diabetes, a disease in which the body does not produce or properly use insulin, becomes more common as we age. In fact, nearly half of all cases are diagnosed after age 55. Atherosclerosis develops earlier and is more aggressive in people who have diabetes. In part, this occurs because diabetes causes the endothelium to produce excessive amounts of superoxide anion, a free radical that destroys nitric oxide. People aged 65 and older who have diabetes are nearly four times more likely than those who don't to develop peripheral vascular disease, a condition that clogs the arteries that carry blood to the legs or arms. And, cardiovascular diseases and stroke are leading causes of diabetes related deaths. If you suspect you have or are at risk for diabetes, check with your doctor. Symptoms include increased thirst, increased hunger, fatigue, increased urination—especially at night, unexplained weight loss, blurred vision, and slow healing of wounds and sores.

Researchers have also found that stress reduction techniques, such as taking a walk, practicing yoga, or deep breathing are important to cardiovascular health. Emotional stress triggers the release of adrenaline from the adrenal gland and noradrenaline from the nerve endings in your heart and blood vessels. These hormones make the heart beat faster and adversely affect blood vessels. Under stress, an older person's blood pressure rises more rapidly and stays higher longer than a younger person's because the older person's blood vessels are stiffer and have lost much of their elasticity.

Exercise: Your Heart's Best Friend

Regular physical exercise is no joke. In fact, it may be the most important thing a person can do to fend off heart disease, stroke, and other age-associated diseases. Emerging scientific evidence suggests that people who exercise regularly not only live longer, they live better.

Scientists have long known that regular exercise causes certain changes in the hearts of younger people: Resting heart rate is lower, heart mass is higher, and stroke volume is higher than in their sedentary counterparts. These differences make the heart a better pump. Evidence now suggests these changes occur even when exercise training begins later in life, at age 60 or 70, for instance. In other words, you don't lose the ability to become better physically conditioned. In addition, several studies have shown that exercise not only helps reduce debilitating symptoms such as breathlessness and fatigue in people who have heart failure, it also prolongs life.

Exercise training may be effective because it appears to improve the function of virtually every cell in the cardiovascular system. Animal studies, for instance, suggest that regular aerobic workouts help heart muscle cells remove calcium from their inner fluid at a faster rate after a contraction. This improved calcium cycling allows the heart to relax more and fill with more blood between beats.

Exercise also improves blood vessel elasticity and endothelial function, in part, by blocking the production of damaging free radicals and maintaining the production of nitric oxide, an important signaling molecule that helps protect the inner layer of the arteries. Together, these changes can slow the progression of atherosclerosis and other age-related cardiovascular conditions.

Endurance exercises such as brisk walking increase your stamina and improve the health of your heart, lungs, and circulatory system. But other exercises are equally important to maintaining health and self-reliance as you get older. Strength exercises, for instance, build muscles and reduce your risk of osteoporosis. Balance exercises help prevent a major cause of disability in older adults: falls. Flexibility or stretching exercises help keep your body limber. As part of a daily routine, these exercises and other physical activities you enjoy can make a difference in your life as you get older.

Metabolic Syndrome Accelerates Aging of Arteries

Many older Americans have high blood pressure or high blood sugar or just a bit too much fat on the belly. While each of these conditions alone is bad enough, having all of these conditions at once—a cluster called metabolic syndrome—magnifies the risk of developing heart disease and stroke. And National Institute on Aging (NIA) scientists may have discovered a reason why: Metabolic syndrome appears to accelerate stiffening and thickening of the arteries.

Metabolic syndrome—also known as syndrome X or insulin resistance syndrome—may affect as many as 47 million Americans, according to the Centers for Disease Control and Prevention (CDC). After age 50, a person has a better than one in three chance of developing this group of medical conditions characterized by insulin resistance and the presence of obesity, abdominal fat, high blood sugar and triglycerides, low HDL (good) blood cholesterol, and high blood pressure.

To determine the effects of metabolic syndrome on aging arteries, NIA researchers studied 471 participants—average age 59—in the Baltimore Longitudinal Study of Aging (BLSA). None of these participants had any detectable signs of cardiovascular disease when initially examined. But those who had three or more conditions associated with metabolic syndrome developed stiffer and thicker arteries at earlier ages than those who didn't have the syndrome.

"It's as if the metabolic syndrome makes your blood vessels older," says Angelo Scuteri, M.D., PhD, an investigator at the NIA's Laboratory of Cardiovascular Science. "If you have metabolic syndrome, when you are 40 your arteries look like they are 55 or 60."

As this work moves forward, scientists hope they can determine how metabolic syndrome promotes accelerated aging in the arteries and perhaps discover ways to prevent or treat it.

Healthy Foods, Healthy Arteries: Is There a Connection?

What you eat can help keep your heart and arteries healthy—or lead to excessive weight, high blood pressure, and high blood cholesterol—three key factors that increase the risk of developing cardiovascular disease, according to the National Heart, Lung, and Blood Institute (NHLBI). Based on the best available scientific evidence, the American Heart Association (AHA) recommends a diet that includes a variety of fruits, vegetables, and grains, while limiting consumption of saturated fat and sodium.

Fruits and vegetables have lots of antioxidants such as vitamin C and vitamin A that neutralize free radicals and may prevent oxidation in the arteries, dietary experts say. Fruits and vegetables also contain plenty of soluble fiber, a substance that has been shown to reduce blood cholesterol levels, which is healthy for the endothelium.

Breads, cereals, and other grain foods, which provide complex carbohydrates, vitamins, minerals, and fiber, are associated with a decreased risk of cardiovascular disease, according to the AHA Dietary Guidelines. However, some studies suggest eating less sugar, breads, and other simple and complex carbohydrates can lower blood insulin levels and decrease body fat and weight—three factors that are linked to an increased risk of heart disease and stroke. In recent years, a number of dietary recommendations based on these findings have become popular and are currently catching the public's awareness. While contentious, these are important issues and long-term studies are required to determine the risks and benefits of such diets, Dr. Lakatta says.

Saturated fats are usually solid at room temperature. These fats are primarily found in animal foods like meat, poultry, and dairy products like butter. Saturated fats tend to raise levels of "bad" low-density lipoprotein (LDL) and increase the risk of atherosclerosis. In fact, within 2 hours of eating a high saturated fat meal, endothelial cells don't work as well. Such meals can cause a temporary 50 percent dip in endothelial function, even in healthy young people who have no risk factors for atherosclerosis, Dr. Lakatta says.

In addition to saturated fats, some scientists are concerned about trans-fatty acids—unsaturated fats that have been artificially solidified by food manufacturers in a process called hydrogenation to make products like margarine and vegetable shortenings. These scientists suspect that trans-fatty acids, which are often described as hydrogenated or partially hydrogenated fats on many food labels, are more damaging to the heart and arteries than saturated fats.

But researchers have found other types of fats may be beneficial. Monounsaturated fats, found mainly in plant foods such as peanuts and olives, help lower LDL cholesterol. Like polyunsaturated fats, monounsaturated fats are usually liquid at room temperature. Polyunsaturated fats, found in fish, nuts, and dark leafy vegetables, have been getting a lot of attention from scientists in the past few years. They've concluded that one type of polyunsaturated fat—omega-3 fatty acid—found in fish may promote several things that improve endothelial function, including increasing nitric oxide production, slashing the production of free radicals and other substances that cause inflammation, and boosting HDL cholesterol levels. Fish such as salmon, herring, and mackerel are good sources of omega-3.

Control over the condition of our arteries may also lie in how much salt we consume. In cultures where little sodium (in the form of salt) is consumed, blood pressures do not rise with age. Cultural differences have also been found in arterial stiffness. One study compared rural and urban populations in China. The urban population consumed much higher levels of sodium than the rural groups. And they had stiffer arteries. Other researchers found that sodium appears to accelerate age-associated stiffening of arteries. In particular, sodium promotes thickening of aging arterial walls, reduces the amount of nitric oxide available to endothelial cells, and promotes the formation of oxygen free radicals. But shifting to a low sodium diet, research suggests, can begin to diminish arterial stiffness in as little as 2 weeks.

Most of the sodium in your diet comes from processed foods. The remaining is added at the table and while cooking. Scientists who study this issue suggest limiting the amount of sodium that you con-sume from all these sources to no more than 1,500 milligrams (mg) each day (an average American adult consumes about 3,300 milligrams daily). They recommend reading food labels carefully and buying foods that say "reduced sodium," "low in sodium," "sodium free," or "no salt added." Some dietitians suggest seasoning foods with herbs and spices like oregano, onion powder, or garlic instead of sodium.

Scientists suspect the more lifestyle changes, including diet and exercise, you can incorporate into your life, the better off your arteries will be, because these interventions work independently as well as in unison to promote the vitality of endothelial cells and contribute to reducing the risk of cardiovascular disease.

Chapter 5

How Aging Affects the Heart and Blood Vessels

Blood Vessels and Aging

Stretched end-to-end, the arteries, veins, and other vessels of the human circulatory system would measure about 60,000 miles. On any given day, the heart pumps about 1,800 gallons of blood through this vast network. In an average lifetime, the heart pumps approximately one million barrels of blood—enough to fill more than 3 supertankers—through the circulatory system.

No doubt about it, the heart and arteries are remarkable. But as we age, the cardiovascular system becomes more susceptible to diseases including high blood pressure and atherosclerosis. Nearly 40 percent of all deaths among those 65 and older can be attributed to heart problems. By age 80, men are nine times more likely to die of chronic heart failure than they were at age 50. Among women, this risk increases 11-fold over the same time period.

Certainly, poor lifestyle—smoking, little or no regular exercise, a diet laden with fat, cholesterol, and sodium—contribute to the development of these cardiovascular disorders. But it is becoming more apparent that like the heart, blood vessels undergo changes with advancing

This chapter includes text excerpted from "Aging Hearts and Arteries: A Scientific Quest," National Institute on Aging (NIA), National Institutes of Health (NIH), July 2014.

age, and these changes, including arterial stiffening and thickening, are major risk factors for these diseases.

This relationship is complex. In fact, studies—in both animals and humans—have found that many of the factors that underlie the age-related changes in the arteries are also implicated in the development of cardiovascular disease. This suggests that there are some common links between these two distinct, but intertwined processes. Based on these and other findings, some investigators theorize that aging is the driving force in a cycle that begins with age-related changes in the blood vessels. These changes create an environment that promotes arterial stiffening, which contributes to development of hypertension (high blood pressure). At the same time, age-related changes also make it easier for fatty deposits to build up on the inside of arteries. This accumulation, part of a process known as atherosclerosis, can accelerate the aging of the arteries, which, in turn, leads to further fatty build up and narrowing of the vessel.

In essence, aging arteries form an alliance with risk factors for atherosclerosis, hypertension, and other precursors of heart disease and stroke to profoundly elevate the risk of developing these conditions. However, as scientists learn more about the changes that occur in aging blood vessels, they are making some key discoveries. For instance, in some people these changes occur at an accelerated rate; in others, they occur much more slowly than average. This suggests that how well your arteries perform as you get older depends on a series of complex interactions among age, disease, lifestyle, and genetics, says Dr. Edward Lakatta, M.D., chief of the Laboratory of Cardiovascular Science at the National Institutes of Health (NIH). In any case, epidemiological studies have consistently shown that people with the greatest amount of arterial stiffening and thickening are at the highest risk for developing stroke, heart attack, and other cardiovascular events.

But investigators also now know that several of these changes, such as arterial stiffening and thickening, don't occur to the same extent in all people. In fact, studies strongly suggest that exercise, good nutrition, and emerging drug therapies can slow the aging of the blood vessels, even among people who are genetically at risk. These interventions could delay or prevent the onset of cardiovascular diseases in many older people.

In Search of a Connection

So, what made scientists think there might be a connection between stiffening and thickening of arteries and heart function? It goes back to what they have learned in the past few decades, partly through National Institute on Aging's (NIA) Baltimore Longitudinal Study of Aging. By comparing younger and older volunteers, scientists have been able to put together a picture of what happens both in the heart and in the blood vessels as people age.

The heart, they have learned, adjusts in many subtle and interconnecting ways: It develops thicker walls, and it fills with blood and pumps the blood out in a different pattern and even by somewhat different mechanisms than when young. But it is also becoming clear that many of these adjustments are made in response to changes in the structure of the aging blood vessels, particularly the arteries. For instance, NIA studies show that among those with the stiffest arteries, heart walls are thicker.

To picture how these and other changes influence cardiovascular health, imagine an animated computer graphic of the arteries at, say, age 25, when the walls are still fairly smooth, slick, and compliant. As the heart contracts, the aortic valve opens and blood is pumped into the aorta, the largest artery in the body, and flows up toward the neck, where the carotid artery branches off to take blood to the head and brain, and then down toward the rest of the body. When the aorta receives the rushing pulse of blood from the heart, it also receives pressure spreading from the walls of the heart to its own walls. This pressure travels along the aorta's walls in wave after wave until it reaches the walls of the smaller branching arteries that take the blood to the rest of the body. There, the speed of these pressure waves—known as pulse wave velocity—slows, and some are sent back through the aorta walls, becoming what are called wave reflections.

Now, add 50 years to this picture. The arteries, including the aorta, grow stiffer and dilate; their walls become thicker, their diameter larger. As a result, the stiffer vessels no longer expand and contract as much as they once did with each heart beat. Eventually, the opposition to the flow of blood by the stiffer aorta walls increases significantly.

Along the walls of the stiffer aorta, the pressure waves move more rapidly, and as a result, the wave reflections occur sooner than they did before. The timing of the wave reflection, in fact, is one of the effects of arterial stiffness that can be measured noninvasively. Epidemiological studies using these measures have determined that high aortic pulse wave velocity (aPWV) is an independent predictor of arterial stiffness and cardiovascular disease and death.

As the walls of the large arteries become stiffer, diastolic blood pressure tends to drop and systolic blood pressure rises. The difference between these two numbers is called pulse pressure. High pulse pressure greater than 60 millimeters of mercury—is associated with

31

greater thickening and stiffening of arterial walls. In turn, arterial stiffening and thickening contribute to increased pulse pressure. Many studies have found that elevated pulse pressure is also an important risk factor for stroke and heart attack.

Next, picture the effects of movement—when a person sits up, stands up, or begins to walk or run—the heart rate increases and blood pressure changes. A group of pressure sensitive nerves in the base of the carotid artery respond by sending a message to the brain. The brain in turn sends a message back to the heart, which changes its rate and strength of contraction. This arterial/brain/heart message system is called the baroreceptor response. Blood vessels also dilate to allow for the extra blood flow. In addition, blood is turned away temporarily from those organs that don't need it (for instance, the stomach), so that more can be delivered to the working muscles.

In the older picture, the baroreceptor response is blunted with age, perhaps as a result of stiffer arteries. Also, at maximum exercise, the large arteries do not dilate as much as in the younger picture. In essence, this age-related stiffening impedes pulsing blood flow from the heart and places an increased workload on the heart.

As the blood moves into the smaller arteries, the hydraulics change. The pulse smoothes out, the flow becomes more steady. The opposition to this steady flow is known as peripheral vascular resistance or PVR; so far studies show that among men, resting PVR does not change with normal aging, but that it does rise somewhat in women. PVR is actually elevated in people who have high diastolic blood pressure, but is also elevated, to a lesser extent, in people who have high systolic and nearly normal diastolic blood pressure. This condition, called systolic hypertension, is so common that a person aged 55 or older has about a 65 percent chance of developing it. However, PVR is not usually directly measured outside of a research laboratory setting because of the complexities involved. Instead, physicians monitor diastolic blood pressure. If it remains steady or increases rather than dropping in the presence of aortic stiffening, it's a sign of elevated PVR.

Inside Every Artery

Scientists are still sorting out why these aging changes in blood pressure and PVR occur and what can be done to prevent them. But one key focal point of research is the inner workings of the arterial wall.

At first glance a large artery resembles a simple rubber tube. But like many first impressions, this is a bit deceiving. The arterial wall is actually comprised of three intricate layers of tissue. The inner-most layer, closest to the blood, is called the intima. The part of the intima nearest to the blood is a single layer of specialized cells, called endothelial cells, which sits atop the sub-endothelial space and a wall called the basement membrane. These endothelial cells act as a barrier to prevent certain substances from entering the vessel wall through the intima. Endothelial cells sense mechanical signals, such as blood pressure and flow, and chemical signals, such as oxygen tension, and temperature. In reaction to these signals, they secrete proteins called cytokines and chemokines as well as growth factors and other sub-stances that help regulate the structure and function of the arteries.

The smooth muscle cells in the media, the middle layer of the artery, are surrounded by a network of fibers primarily made of two proteins, collagen and elastin. The elastin forms concentric rings within the ves-sel wall. The outermost layer, the adventitia, is composed of connective tissue and small blood vessels that feed the walls of large arteries. Together, these three layers of artery wall surround the lumen, the opening that blood flows through on its journey throughout the body. With age, each of these layers change in complex ways.

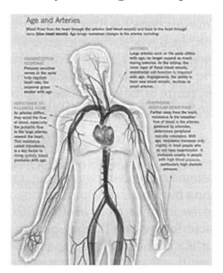

Figure 5.1. *Age and Arteries Diagram*

Time Takes Its Toll

Aging, for instance, triggers thickening of the intima and stiffening of the arterial walls. This occurs, in part, because of a fierce molecular struggle.

Healthy endothelial cells produce nitric oxide, an important signaling molecule that helps keep arteries supple. When nitric oxide enters a cell, it stimulates a biochemical process that relaxes and dilates blood vessels. Nitric oxide also helps keep atherosclerosis in check by preventing platelets and white blood cells from sticking to the blood vessel walls. The molecule also can curb the abnormal growth of vascular muscle, which can thicken blood vessel walls.

But unhealthy endothelial cells are a different story. In these cells, nitric oxide regulation is impaired. To make nitric oxide, endothelial cells need L-arginine, an amino acid that is one of the basic building blocks of proteins, and an enzyme called nitric oxide synthase (NOS). Normally, endothelial cells have plenty of L-arginine and NOS. But NOS is often in short supply in aging blood vessels. In addition, people who have heart disease or who are at high risk of developing it produce a modified amino acid called asymmetric dimethylarginine (ADMA). ADMA blocks the production of nitric oxide from L-arginine. Even if sufficient amounts of nitric oxide are produced, it can be inactivated by oxygen free radicals, unstable molecules that injure vascular tissue. In any case,without adequate levels of biologically available nitric oxide, endothelial cells in the intima can't function properly. In fact, some researchers consider decreased availability of nitric oxide in the endothelium as one of the earliest signs of arterial aging and a pathological sign of atherosclerosis and high blood pressure. However, much of this complex process remains a mystery and scientists continue to explore precisely how nitric oxide production and bioavailability affect blood vessels.

But they do know that endothelial cells depend on nitric oxide to help subdue the production of oxygen free radicals. Nitric oxide molecules can eradicate some of these free radicals, but in the process they also destroy themselves. This leaves less nitric oxide available to help endothelial cells keep arteries in tiptop shape.

Angiotensin II, a growth factor involved in this process, is more prevalent in aging arteries. In addition to increasing free radical production, angiotensin II decreases nitric oxide production and stimulates blood vessel inflammation. It also can cause vessels to tighten and raise blood pressure, forcing the heart to work harder.

Much of angiotensin II's damage is done in partnership with an enzyme called NADPH oxidase, the primary source of free radicals in the arteries. After angiotensin II activates it, NADPH oxidase causes an increase in production of superoxide, a free radical. Superoxide binds with nitric oxide to create an even more potent free radical called peroxynitrite. Peroxynitrite then binds to proteins and nitrites, harming them. Like other free radical processes, this chain of events steals bioavailable nitric oxide away from endothelial cells, leaving them more vulnerable to damage. But the impact of angiotensin II isn't limited to the intima. It also has an important role in age-associated alterations of the media, the middle layer of the arterial wall.

In addition to depleting nitric oxide, free radicals can damage the membranes and DNA of endothelial cells in the intima and smooth muscle cells in the media. Free radical damage is one of many things that can induce some of these cells to stop functioning, shrink, and ultimately die in a process known as apoptosis. Apoptosis may contribute to the decline in cardiovascular health as we age. Free radicals also can oxidize proteins, altering their structure and function. As a result, these proteins can't work properly, and this can trigger a cascade of cellular alterations that promote stiffening and thickening of arterial walls and contribute to atherosclerotic plaque build up.

Stuck in the Middle with You

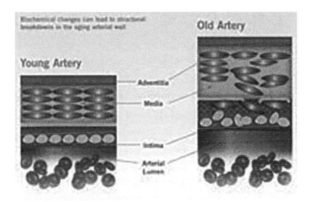

Figure 5.2. *Arteries: Young and Old*

With age, some smooth muscle cells in the media die causing the remaining ones to work harder and grow larger. Over time, other alterations cause some smooth muscle cells to stop contracting as usual. Instead, these cells begin producing excessive amounts of proteins and other matrix substances, creating an imbalance of elastin and collagen in the media. As the amount of collagen increases in the blood vessel wall, it tends to bind to glucose molecules, forming crosslinks known as advanced glycation end products (AGES). This process, which has been compared to what happens as turkey is roasted in an oven, is slow and complex. But as more AGES form, the collagen strands in the media turn brown, become crosslinked, and become less supple. Age takes its toll on elastin, too. It becomes overloaded with calcium, stretches out, and eventually ruptures, further eroding an artery's flexibility.

Scientists studying this process are particularly intrigued by matrix metalloprotease-2 (MMP2), an enzyme activated by angiotensin II as well as many other signals. Although many of its functions are unclear, studies in rodents, monkeys, and humans suggest MMP2 helps break down key components of the basement membrane, the barrier that separates the intima from the media in artery walls. MMP2, in conjunction with angiotensin II, also activates other growth factors, such as transforming growth factor, which might stimulate collagen and cell growth, the development of fibrous tissue, and contribute to thickening of the intima. In addition, this combination of MMP2 and angiotensin II activates PDGF-B, a growth factor, which acts as an attractant that lures smooth muscle cells to migrate from the media to the intima.

But in smaller blood vessels, the activity of PDGF-B and other growth factors, such as vascular endothelial growth factor (VEGF), tend to decline with age. These growth factors play an important role in a process called angiogenesis that leads to the development of new small blood vessels. In some cases, angiogenesis can stimulate the growth of new collateral small vessels around narrow spots or blockages in the arteries that threaten to reduce blood flow to the heart. As we age, however, this process switches off. Enzymes that break down collagen also seem to be involved in this process and are less active as we get older. Scientists are still unraveling why this happens, but as age-associated changes and damage accumulate in endothelial cells, they secrete less of the critical growth factors needed for angiogenesis. Angiogenesis also depends, in part, on the availability of nitric oxide, which declines with age. In addition, there appears to be an age-associated decrease in the number of endothelial progenitor cells. These adult stem cells are produced in the bone marrow and circulate in the bloodstream.

Under certain circumstances, endothelial progenitor cells can differentiate into endothelial cells, which are needed to form new blood vessels or repair damaged ones. In essence, progenitor cells are the "mothers" of "daughter" endothelial cells. As the number of progenitor cells declines, angiogenesis is less likely to occur. Researchers are investigating ways, such as gene and cell therapy, to reactivate angiogenesis in older people who have cardiovascular disease. But scientists have much to learn about the safety and efficacy of these techniques.

From Balloon to Bicycle Tire

Scientists are still piecing together how, or even if, many of these various processes interact. But they do know that, as the result of these and other age associated changes in large arteries, the endothelial barrier in the intima becomes more porous. Some of the signals these cells transmit to the smooth muscle cells in the media become garbled. In turn, these smooth muscle cells can mistakenly perceive that an injury has occurred. They move into the intima, multiply, and produce collagen and other molecules. In reaction, the endothelial cells produce substances that send signals to circulating blood cells to help out in the repair process. Unfortunately, in their effort to help, blood cells stick to endothelial cells instead of flowing smoothly through the blood vessel. The net impact of these interactions is that the intimal-media layer thickens, contributes to arterial stiffness, and creates a fertile environment for the development of atherosclerosis in aging arteries.

The cumulative effect of all these age-related changes can be boiled down to this: the ability of larger blood vessels to expand and contract diminishes, the lumen enlarges, and the arterial walls thicken. The result is "hardened"or stiffened arteries that set the stage for the onset of high blood pressure, elevated pulse wave velocity, atherosclerosis, and other precursors of cardiovascular disease. The more severe the effects of aging are on the blood vessels, the easier it is for atherosclerosis, hypertension, and other processes to do damage and, in turn, have an effect on the rate of aging in the vessels. Smoking, lack of exercise, a poor diet, and obesity also can exacerbate these effects.

It's this cycle, with age as the principal instigator, which gradually helps change youthful and healthy blood vessels into old and potentially diseased ones. In a sense, this progression transforms a young person's arteries, which are like soft latex balloons, into the equivalent of rigid, bulky bicycle tires in later life.

However, arterial stiffness and intimal-media thickening occur at varying rates in different people. Studies suggest that the rate of both of these age related changes predict stroke, heart disease, and other cardiovascular problems. For example, in one large study that followed healthy volunteers who had no previous symptoms of heart disease, those who had the greatest amount of intimal-media thickening were four times more likely to develop cardiovascular conditions over the next 7 years compared to those with the least arterial thickening. Similarly, studies have shown that healthy people with the stiffest blood vessels were three times more apt to develop high blood pressure over a 5-year span than those with more pliable vessels. In yet another large-scale study, involving 3,075 healthy older people, those who had the highest pulse wave velocity (PWV)—a measure of arterial stiffness—were three times more likely to die of cardiovascular disease than those who had the lowest PWVs.

Can Gene Therapy Be Used to Treat Heart Problems?

In the future, an experimental technique, called gene therapy, may allow doctors to treat heart disease and other cardiovascular disorders by inserting a gene into a patient's cells instead of using drugs or surgery. Investigators are testing several approaches to gene therapy including:

- Replacing a mutated gene that causes disease with a healthy copy of the gene

- Inactivating or "knocking out" a mutated gene that is functioning improperly, or

- Introducing a new gene into the body to help fight a disease.

The NIH has been on the cutting edge of this research. More than a decade ago, for instance, cardiovascular investigators began experimenting with ways to increase the supply of certain growth factors through gene therapy. If more growth factors could be produced, scientists theorized they might stimulate angiogenesis—the growth of new small blood vessels called capillaries.

Knowing the genes that code for the growth factors, the investigators found ways to add copies of these genes to heart muscle. To get genes to the myocytes, they engineered molecular delivery trucks called vectors for the genes. These vectors, made from inactivated adenoviruses—the same viral culprits that cause the common cold—were injected into rats. Scientists hoped the vectors would unload their DNA cargo, which then would begin producing the proteins needed to induce capillary growth. And in this experiment, that's exactly what happened. One of the vectors worked.

More recently, scientists successfully used gene therapy in older rats to increase the activity of the gene that produces calcium pump proteins on sarcoplasmic reticulum, the cellular storage bin for calcium. This therapy significantly improved heart muscle contraction in these rodents. In another animal study, researchers at The Johns Hopkins School of Medicine in Baltimore used gene therapy to convert a small region of guinea pig heart muscle tissue into specialized pace making cells. Potentially, this technique could one day lead to the development of genetically engineered, biological pacemakers to replace implantable electronic devices. However, scientists must overcome many technical challenges before gene therapy will be a practical approach to treating disease.

New Blood Test May Help Doctors Detect Emerging Heart Disease

Blood often tells the story of our lives. Tests that measure blood cholesterol levels and other cardiovascular risk factors have become a routine part of health screenings. And in the future, doctors may check yet another blood test—one that measures inflammation—that may help them better assess the risk of disease in the aging heart and arteries.

The test measures levels of C-reactive protein (CRP), a substance produced in the liver, which is often elevated in people who have rheumatoid arthritis and other diseases that cause chronic inflammation. Several studies have indicated that increased blood levels of CRP in otherwise healthy people are associated with an increased risk of heart attack, stroke, and other cardiovascular problems.

Scientists are still investigating whether CRP is merely an indicator of inflammation or if it has an active role in this process. In any case, cardiovascular risk factors such as excessive weight, diabetes, and a sedentary lifestyle are associated with high CRP blood levels. Healthy people with CRP levels less than 1 milligram per liter of blood are considered at the lowest risk of a cardiovascular event in the next 10 years. Depending on medical history and other factors, a person at intermediate risk—1 to 3 milligrams of CRP per liter of blood—could have up to a 20 percent risk of having a heart attack in the next decade. Those with CRP levels of 3 milligrams or more per liter have the highest risk.

However, researchers stress that inflammation is just one of many factors that could increase your risk of cardiovascular disease as you get older. To date no evidence has emerged to suggest that treating people for elevated CRP alone improves survival or reduces cardiovascular complications. For now, detection and treatment of more well-established risk factors, such as high blood pressure and high blood cholesterol, remains a greater priority.

But some treatments for these other risk factors could help lower CRP. The same lifestyle changes, for instance, that help lower cholesterol—regular exercise, a healthy diet, weight loss, and quitting smoking—can also help reduce inflammation. Aspirin and other drugs, including cholesterol-lowering medications such as statins, can decrease CRP levels as well.

Part Two

Diagnosing and Treating Blood and Circulatory Disorders

Chapter 6

Blood Tests

Chapter Contents

Section 6.1

Blood Typing

"Blood Typing," © 2016 Omnigraphics. Reviewed July 2016.

Blood typing is a classification system used to sort human blood according to the kinds of antigens (blood proteins) found on red blood cells. There are four primary types of blood: A, B, AB, and O. Each blood type is further classified by an Rh positive or negative designation. Rh refers to Rhesus factor and indicates the presence (positive) or absence (negative) of a specific protein found on the surface of red blood cells. Blood type is an inherited trait.

Blood typing is important because not all blood types are compatible with each other. Giving the wrong blood type to a person through a blood transfusion can result in serious complications and even death. Blood typing is especially important for pregnant women. If the expectant mother is Rh-negative and the expectant father is Rh-positive, the mother will need to receive treatment to help protect the fetus from complications that could arise from a mix of incompatible blood types.

Testing Blood Type

Blood type tests are performed for a variety of reasons. Some of the most common include:

- Classification of donated blood

- Preparation for a blood transfusion or any surgery

- Preparation for organ transplant

- When a woman is pregnant or plans to become pregnant

- Identification of individuals (for example, determining blood relations)

The two most common blood typing tests are the ABO and the Rh tests.

The ABO test examines red blood cells in order to classify the blood as A, B, AB, or O. Blood that is type A contains the A antigen, and type B contains the B antigen. These two blood types are incompatible. Each contains antibodies that will attack and destroy the cells of the other. Type AB blood contains both A and B antigens, meaning that it is compatible with both A and B blood types. People with type AB blood can receive blood from anyone of any blood type, making type AB the "universal recipient." Type O blood contains no antigens, and can be given to anyone of any blood type. For this reason, type O blood is known as the "universal donor."

To test for blood type, a small amount of blood is mixed with serum containing blood antibodies and observed to see if the sample blood cells agglutinate (stick together). Blood cells that stick together when mixed with Anti-A serum is classified as type A. Type B blood cells stick together when mixed with Anti-B serum. Type AB blood cells stick together when mixed with both Anti-A and Anti-B serums. Blood cells that do not stick together when mixed with Anti-A or Anti-B serums is classified as type O.

A second blood type test is performed to verify the results of the first test. In the second test, known as back-typing, a small amount of the blood being tested is mixed with a small amount of blood that has already been classified as type A or type B and observed for agglutination (sticking together). If the sample blood cells stick together when mixed with type B blood, the sample is identified as type A. Conversely, if the sample blood cells stick together when mixed with type A blood, the sample is identified as type B. If the sample blood cells stick together when mixed with either type A or type B blood, the sample is identified as type O. If the sample blood cells do not stick together when mixed with type A or type B blood, the sample is identified as type AB.

The Rh test is performed by mixing a small blood sample with a serum that contains anti-Rh serum. If the sample blood cells stick together when mixed with anti-Rh serum, the blood is Rh-positive. If the sample blood cells do not stick together when mixed with anti-Rh serum, the blood is Rh-negative. People with Rh-negative blood can only receive Rh-negative blood; people with Rh-positive blood can receive either Rh-positive or Rh-negative blood.

The results of both kinds of blood type testing are used for complete identification of blood type. For example, type A blood that is Rh-positive is A-positive, type B blood that is Rh-negative is B-negative, and so on.

Blood Type Compatibility

- A person with A-negative blood can receive types A-negative and O-negative blood.

- A person with A-positive blood can receive types A-negative, A-positive, O-negative, and O-positive blood.

- A person with B-negative blood can receive types B-negative and O-negative blood.

- A person with B-positive blood can receive types B-negative, B-positive, O-negative, and O-positive blood.

- A person with AB-negative blood can receive types AB-negative and O-negative blood.

- A person with AB-positive blood can receive any type of blood.

- A person with O-negative blood can only receive type O-negative blood.

- A person with O-positive blood can receive O-negative or O-positive blood.

References

1. Gersten, Todd. "Blood Typing," MedlinePlus, February 24, 2014.

2. "Blood Type Test," WebMD, September 9, 2014.

Section 6.2

Complete Blood Count

This section includes text excerpted from "Understanding Your Complete Blood Count (CBC) and Common Blood Deficiencies," National Institutes of Health (NIH), May 2015.

What Is a Complete Blood Count (CBC)?

A complete blood count (CBC) is a common blood test that gives doctors information about five major parts of your blood: three types of cells (red blood cells, white blood cells, and platelets) and two values (hemoglobin and hematocrit values). Normal ranges may be slightly different for men and women. The five parts of a CBC are:

White blood cell (WBC) count

White blood cells help your body fight off infections. The normal range for WBC is 5 to 10 K/uL. Your CBC will also measure what is called the ANC (absolute neutrophil count). That is the specific number of white blood cells in your blood that fight infection.

Red blood cell (RBC) count

Red blood cells carry oxygen and remove waste from your body. These cells also have a protein in them called hemoglobin, which is what makes red blood cells the color red. The normal range for RBC is 4 to 5.5 M/uL.

Hemoglobin (HGB) value

Hemoglobin carries oxygen from your lungs to the rest of your body and also moves carbon dioxide (waste) to your lungs so that you breathe it out. The normal range for HGB is 12 to 17.4 g/dL.

Hematocrit (HCT) value

The hematocrit value measures how much of your total blood count is made up of red blood cells. The normal range for HCT is 36% to 52%.

Platelet count

Platelets help stop bleeding by sticking together to form blood clots, which "plug" cuts and wounds. A normal platelet count range is 140 to 400 K/uL.

Blood Disorders

Sometimes, your CBC may show that your counts or values are too low. For example, you might not have enough white blood cells, or your platelet count could be lower than normal. When this happens, it can cause health problems.

Neutropenia (Low White Blood Cell Count)

If you have neutropenia, then you do not have enough white blood cells (called neutrophils) that fight off infection. In other words, your ANC (absolute neutrophil count) is too low.

The lower your ANC is, the more likely that you are to have health problems:

- If your ANC is lower than 1,000 (1.0K/uL), then you have a higher risk of getting an infection.

- If your ANC is lower than 500, then you have a higher risk of getting a more serious infection.

You can pick up these infections through the air, blood, sweat, and saliva. And, some germs can get into your body when you touch something with germs on it and then touch your eyes, nose, or mouth.

The steps below will help you avoid germs and help keep you safe while your white blood cell count is low.

- Wash your hands often, including before you eat and after you:

  - use the bathroom

  - cough, sneeze, or blow your nose

  - shake someone's hand

  - touch anything handled by others

- Take a shower or bath every day.

- If your skin gets dry, use unscented lotion or oils. This will help stop your skin from cracking, which can let in germs.

- If you cut or scrape yourself, clean the area with soap and warm water right away. Then cover it with a bandage.

- Always wear shoes in the hospital and at home.

- Rinse your mouth out with water after you eat and before you go to bed.

- Use an ultra-soft toothbrush, and only floss if your ANC is higher than 500 and your platelet count is 50,000 or higher.

- Use lip balm (like ChapStick) on your lips to prevent chapping.

- If you wear dentures, make sure that they fit well.

- Check with your doctor before you see the dentist.

- Ask someone else to clean around the house, especially litter boxes, birdcages, and fish tanks.

- Do not touch fresh flowers, houseplants, dirt or soil, or stagnant (still) water, and do not keep any plants in your home, not even dried flowers. Ask your doctor about when it is safe to have plants or flowers near you.

- Avoid crowded places, and stay away from people who are sick.

- Never swim in lakes, ponds, rivers, or oceans. If you want to swim, talk it over with your doctor or nurse first, and swim only in a pool that is treated with chlorine to kill germs. Also, stay out of hot tubs and Jacuzzis.

- Keep away from construction sites, since germs can hide in dirt and dust.

- Use an electric shaver instead of a razor, and do not get a manicure, pedicure, or fake nails (or nail tips).

- Prevent cuts and tears in your rectum by avoiding enemas, rectal thermometers, or suppositories (medicines that you put in your anus).

- Women need to avoid tampons, vaginal suppositories (like for a yeast infection), and douches.

- Be sure not to get any vaccines (like a flu shot) unless your doctor tells you to.

- Use a water-based lubricant during sex.

- Avoid anal sex. It is more likely than vaginal sex to cause cuts and tears.

When you have neutropenia, you need to watch for signs of infection. Check your temperature at least once a day. Your doctor or nurse may tell you to check it more often. If you have a fever, that is a sign that you might have an infection.

- Call your doctor or nurse right away if:

- Your temperature is between 100.4 and 100.9°F two or more times in one day.

- Your temperature ever reaches 101.0°F or above.

- You are:
  - short of breath or having chest pain
  - experiencing chills or have flushed skin
  - sweating
  - urinating (peeing) often

- feeling burning when you urinate
- red, tender, or have pain anywhere on your body
- feeling run down or having other flu-like symptoms, like:
  - sore throat
  - sneezing
  - runny nose
  - coughing
  - stomach problems (feeling sick, throwing up, diarrhea)

Your doctor and nurse can look for signs of infection by testing your blood and urine. They may also do a chest X-ray. If you have an infection, your doctor will give you medicine to fight it.

Anemia

If you have anemia, then you do not have enough red blood cells in your blood, and your hematocrit and hemoglobin levels are too low. Many different things, like medicines, low vitamin levels, and diseases, can cause anemia. Your doctor will run tests to find out the cause and figure out the best treatment. People with serious cases of anemia may need a blood transfusion to keep them safe.

When you are anemic, you may feel weak and tired. You may also experience dizziness, shortness of breath, racing heartbeat (heart palpitations), pounding in your head, and ringing in your ears.

To prevent symptoms of anemia, rest often during the day, especially between activities; make sure that you get enough sleep at night; and get up slowly if you have been sitting or lying down. This can help you feel less dizzy.

Thrombocytopenia

If you have thrombocytopenia, then you do not have enough platelets in your blood, and your blood will not clot normally.

When you have thrombocytopenia, you may bruise easily. You may also experience:

- tiny red or purple spots on your skin (petechiae)
- nose bleeds
- bleeding gums

- cuts that keep bleeding
- black or bloody stool (poop)
- brown or red urine (pee)
- heavy periods (increased bleeding from the vagina)

There are lots of over-the-counter (OTC) medicines that can keep your platelets from working the way that they are supposed to, especially medicines that have aspirin in them. So when your platelet count is low, talk with your doctor or nurse before you take any new medicines.

- Never take any medicine that has aspirin in it.
- You will also need to avoid some other common OTC medicines, including:
  - Ibuprofen (Motrin, Advil, Midol, Pediacare Fever).
  - Naproxen (Naprosyn, Naprelan, Aleve, Anaprox).

Make safe choices for personal care:

- Use an ultra-soft toothbrush to keep your gums from bleeding. If your gums bleed when you brush your teeth, use Toothettes (special mouth swabs) instead of a toothbrush.
- Only floss your teeth if your platelet count is 50,000 or higher.
- Use an electric shaver rather than a razor, especially if your platelet count is lower than 20,000.
- When you blow your nose, be gentle.
- Never use enemas, rectal thermometers (thermometers that go in the anus), and suppositories.
- Women should not douche or use tampons or vaginal suppositories (like for a yeast infection).
- If you have sex, use water-based lubricants. If your platelet count is too low, sex may not be safe. Check with your doctor.
- Eat a balanced diet, so that you do not become constipated.
- Avoid eating foods that might upset your stomach, like popcorn or apple peels.
- Choose loose-fitting clothing and avoid anything with tight waistbands.

- Wear shoes in the hospital and at home.

- Ask your doctor before gardening. If your doctor says it is safe, then you can garden with gloves on.

- Avoid certain activities, including using sharp knives or blades and contact sports, such as football and hockey.

Call your doctor or nurse right away if you have any of the following symptoms:

- new tiny red or purple spots on your skin (about the size of a pinpoint or larger)

- new bruises on your body

- nosebleeds

- bleeding gums

- bleeding from an area where you had a procedure (like where you got a catheter)

- blood in your urine or stool

- headaches

- feeling very tired

- confusion

- falling down

Section 6.3

Fibrinogen Test

"Fibrinogen Test," © 2016 Omnigraphics. Reviewed July 2016.

A fibrinogen test, also known as a Factor I test, measures the level of fibrinogen in a person's blood. Fibrinogen is a blood plasma protein that is produced by the liver. It is one of 13 blood elements that help to form blood clots to stop bleeding after an injury. Low fibrinogen affects the body's ability to form blood clots, which can result in excessive bleeding.

Fibrinogen tests are usually performed on people who experience problems with blood clotting, excessive bleeding, or excessive bruising after an injury. Fibrinogen tests are also performed on people who experience blood in their urine or stool, or have had a ruptured spleen or gastrointestinal tract hemorrhage. The test is an important tool in the diagnosis of disseminated intravascular coagulation, a condition in which small blood clots form inside the blood vessels throughout the body.

Testing for elevated levels of fibrinogen is also used to help diagnose or determine the risk of cardiovascular disease (heart disease) or brain aneurysm (stroke). Elevated fibrinogen levels can result from certain health conditions including acute infections, cancer, coronary heart disease, heart attack, stroke, rheumatoid arthritis, kidney disease, liver disease, peripheral artery disease, and pregnancy. Receiving a blood transfusion, taking certain drugs, and smoking can also cause elevated fibrinogen levels in the body.

Methods

Fibrinogen tests can be conducted using one of four methods. In the Clauss method, plasma drawn from the person being tested is mixed with concentrated thrombin (an enzyme in blood plasma) and analyzed. The time it takes for the blood clot to form is noted and compared against standard measures. Automated equipment senses when the blood clot has formed based on the optical density of the plasma/thrombin mixture.

In PT-derived fibrinogen tests, a baseline measurement for known fibrinogen levels in various diluted plasma samples (the control group) is compared to the fibrinogen levels found in equivalent plasma dilutions created from the blood plasma being tested.

Immunological fibrinogen tests are conducted to measure the fibrinogen protein concentration in blood, rather than fibrinogen function.

Gravimetric fibrinogen tests are used to measure the weight of a clot produced using the Clauss method, instead of measuring the optical density of the clot. Another type of gravimetric fibrinogen test measures the amount of fibrinogen protein present in a blood clot created using the Clauss method.

Results

A normal fibrinogen blood level is typically between 1.5 to 3.0 grams per liter.

Normal reference ranges are usually as follows:
Adult: 200 mg/dl–400 mg/dl
New born: 125 mg/dl–300 mg/dl
Fibrinogen levels are considered abnormal if the level is higher or lower than the normal range. An abnormal result may be due to an inherited or acquired condition such as:

- Afibrinogenemia—absence of fibrinogen in the body

- Disseminated Intravascular Coagulation—too much fibrinogen used by the body

- Dysfibrinogenemia—fibrinogen performance malfunction

- Fibrinolysis—excessive breakdown of fibrinogen in the body

- Hemorrhage—excessive bleeding

- Hypofibrinogenemia—too little fibrinogen in the body

- Placenta Abruptio—the placenta separates from the uterus wall during pregnancy

Spontaneous bleeding will occur when the fibrinogen level falls below 100mg/dl.

Treatment

Fibrinogen deficiency is treatable through the use of blood products that act as a replacement or substitute for the fibrinogen protein in the body. Fibrinogen concentrate may be used to prevent excessive bleeding in people during surgery, during or after childbirth, before dental surgery, or after traumatic injury.

References

1.   Chen, Yi-Bin. "Fibrinogen Blood Test," MedlinePlus, January 27, 2015.

2.   Underwood, Corinna. "Fibrinogen," HealthLine, January 4, 2016.

3.   "Fibrinogen," American Association for Clinical Chemistry, April 10, 2014.

4.   "Fibrinogen Assays," Practical Haemostasis, n.d.

Section 6.4

Reticulocyte Count

What Is Reticulocyte Count?

Reticulocytes are immature red blood cells (RBCs). They're made in the bone marrow (the spongy material inside bone) and are released into the bloodstream, where they circulate for about 1–2 days before developing into mature red blood cells. Normally, only about 1% of all red blood cells in the bloodstream are reticulocytes.

A reticulocyte count measures how many of these immature red blood cells are in the bloodstream. This gives an idea of the rate at which these cells are made in the bone marrow.

Why It's Done

A reticulocyte count is helpful when a doctor needs more information about someone's anemia (a low number of RBCs). For example, the number of reticulocytes in the blood can be low if anemia is occurring because fewer reticulocytes are being produced by the bone marrow.

The count can be high because more reticulocytes are being produced to replace mature RBCs being destroyed by disease or if there is bleeding. The test also can be used to monitor whether treatment for anemia is working.

Preparation

No special preparations are needed. On the day of the test, having your child wear a T-shirt or short-sleeved shirt can make things easier for the technician drawing the blood.

Let the doctor know if your child has had a blood transfusion in the past 3 months because this can affect the reticulocyte count.

The Procedure

A health professional will usually draw the blood from a vein, after cleaning the skin surface with antiseptic and placing an elastic band (tourniquet) around the upper arm to apply pressure and cause veins to swell with blood. A needle is inserted into a vein (usually in the arm inside of the elbow or on the back of the hand) and blood is withdrawn and collected in a vial or syringe.

After the procedure, the elastic band is removed. Once the blood has been collected, the needle is removed and the area is covered with cotton or a bandage to stop the bleeding. Collecting blood for this test will only take a few minutes.

What to Expect

Collecting a sample of blood is only temporarily uncomfortable and can feel like a quick pinprick. Afterward, there may be some mild bruising, which should go away in a few days.

Getting the Results

The blood sample will be processed by a machine and the results are usually available after a few hours or the next day.

If the reticulocyte count is abnormal, further testing may be necessary to determine what's causing the problem and how to treat it.

Risks

The reticulocyte count is considered a safe procedure. However, as with many medical tests, some problems can occur with having blood drawn, like:

- fainting or feeling lightheaded

- hematoma (blood accumulating under the skin causing a lump or bruise)

- pain associated with multiple punctures to locate a vein

Chapter 7

Bone Marrow Tests

What Are Bone Marrow Tests?

Bone marrow tests are used to check whether your bone marrow is healthy. These tests also show whether your bone marrow is making normal amounts of blood cells.

Bone marrow is the sponge-like tissue inside the bones. It contains stem cells that develop into the three types of blood cells that the body needs:

- red blood cells carry oxygen through the body

- white blood cells fight infection

- platelets stop bleeding

Another type of stem cell, called an embryonic stem cell, can develop into any type of cell in the body. These cells aren't found in bone marrow.

Who Needs Bone Marrow Tests?

Your doctor may recommend bone marrow tests if he or she thinks you have a blood or bone marrow disease or condition, such as:

- **Myelodysplastic syndrome.** This is a group of diseases in which your bone marrow doesn't make enough normal blood cells.

This chapter includes text excerpted from "Bone Marrow Tests," National Heart, Lung, and Blood Institute (NHLBI), December 12, 2011. Reviewed July 2016.

- **Neutropenia.** This is a condition in which you have a lower than normal number of white blood cells in your blood.

- **Anemia.** Anemia occurs if you have a lower than normal number of red blood cells. The condition also can occur if your red blood cells don't have enough of an iron-rich protein that carries oxygen from the lungs to the rest of the body.

- **Aplastic anemia.** This type of anemia occurs if your bone marrow doesn't make enough new blood cells (red blood cells, white blood cells, and platelets). Aplastic anemia is a rare, but serious condition.

- **Myelofibrosis.** This is a serious bone marrow disorder that disrupts normal production of blood cells and leads to severe anemia.

- **Thrombocytopenia.** This is a group of conditions in which your body doesn't make enough platelets and your blood doesn't clot as it should.

- **Essential thrombocythemia.** This is a disease in which your bone marrow makes too many blood cells, especially platelets.

- **Leukemia.** This is a cancer of the white blood cells. Types of leukemia include acute and chronic leukemias and multiple myeloma.

Your doctor also may recommend bone marrow tests if you have another type of cancer. Examples include breast cancer that has spread to the bone or Hodgkin and non-Hodgkin lymphomas (cancers of a certain type of white blood cell).

Bone marrow tests help show what stage the cancer is in. That is, the tests help doctors know how serious the cancer is and how much it has spread in the body.

Bone marrow tests also can show what's causing a fever. Doctors may recommend the tests for people who have diseases that affect the immune system. The tests also are used for patients who may have uncommon bacterial infections.

What to Expect before Bone Marrow Tests

Before having bone marrow tests, a doctor, nurse, or physician assistant will explain the testing process and procedure and answer questions you might have.

Let your healthcare team know:

- whether you're allergic to any medicines

- whether you have a bleeding disorder

- what medicines you're taking (you might have to stop taking some medicines, such as blood-thinning medicines, before having bone marrow tests)

- whether you're pregnant

Before the tests, you may be given medicine to help you relax. This medicine makes you sleepy, so you likely won't be able to drive after the test. Thus, your healthcare team may advise you to arrange a ride home.

What to Expect during Bone Marrow Tests

Bone marrow tests usually take about 30 minutes. The tests can be done in a hospital, doctor's office, or other healthcare facility.

Bone marrow tests generally are done on the pelvic bone. In most people, part of this bone is accessible on the lower back. If your doctor uses that part of the pelvic bone, you'll lie on your side or stomach for the test. Aspiration might be done on the breastbone.

Medicine will be used to numb the area where your doctor will insert the needle. Although you'll be awake during the tests, the medicine helps reduce pain.

If you're very nervous or anxious, your doctor may give you medicine to help you relax or sleep. If so, your healthcare team will closely check your breathing, heart rate, and blood pressure during the tests.

The area on your body where your doctor will insert the needle is cleaned and draped with a cloth. Your doctor will see only the site where the needle is inserted. He or she will make a small incision (cut) in your skin. This makes it easier to insert the needle into the bone. After the test, you might need stitches to close the cut.

For bone marrow aspiration, your doctor will insert the needle into the marrow and remove a sample of fluid bone marrow. You may feel a brief, sharp pain. The fluid that's removed from the bone marrow will be taken to a laboratory and studied under a microscope.

If your doctor decides to do a bone marrow biopsy, it will be done after the aspiration. For the biopsy, your doctor will use a needle to remove a sample of bone marrow tissue. Thin sections of this tissue will be studied under a microscope.

During both tests, it's important for you to remain still and as relaxed as possible (if you're awake).

What to Expect after Bone Marrow Tests

After the bone marrow tests, a nurse will hold a bandage on the site where the needle was inserted until the bleeding stops. Then he or she will put a smaller bandage on the site.

Most people can go home the same day as the tests. If you received medicine to help you relax during the tests, you may need to arrange a ride home.

After 24 hours, you can take off the bandage. Call your doctor if you develop a fever, have a lot of pain, or see redness, swelling, or discharge at the site. These are signs of infection.

Expect mild discomfort for about a week. Your doctor may tell you to take an over-the-counter pain medicine.

What Do Bone Marrow Tests Show?

Bone marrow tests show whether your bone marrow is making enough healthy blood cells. If it's not, the results can tell your doctor which cells are unhealthy and why.

Bone marrow tests are an important medical tool. They're used to diagnose many blood and bone marrow disorders, including anemia and certain kinds of cancer.

Bone marrow tests also are used to find out how severe cancer is and how much it has spread throughout the body. The tests also help doctors find the cause of fevers and infections.

Your doctor will combine information from your bone marrow tests with information from a physical exam, blood tests, and other tests, such as imaging scans and X-rays.

What Are the Risks of Bone Marrow Tests?

Bone marrow tests are safe for most people. Complications are rare, but can occur. For example, some people develop bleeding or infections.

To prevent bleeding from the site where the needle was inserted, don't do any heavy lifting or vigorous exercise for a few days after the tests.

To prevent infections, don't shower or bathe for the first day after the tests.

Bone marrow tests might not be safe for people who have certain bleeding disorders, such as hemophilia. Your doctor can tell you whether bone marrow tests are safe for you.

Chapter 8

Bleeding and Clotting Tests

Chapter Contents

Section 8.1

Bleeding Time

"Bleeding Time," © 2016 Omnigraphics.
Reviewed July 2016.

Bleeding Time Test

When a person is injured and begins to bleed, blood platelets immediately begin forming clots to seal the wound and prevent further blood loss. This process is known as hemostasis. A bleeding time test measures platelet function during hemostasis, or the amount of time it takes to stop bleeding after an injury. This test is performed to help diagnose problems with bleeding and blood clotting. Bleeding time tests are most often performed on people who experience excessive bleeding, particularly after minor injuries such as small cuts or punctures. A bleeding time test may also be performed on people who have a family history of bleeding disorders. It is sometimes performed before surgery to assess a person's risk of excessive bleeding during or after surgery.

To conduct a bleeding time test, a health professional inflates a blood pressure cuff around a person's upper arm. With the cuff inflated, the health professional makes two small cuts on the person's lower arm. These cuts are superficial, similar to a scratch, and just deep enough to cause a very small amount of bleeding. After the cuts are made, the blood pressure cuff is deflated. Special blotting paper is pressed on the cuts every 30 seconds until no more blood is absorbed by the paper, indicating that bleeding has stopped. The health professional notes the length of time it takes for the person to stop bleeding.

Results

During a bleeding time test, healthy people typically stop bleeding within one to nine minutes. A longer bleeding time can indicate blood platelet malfunction. This can mean either the body is producing too many or too few platelets, or the blood platelets may not be working properly. A longer bleeding time can also indicate a blood vessel defect, meaning that there may be a problem in the body's ability to deliver blood throughout the body.

Bleeding time tests are important tools in the diagnosis of certain blood disorders such as hemophilia, thrombocythemia, and von Willebrand's disease. Hemophilia is a genetic platelet malfunction that is present at birth. People who live with hemophilia experience excessive bleeding after injury because their bodies have difficulty forming blood clots in deep tissue (for example, in joints and muscles). von Willebrand's disease is an inherited condition affecting the body's ability to form blood clots after injuries to skin or mucous membranes (for example, inside the nose, mouth, and intestines). Thrombocythemia is a condition in which the body produces too few blood platelets. Some people develop platelet malfunction due to chronic illness.

References

1. Chen, Yi-Bin. "Bleeding Time," MedlinePlus, January 2, 2015.

2. Krans, Brian. "Bleeding Time Test," HealthLine, December 21, 2015.

Section 8.2

Partial Thromboplastin Time

This section includes text excerpted from "Blood Test: Partial Thromboplastin Time (PTT)," © 1995–2016. The Nemours Foundation/KidsHealth®. Reprinted with permission.

What Is Partial Thromboplastin Time?

A partial thromboplastin time (PTT) test measures how long it takes for a clot to form in a blood sample. A clot is a thick lump of blood that the body produces to seal leaks, wounds, cuts, and scratches and prevent excessive bleeding.

The blood's ability to clot involves platelets (also called thrombocytes) and proteins called clotting factors. Platelets are oval-shaped cells made in the bone marrow. Most clotting factors are made in the liver.

When a blood vessel breaks, platelets are first to the area to help seal off the leak and temporarily stop or slow the bleeding. But for the clot to become strong and stable, the action of clotting factors is required.

The body's clotting factors are numbered using the Roman numerals I through XII. They work together in a specialized sequence, almost like pieces of a puzzle. When the last piece is in place, the clot develops—but if even one piece is missing or defective, the clot can't form.

The PTT test is used to evaluate the ability of a person's blood to clot. If it takes an abnormally long time for the blood to clot, it can indicate a problem with one or more of several different clotting factors. This may be a sign of:

- a missing, deficient, or defective clotting factor or factors

- liver disease (because many clotting factors are made in the liver)

- treatment with heparin, a blood-thinning medication

Why It's Done

Doctors may order the PTT test as part of an evaluation for a bleeding disorder such as hemophilia or von Willebrand disease. Symptoms of a bleeding disorder can include easy bruising, nosebleeds that won't stop, excessive bleeding after dental procedures, gums bleeding easily, heavy menstrual periods, blood in the urine, or swollen or painful joints.

Even in the absence of symptoms, doctors may use the test to ensure that clotting ability is normal before a patient undergoes a major procedure such as surgery.

The PTT test is especially useful in monitoring the effects of the blood-thinning medication heparin. Blood thinners are frequently given to prevent clots in patients who've had a heart attack or stroke, or who have an artificial heart valve. Because dosing is critical—enough medication must be given to prevent dangerous clots, but not so much so as to cause excessive bleeding—close monitoring is necessary.

In many cases, the PTT test is performed with a prothrombin time (PT) test to give doctors a more complete picture of clotting factor function.

Preparation

No special preparations are needed for this test. If your child takes blood-thinning medication, antihistamines, or aspirin, you should tell the doctor because these can affect test results.

On the day of the test, having your child wear a T-shirt or short-sleeved shirt can make things easier for the technician drawing the blood.

The Procedure

A health professional will clean the skin surface with antiseptic, and place an elastic band (tourniquet) around the upper arm to apply pressure and cause the veins to swell with blood. Then a needle is inserted into a vein (usually in the arm inside of the elbow or on the back of the hand) and blood is withdrawn and collected in a vial or syringe.

After the procedure, the elastic band is removed. Once the blood has been collected, the needle is removed and the area is covered with cotton or a bandage to stop the bleeding. Collecting the blood for the test will only take a few minutes.

What to Expect

Collecting a sample of blood is only temporarily uncomfortable and can feel like a quick pinprick. Afterward, there may be some mild bruising, which should go away in a day or so.

Getting the Results

Partial thromboplastin time is measured in seconds. PTT test results are compared with the average clotting time of healthy people.

The time is longer in people who take blood thinners. The blood sample will be processed by a machine and the results are usually available after a few hours or the next day.

Risks

The PTT test is considered a safe procedure. However, as with many medical tests, some problems can occur with having blood drawn. These include:

- fainting or feeling lightheaded

- hematoma (blood accumulating under the skin causing a lump or bruise)

- pain associated with multiple punctures to locate a vein

Chapter 9

Tests Used in the Assessment of Vascular Disease

How Is Heart Disease Diagnosed?

Your doctor will diagnose coronary heart disease (CHD) based on your medical and family histories, your risk factors, a physical exam, and the results from tests and procedures.

No single test can diagnose CHD. If your doctor thinks you have CHD, he or she may recommend one or more of the following tests.

EKG (Electrocardiogram)

An EKG is a simple, painless test that detects and records the heart's electrical activity. The test shows how fast the heart is beating and its rhythm (steady or irregular). An EKG also records the strength and timing of electrical signals as they pass through the heart.

An EKG can show signs of heart damage due to CHD and signs of a previous or current heart attack.

This chapter includes text excerpted from "Heart Disease in Women," National Heart, Lung, and Blood Institute (NHLBI), April 21, 2014.

Stress Testing

During stress testing, you exercise to make your heart work hard and beat fast while heart tests are done. If you can't exercise, you may be given medicines to increase your heart rate.

When your heart is working hard and beating fast, it needs more blood and oxygen. Plaque-narrowed coronary (heart) arteries can't supply enough oxygen-rich blood to meet your heart's needs.

A stress test can show possible signs and symptoms of CHD, such as:

- Abnormal changes in your heart rate or blood pressure

- Shortness of breath or chest pain

- Abnormal changes in your heart rhythm or your heart's electrical activity

If you can't exercise for as long as what is considered normal for someone your age, your heart may not be getting enough oxygen-rich blood. However, other factors also can prevent you from exercising long enough (for example, lung diseases, anemia, or poor general fitness).

As part of some stress tests, pictures are taken of your heart while you exercise and while you rest. These imaging stress tests can show how well blood is flowing in your heart and how well your heart pumps blood when it beats.

Echocardiography

Echocardiography (echo) uses sound waves to create a moving picture of your heart. The test provides information about the size and shape of your heart and how well your heart chambers and valves are working.

Echo also can show areas of poor blood flow to the heart, areas of heart muscle that aren't contracting normally, and previous injury to the heart muscle caused by poor blood flow.

Chest X-Ray

A chest X-ray creates pictures of the organs and structures inside your chest, such as your heart, lungs, and blood vessels.

A chest X-ray can reveal signs of heart failure, as well as lung disorders and other causes of symptoms not related to CHD.

Blood Tests

Blood tests check the levels of certain fats, cholesterol, sugar, and proteins in your blood. Abnormal levels may be a sign that you're at risk for CHD. Blood tests also help detect anemia, a risk factor for CHD.

During a heart attack, heart muscle cells die and release proteins into the bloodstream. Blood tests can measure the amount of these proteins in the bloodstream. High levels of these proteins are a sign of a recent heart attack.

Coronary Angiography and Cardiac Catheterization

Your doctor may recommend coronary angiography if other tests or factors suggest you have CHD. This test uses dye and special X-rays to look inside your coronary arteries.

To get the dye into your coronary arteries, your doctor will use a procedure called cardiac catheterization.

A thin, flexible tube called a catheter is put into a blood vessel in your arm, groin (upper thigh), or neck. The tube is threaded into your coronary arteries, and the dye is released into your bloodstream.

Special X-rays are taken while the dye is flowing through your coronary arteries. The dye lets your doctor study the flow of blood through your heart and blood vessels.

Coronary angiography detects blockages in the large coronary arteries. However, the test doesn't detect coronary microvascular disease (MVD). This is because coronary MVD doesn't cause blockages in the large coronary arteries.

Even if the results of your coronary angiography are normal, you may still have chest pain or other CHD symptoms. If so, talk with your doctor about whether you might have coronary MVD.

Your doctor may ask you to fill out a questionnaire called the Duke Activity Status Index. This questionnaire measures how easily you can do routine tasks. It gives your doctor information about how well blood is flowing through your coronary arteries.

Your doctor also may recommend other tests that measure blood flow in the heart, such as a cardiac MRI (magnetic resonance imaging) stress test.

Cardiac MRI uses radio waves, magnets, and a computer to create pictures of your heart as it beats. The test produces both still and moving pictures of your heart and major blood vessels.

Other tests done during cardiac catheterization can check blood flow in the heart's small arteries and the thickness of the artery walls.

Tests Used to Diagnose Broken Heart Syndrome

If your doctor thinks you have broken heart syndrome, he or she may recommend coronary angiography. Other tests are also used to diagnose this disorder, including blood tests, EKG, echo, and cardiac MRI.

Chapter 10

Commonly Used Medications for Cardiovascular Health

Chapter Contents

Section 10.1

Blood Thinner Pills: Your Guide to Using Them Safely

This section includes text excerpted from "Blood Thinner Pills: Your Guide to Using Them Safely," Agency for Healthcare Research and Quality (AHRQ), September 2015.

About Your Blood Thinner

Your doctor has prescribed a medicine called a blood thinner to prevent blood clots. Blood clots can put you at risk for heart attack, stroke, and other serious medical problems. A blood thinner is a kind of drug called an anticoagulant. "Anti" means against and "coagulant" means to thicken into a gel or solid.

Blood thinner drugs work well when they are used correctly.

Depending on where you receive care, you may be seen by a doctor, nurse, physician's assistant, nurse practitioner, pharmacist, or other healthcare professional. The term "doctor" is used in this section to refer to the person who helps you manage your blood thinner medicine.

You and your doctor will work together as a team to make sure that taking your blood thinner does not stop you from living well and safely.

There are different types of blood thinners. The most common blood thinner that doctors prescribe is warfarin (Coumadin®). Your doctor may also discuss using one of the newer blood thinners depending on your individual situation.

How to Take Your Blood Thinner

Always take your blood thinner as directed. For example, some blood thinners need to be taken at the same time of day, every day.

Never skip a dose, and never take a double dose.

If you miss a dose, take it as soon as you remember. If you don't remember until the next day, call your doctor for instructions. If this happens when your doctor is not available, skip the missed dose and start again the next day. Mark the missed dose in a diary or on a calendar.

A pillbox with a slot for each day may help you keep track of your medicines.

Check Your Medicine

Check your medicine when you get it from the pharmacy.

- Does the medicine seem different from what your doctor prescribed or look different from what you expected?

- Does your pill look different from what you used before?

- Are the color, shape, and markings on the pill the same as what you were given before?

If something seems different, ask the pharmacist to double check it. Many medication errors are found by patients.

Using Other Medicines

Tell your doctor about every medicine you take. The doctor needs to know about all your medicines, including medicines you used before you started taking a blood thinner.

Other medicines can change the way your blood thinner works. Your blood thinner can also change how other medicines work.

It is very important to talk with your doctor about all the medicines you take, including other prescription medicines, over-the-counter medicines, vitamins, and herbal products.

Products that contain aspirin may lessen the blood's ability to form clots and may increase your risk of bleeding when you also are taking a blood thinner. **If you are taking a blood thinner, talk to your doctor before taking any medication that has aspirin in it.**

Medicines you get over the counter may also interact with your blood thinner. Following is a list of some common medicines that you should talk with your doctor or pharmacist about before using.

Pain relievers, cold medicines, or stomach remedies, such as:

- Advil®

- Aleve®

- Alka-Seltzer®

- Excedrin®

- ex-lax®

- Midol®

- Motrin®

- Nuprin®

- Pamprin HB®

- Pepto Bismol®

- Sine-Off®

- Tagamet HB®

- Tylenol®

Vitamins and herbal products, such as:

- Centrum®, One a Day®, or other multivitamins

- Garlic

- Ginkgo biloba

- Green tea

Talk to your doctor about every medication and over-the-counter product that you take.

Talk to Your Other Doctors

Because you take a blood thinner, you will be seen regularly by the doctor who prescribed the medicine. You may also see other doctors for different problems. When you see other doctors, it is very important that you tell them you are taking a blood thinner. You should also tell your dentist and the person who cleans your teeth.

If you use different pharmacies, make sure each pharmacist knows that you take a blood thinner.

Blood thinners can interact with medicines and treatments that other doctors might prescribe for you. If another doctor orders a new medicine for you, tell the doctor who ordered your blood thinner because dose changes for your blood thinner may be needed.

Tell all your doctors about every medication and over-the-counter product that you take.

Possible Side Effects

When taking a blood thinner it is important to be aware of its possible side effects. Bleeding is the most common side effect.

Call your doctor immediately if you have any of the following signs of serious bleeding:

- menstrual bleeding that is much heavier than normal
- red or brown urine
- bowel movements that are red or look like tar
- bleeding from the gums or nose that does not stop quickly
- vomit that is brown or bright red
- anything red in color that you cough up
- severe pain, such as a headache or stomachache
- unusual bruising
- a cut that does not stop bleeding
- a serious fall or bump on the head
- dizziness or weakness

Stay Safe While Taking Your Blood Thinner

Call your doctor and go to the hospital immediately if you have had a fall or hit your head, even if you are not bleeding. You can be bleeding but not see any blood. For example, if you fall and hit your head, bleeding can occur inside your skull. Or, if you hurt your arm during a fall and then notice a large purple bruise, this means you are bleeding under your skin.

Because you are taking a blood thinner, you should try not to hurt yourself and cause bleeding. You need to be careful when you use knives, scissors, razors, or any sharp object that can make you bleed.

You also need to avoid activities and sports that could cause injury. Swimming and walking are safe activities. If you would like to start a new activity that will increase the amount of exercise you get every day, talk to your doctor.

You can still do many things that you enjoy. If you like to work in the yard, you still can. Just be sure to wear sturdy shoes and gloves to protect yourself. If you like to ride your bike, be sure you wear a helmet.

To prevent injury indoors:

- Be very careful using knives and scissors.
- Use an electric razor.

- Use a soft toothbrush.

- Use waxed dental floss.

- Do not use toothpicks.

- Wear shoes or non-skid slippers in the house.

- Be careful when you trim your toenails.

- Do not trim corns or calluses yourself.

  To prevent injury outdoors:

- Always wear shoes.

- Wear gloves when using sharp tools.

- Avoid activities and sports that can easily hurt you.

- Wear gardening gloves when doing yard work.

Food and Your Blood Thinner

If your doctor has prescribed warfarin, the foods you eat can affect how well your blood thinner works for you. High amounts of vitamin K can work against warfarin. Other blood thinners are not affected by vitamin K. Ask your doctor if your diet can affect how well your blood thinner works.

If you are taking a blood thinner, you should avoid drinking alcohol.

Call your doctor if you are unable to eat for several days, for whatever reason. Also call if you have stomach problems, vomiting, or diarrhea that lasts more than 1 day. These problems could affect your blood thinner dose.

Blood Tests

You will have to have your blood tested often if you are taking warfarin. The blood test helps your doctor decide how much medicine you need.

The International Normalized Ratio (INR) blood test measures how fast your blood clots and lets the doctor know if your dose needs to be changed. Testing your blood helps your doctor keep you in a safe range. If there is too much blood thinner in your body, you could bleed too much. If there is not enough, you could get a blood clot.

Regular blood tests are not needed for some of the newer blood thinners.

Section 10.2

Facts about Using Aspirin

This section includes text excerpted from "Aspirin for Reducing
Your Risk of Heart Attack and Stroke: Know the Facts," U.S. Food
and Drug Administration (FDA), May 2, 2014.

You can walk into any pharmacy, grocery or convenience store and
buy aspirin without a prescription. The Drug Facts label on medication
products, will help you choose aspirin for relieving headache, pain,
swelling, or fever. The Drug Facts label also gives directions that will
help you use the aspirin so that it is safe and effective.

But what about using aspirin for a different use, time period, or in
a manner that is not listed on the label? For example, using aspirin to
lower the risk of heart attack and clot-related strokes. In these cases,
the labeling information is not there to help you with how to choose
and how to use the medicine safely. **Since you don't have the labeling directions to help you, you need the medical knowledge of
your doctor, nurse practitioner or other health professional.**

You can increase the chance of getting the good effects and decrease
the chance of getting the bad effects of any medicine by choosing and
using it wisely.

Know the Facts and Work with Your Health Professional

FACT: Daily Use of Aspirin Is Not Right for Everyone

Aspirin has been shown to be helpful when used daily to lower the
risk of heart attack, clot-related strokes and other blood flow problems
in patients who have cardiovascular disease or who have already had
a heart attack or stroke. Many medical professionals prescribe aspirin
for these uses. There may be a benefit to daily aspirin use for you if you
have some kind of heart or blood vessel disease, or if you have evidence
of poor blood flow to the brain. However, the risks of long-term aspirin
use may be greater than the benefits if there are no signs of, or risk
factors for heart or blood vessel disease.

Every prescription and over-the-counter medicine has benefits and risks—even such a common and familiar medicine as aspirin. Aspirin use can result in serious side effects, such as stomach bleeding, bleeding in the brain, kidney failure, and some kinds of strokes. No medicine is completely safe. By carefully reviewing many different factors, your health professional can help you make the best choice for you.

When You Don't Have the Labeling Directions to Guide You, You Need the Medical Knowledge of Your Doctor, Nurse Practitioner, or Other Health Professional.

FACT: Daily Aspirin Can Be Safest When Prescribed by a Medical Health Professional

Before deciding if daily aspirin use is right for you, your health professional will need to consider:

- Your medical history and the history of your family members

- Your use of other medicines, including prescription and over-the-counter

- Your use of other products, such as dietary supplements, including vitamins and herbals

- Your allergies or sensitivities, and anything that affects your ability to use the medicine

- What you have to gain, or the benefits, from the use of the medicine

- Other options and their risks and benefits

- What side effects you may experience

- What dose, and what directions for use are best for you

- How to know when the medicine is working or not working for this use

Make Sure to Tell Your Health Professional All the Medicines (Prescription and Over-The-Counter) and Dietary Supplements, including Vitamins and Herbals, That You Use—Even If Only Occasionally

FACT: Aspirin Is a Drug

If you are at risk for heart attack or stroke your doctor may prescribe aspirin to increase blood flow to the heart and brain. But any drug—including aspirin—can have harmful side effects, especially when mixed with other products. In fact, the chance of side effects increases with each new product you use.

New products includes prescription and other over-the-counter medicines, dietary supplements (including vitamins and herbals), and sometimes foods and beverages. For instance, people who already use a prescribed medication to thin the blood should not use aspirin unless recommended by a health professional. There are also dietary supplements known to thin the blood. Using aspirin with alcohol or with another product that also contains aspirin, such as a cough-sinus drug, can increase the chance of side effects.

Your health professional will consider your current state of health. Some medical conditions, such as pregnancy, uncontrolled high blood pressure, bleeding disorders, asthma, peptic (stomach) ulcers, liver and kidney disease, could make aspirin a bad choice for you.

Make Sure That All Your Health Professionals Are Aware That You Are Using Aspirin to Reduce Your Risk of Heart Attack and Clot-Related Strokes.

FACT: Once Your Doctor Decides That Daily Use of Aspirin Is for You, Safe Use Depends on Following Your Doctor's Directions

There are no directions on the label for using aspirin to reduce the risk of heart attack or clot-related stroke. You may rely on your health professional to provide the correct information on dose and directions for use. Using aspirin correctly gives you the best chance of getting the greatest benefits with the fewest unwanted side effects. Discuss with your health professional the different forms of aspirin products that might be best suited for you.

Aspirin has been shown to lower the risk of heart attack and stroke in patients who have cardiovascular disease or who have already had a heart attack or stroke, but not all over-the-counter pain and fever reducers do that. Even though the directions on the aspirin label do not apply to this use of aspirin, you still need to read the label to confirm that the product you buy and use contains aspirin at the correct dose. Check the Drug Facts label for "active ingredients: aspirin" or "acetylsalicylic acid" at the dose that your health professional has prescribed.

Remember, if you are using aspirin everyday for weeks, months or years to prevent a heart attack, stroke, or for any use not listed on the label—without the guidance from your health professional—you could be doing your body more harm than good.

Section 10.3

Anticoagulants and Antiplatelet Agents

This section includes text excerpted from "Antithrombotic
Agents: Anticoagulants and Antiplatelet Agents," LiverTox®,
National Institutes of Health (NIH), June 28, 2016.

Overview: Antithrombotic Agents

Antithrombotic agents are separated into those drugs that decrease
the synthesis of coagulation factors or interrupt the coagulation cascade (anticoagulants) and those that inhibit platelet function (antiplatelet agents). A third class of agents are the thrombolytic drugs,
which act to promote dissolution of thromboses after they have formed.
The antithrombotic agents are rare causes of clinically apparent acute
liver injury.

Anticoagulants are used largely for the prevention and treatment
of venous thromboses, although they have some activity against arterial thromboses. Their major clinical use is prevention and treatment
of deep vein thrombosis in high risk persons (such as after hip or knee
replacement surgery or with prolonged immobilization), prevention
and treatment of pulmonary embolism, and prevention of arterial
embolism in patients with atrial fibrillation.

Antiplatelet agents are effective for the prevention and treatment of arterial thromboses (which are platelet rich). Aspirin is an
irreversible inhibitor of cyclooxygenase 1, which blocks platelet activation and aggregation for the life of the platelet. Aspirin is an irreversible inhibitor of cyclooxygenase 1, which blocks platelet activation
and aggregation for the life of the platelet. Aspirin is commonly used
for treatment and prevention of coronary, cerebrovascular and other
arterial thromboses (myocardial infarction, stroke, peripheral vascular disease). Dipyridamole blocks adenosine uptake which results
in inhibition of platelet aggregation; it is used with or without aspirin for secondary prevention of myocardial infarction or stroke. The
thienopyridines inhibit the major adenosine diphosphate receptor on
platelets which blocks their activation and aggregation; these agents

are also used for secondary prevention of coronary and cerebrovascular thrombosis. Ticagrelor is a platelet aggregation inhibitor with activity similar to the thienopyridines that is used with aspirin (<100 mg daily) as secondary prevention of arterial thrombosis with acute coronary syndrome. Finally, the glycoprotein IIb/IIIa receptor blockers have an immediate effect in preventing platelet aggregation blocking the action of fibrinogen and von Willebrand factor on these platelet receptors; these agents are administered intravenously and are used to attain immediate platelet inhibition in acute coronary syndrome or percutaneous coronary artery intervention.

Thrombolytic drugs include tissue plasminogen activators (tPA: alteplase, reteplase and tenecteplase), anistreplase, streptokinase and urokinase. These agents are administered intravenously immediately or soon after after arterial or venous thromboses or emboli. These agents have not been definitely linked to instances of acute liver injury.

Chapter 11

Commonly Used Medications for Anemia

Chapter Contents

Section 11.1

Iron Supplements

This section contains text excerpted from the following sources:
Text in this chapter begins with excerpts from "How Is Iron-
Deficiency Anemia Treated?" National Heart, Lung, and Blood
Institute (NHLBI), March 26, 2014; Text beginning with the heading
"Dietary Supplements" is excerpted from "Iron," Office of Dietary
Supplements (ODS), February 11, 2016.

You may need iron supplements to build up your iron levels as quickly as possible. Iron supplements can correct low iron levels within months. Supplements come in pill form or in drops for children.

Large amounts of iron can be harmful, so take iron supplements only as your doctor prescribes. Keep iron supplements out of reach from children. This will prevent them from taking an overdose of iron.

Iron supplements can cause side effects, such as dark stools, stomach irritation, and heartburn. Iron also can cause constipation, so your doctor may suggest that you use a stool softener.

Your doctor may advise you to eat more foods that are rich in iron. The best source of iron is red meat, especially beef and liver. Chicken, turkey, pork, fish, and shellfish also are good sources of iron.

The body tends to absorb iron from meat better than iron from nonmeat foods. However, some nonmeat foods also can help you raise your iron levels. Examples of nonmeat foods that are good sources of iron include:

- iron-fortified breads and cereals

- peas; lentils; white, red, and baked beans; soybeans; and chickpeas

- tofu

- dried fruits, such as prunes, raisins, and apricots

- spinach and other dark green leafy vegetables

- prune juice

The Nutrition Facts labels on packaged foods will show how much iron the items contain. The amount is given as a percentage of the total amount of iron you need every day.

Vitamin C

Vitamin C helps the body absorb iron. Good sources of vitamin C are vegetables and fruits, especially citrus fruits. Citrus fruits include oranges, grapefruits, tangerines, and similar fruits. Fresh and frozen fruits, vegetables, and juices usually have more vitamin C than canned ones.

If you're taking medicines, ask your doctor or pharmacist whether you can eat grapefruit or drink grapefruit juice. Grapefruit can affect the strength of a few medicines and how well they work.

Other fruits rich in vitamin C include kiwi fruit, strawberries, and cantaloupes.

Vegetables rich in vitamin C include broccoli, peppers, Brussels sprouts, tomatoes, cabbage, potatoes, and leafy green vegetables like turnip greens and spinach.

Treatment to Stop Bleeding

If blood loss is causing iron-deficiency anemia, treatment will depend on the cause of the bleeding. For example, if you have a bleeding ulcer, your doctor may prescribe antibiotics and other medicines to treat the ulcer.

If a polyp or cancerous tumor in your intestine is causing bleeding, you may need surgery to remove the growth.

If you have heavy menstrual flow, your doctor may prescribe birth control pills to help reduce your monthly blood flow. In some cases, surgery may be advised.

Treatments for Severe Iron-Deficiency Anemia

Blood Transfusion

If your iron-deficiency anemia is severe, you may get a transfusion of red blood cells. A blood transfusion is a safe, common procedure in which blood is given to you through an intravenous (IV) line in one of your blood vessels. A transfusion requires careful matching of donated blood with the recipient's blood.

A transfusion of red blood cells will treat your anemia right away. The red blood cells also give a source of iron that your body can reuse. However, a blood transfusion is only a short-term treatment. Your doctor will need to find and treat the cause of your anemia.

Blood transfusions are usually reserved for people whose anemia puts them at a higher risk for heart problems or other severe health issues.

Iron Therapy

If you have severe anemia, your doctor may recommend iron therapy. For this treatment, iron is injected into a muscle or an IV line in one of your blood vessels.

IV iron therapy presents some safety concerns. It must be done in a hospital or clinic by experienced staff. Iron therapy is usually given to people who need iron long-term but can't take iron supplements by mouth. This therapy is also given to people who need immediate treatment for iron-deficiency anemia.

Dietary Supplements

Iron is available in many dietary supplements. Multivitamin/multimineral supplements with iron, especially those designed for women, typically provide 18 mg iron (100% of the Daily Value (DV)). Multivitamin/multimineral supplements for men or seniors frequently contain less or no iron. Iron-only supplements usually deliver more than the DV, with many providing 65 mg iron (360% of the DV).

Frequently used forms of iron in supplements include ferrous and ferric iron salts, such as ferrous sulfate, ferrous gluconate, ferric citrate, and ferric sulfate. Because of its higher solubility, ferrous iron in dietary supplements is more bioavailable than ferric iron. High doses of supplemental iron (45 mg/day or more) may cause gastrointestinal side effects, such as nausea and constipation. Other forms of supplemental iron, such as heme iron polypeptides, carbonyl iron, iron amino-acid chelates, and polysaccharide-iron complexes, might have fewer gastrointestinal side effects than ferrous or ferric salts.

The different forms of iron in supplements contain varying amounts of elemental iron. For example, ferrous fumarate is 33 percent elemental iron by weight, whereas ferrous sulfate is 20 percent and ferrous gluconate is 12 percent elemental iron. Fortunately, elemental iron is listed in the Supplement Facts panel, so consumers do not need to calculate the amount of iron supplied by various forms of iron supplements.

Approximately 14 percent to 18 percent of Americans use a supplement containing iron. Rates of use of supplements containing iron vary by age and gender, ranging from 6 percent of children aged 12 to 19 years to 60 percent of women who are lactating and 72 percent of pregnant women.

Calcium might interfere with the absorption of iron, although this effect has not been definitively established. For this reason, some experts suggest that people take individual calcium and iron supplements at different times of the day.

Interactions with Medications

Iron can interact with certain medications, and some medications can have an adverse effect on iron levels. A few examples are provided below. Individuals taking these and other medications on a regular basis should discuss their iron status with their healthcare providers.

Levodopa

Some evidence indicates that in healthy people, iron supplements reduce the absorption of levodopa (found in Sinemet® and Stalevo®), used to treat Parkinson's disease and restless leg syndrome, possibly through chelation. In the United States, the labels for levodopa warn that iron-containing dietary supplements might reduce the amount of levodopa available to the body and, thus, diminish its clinical effectiveness.

Levothyroxine

Levothyroxine (Levothroid®, Levoxyl®, Synthroid®, Tirosint®, and Unithroid®) is used to treat hypothyroidism, goiter, and thyroid cancer. The simultaneous ingestion of iron and levothyroxine can result in clinically significant reductions in levothyroxine efficacy in some patients. The labels for some of these products warn that iron supplements can reduce the absorption of levothyroxine tablets and advise against administering levothyroxine within 4 hours of iron supplements.

Proton Pump Inhibitors

Gastric acid plays an important role in the absorption of nonheme iron from the diet. Because proton pump inhibitors, such as lansoprazole (Prevacid®) and omeprazole (Prilosec®), reduce the acidity of stomach contents, they can reduce iron absorption. Treatment with proton pump inhibitors for up to 10 years is not associated with iron depletion or anemia in people with normal iron stores. But patients with iron deficiency taking proton pump inhibitors can have suboptimal responses to iron supplementation.

Section 11.2

Erythropoiesis-Stimulating Agents

This section contains text excerpted from the following sources: Text under the heading "Overview of Erythropoiesis" is excerpted from "Epoetin and Darbepoetin for Managing Anemia in Patients Undergoing Cancer Treatment: Comparative Effectiveness Update," Agency for Healthcare Research and Quality (AHRQ), April 2013; Text under the heading "Erythropoiesis-Stimulating Agents" is excerpted from "Effect of Erythropoiesis-Stimulating Agent Policy Decisions on Off-Label Use in Myelodysplastic Syndromes," Centers for Medicare and Medicaid Services (CMS), 2014.

What Is Erythropoiesis?

Anemia, a deficiency in the concentration of hemoglobin-containing red blood cells, is prevalent among cancer patients, depending on the type of malignancy and treatment. Transfusion is one option for treating anemia related to cancer and cancer treatment. Transfusion carries a very low risk of infection and other adverse events, including transfusion reactions, alloimmunization, overtransfusion, and immune modulation with theoretically possible adverse effects on tumor growth.

Erythropoietin, a hormone produced in the kidney, is the major regulator of red blood cell production (erythropoiesis). Commercially produced recombinant human erythropoietins have been extensively studied and used clinically for more than a decade to treat anemia in association with various diseases, reducing the need for transfusion. These include epoetin alfa (Epogen®, Procrit®) and epoetin beta (not available in the United States); they have similar clinical efficacy. Darbepoetin alfa (Aranesp®), more recently developed, produces a similar physiologic response and is commercially available in the United States. All erythropoietic-stimulating agents (ESAs) increase the number of red blood cells within about 2 to 3 weeks when given to individuals with functioning erythropoiesis.

Erythropoiesis-Stimulating Agents

The erythropoiesis-stimulating agents (ESAs) epoetin alfa and darbepoetin are indicated for the treatment of anemia caused by end-stage renal disease (ESRD), zidovudine therapy in patients with HIV, chemotherapy in cancer patients, and also to reduce transfusion need in patients scheduled for noncardiac major surgery. In addition to the approved indications, ESAs are used off label in patients with myelodysplastic syndromes (MDS). MDS are a group of hematopoietic stem cell neoplasms characterized by ineffective hematopoiesis. Approximately 80 percent of MDS patients experience symptomatic anemia. ESA use is a central component of the strategy for reducing dependence on red blood cell transfusions. Clinical trial results indicate that approximately 40 percent of selected patients have a clinically meaningful hemoglobin response to ESAs, with a median response duration of two years.

Several studies, published beginning in 2003, raised concerns about the safety of ESAs. Associations were found between ESA use in cancer patients and venous thromboembolic events, tumor progression, and reduced overall survival. Consequently, the U.S. Food and Drug Administration (FDA) issued safety alerts in 2006 and required pharmaceutical companies to add safety warnings to ESA labels (i.e., "black box" warnings) in 2007–2008.

Chapter 12

Blood Transfusion

Blood transfusions save lives every day. Hospitals use blood trans-fusions to help people who are injured, having surgery, getting cancer treatments, or being treated for other diseases that affect the blood, like sickle cell anemia. In fact, about 5 million people each year in the United States get blood transfusions.

A Bit about Blood

As blood moves throughout the body, it carries oxygen and nutrients to all the places they're needed. Blood also collects waste products, like carbon dioxide, and takes them to the organs responsible for making sure wastes leave the body.

Blood is a mixture of cells and liquid. Each has a specific job:

- **Red blood cells** carry oxygen to the body's tissues and remove carbon dioxide. Red blood cells make up about 40%–45% of a person's blood and live for 120 days.

- **White blood cells** are part of the immune system, and its main defense against infection. White blood cells make up less than 1% of a person's blood.

- **Platelets** are cell fragments that help blood clot, which helps to prevent and control bleeding. A person's blood has about 1 plate-let for every 20 red blood cells.

This chapter includes text excerpted from "Blood Transfusion," © 1995–2016. The Nemours Foundation/KidsHealth®. Reprinted with permission.

- **Plasma** is a pale yellow liquid mixture of water, proteins, electrolytes, carbohydrates, cholesterol, hormones, and vitamins. About 55% of our blood is plasma.

Blood cells are made in the bone marrow (a spongy material inside many of the bones in the body). A full-grown adult has about 10 pints of blood (almost 5 liters) in his or her body.

What Is a Blood Transfusion?

A transfusion is a simple medical procedure that doctors use to make up for a loss of blood—or for any part of the blood, such as red blood cells or platelets.

A person usually gets a blood transfusion through an intravenous line, a tiny tube that is inserted into a vein with a small needle. The whole process takes about 1 to 4 hours, depending on how much blood is needed.

Blood from a donor needs to match the blood type of the person receiving it. There are eight main blood types:

1. O positive

2. O negative

3. A positive

4. A negative

5. B positive

6. B negative

7. AB positive

8. AB negative

In emergencies, there are exceptions to the rule that the donor's blood type must match the recipient's exactly. Blood type O negative is the only type of blood that people of all other blood types can receive. Medical teams use it in situations when patients need a transfusion but their blood type is unknown. Because of this, O negative donors are called "universal donors." People who have type AB blood are called "universal recipients" because they can safely receive any type of blood.

A blood transfusion usually isn't whole blood—it could be any one of the blood's components. For example, chemotherapy can affect how bone marrow makes new blood cells. So some people getting treatment for cancer might need a transfusion of red blood cells or platelets.

Other people might need plasma or only certain parts of plasma. People who have hemophilia, a disease that affects the blood's ability to clot, need plasma or the clotting factors contained in plasma to help their blood clot and prevent internal bleeding.

Where Does the Blood Come From?

In the United States, the blood supply for transfusions comes from people who volunteer to donate their blood. Donors give blood at local blood banks, at community centers during blood drives, or through the American Red Cross.

When people know they are going to have an operation that might include a blood transfusion, they may choose to receive blood from one of several different places. Most patients choose to receive blood from the donated supply, but some decide to use their own blood. Providing your own blood before surgery is called **autologous** blood donation.

Another option for blood transfusions is called **directed donation**. This is when a family member or friend donates blood specifically to be used by a designated patient. For directed donation, the donor must have a blood type that is compatible with the recipient's. He or she must also meet all the requirements of a regular volunteer blood donor. There is no medical or scientific evidence that blood from directed donors is safer or better than blood from volunteer donors.

How Safe Is Donated Blood?

Some people worry about getting diseases from infected blood, but the United States has one of the safest blood supplies in the world. Many organizations, including community blood banks and the federal government, work hard to ensure that the blood supply is safe.

All blood donors must provide a detailed history, including recent travel, infections, medicines, and health problems. In addition, the American Red Cross and other donation groups test donated blood for viruses like HIV (the virus that causes AIDS), hepatitis B, hepatitis C, syphilis, and West Nile virus. Since blood can also be infected with bacteria or parasites, some blood components also get tested for these. If any of these things are found, the blood is destroyed.

The U.S. Food and Drug Administration (FDA) regulates U.S. blood banks. All blood centers must pass regular inspections in order to continue their operations.

Do People Get Sick from Transfusions?

Most people's bodies handle blood transfusions very well. But, like any medical procedure, there are some risks, including:

- **Fever**. Patients can have a fever with a blood transfusion, sometimes along with chills, a headache, or nausea. These symptoms can be caused by a reaction between the recipient's immune system and immune cells in the donor blood. When this happens, doctors will stop the transfusion and give the patient fever-reducing medicine. When the patient's temperature is back to normal, the transfusion usually can continue.

- **Allergic reaction**. Allergic reactions to blood transfusions (like hives or itching) happen because of a reaction between the recipient's immune system and proteins in the donated blood. In a few rare cases, an allergic reaction can be severe (a condition called anaphylaxis). Stopping the transfusion and giving the patient medications for allergy, including antihistamines and steroids, can treat these reactions. If the reaction is mild, the transfusion can start again. If it is more serious, doctors may have to take other measures before the patient can be given a transfusion again.

- **Hemolytic reaction**. A hemolytic reaction can be life-threatening. It happens when the patient's blood and the donated blood do not match. When the types don't match, the recipient's immune system attacks the red blood cells in the donated blood and destroys them. (The word hemolysis means the destruction of red blood cells.)

If a hemolytic reaction happens, doctors stop the transfusion and treat the symptoms. Hemolytic reaction is very rare, though, as healthcare professionals take many precautions to confirm a patient's and donor's blood are compatible before giving a transfusion.

In almost every situation, the benefits of having a blood transfusion far outweigh the risks.

Chapter 13

Bone Marrow and Stem Cell Transplants

Understanding Bone Marrow and Cord Blood Transplants

What Is a Bone Marrow Transplant?

A bone marrow transplant is a potentially life-saving treatment for people with leukemia, lymphoma and many other diseases. Patients undergo chemotherapy and sometimes radiation to destroy their diseased marrow. Then a donor's healthy blood-forming cells are given directly into the patient's bloodstream, where they can begin to multiply and function.

For a patient's body to accept these healthy cells, the donor's tissue type needs to match the patient's type as closely as possible. Patients who do not have a suitably matched donor in their family may search for an unrelated bone marrow donor or donated umbilical cord blood unit through the registry of the C.W. Bill Young Cell Transplantation Program, also called the Be The Match Registry®. The registry is a listing of potential bone marrow donors and donated cord blood units and is operated under Federal contracts by the National Marrow Donor Program®.

This chapter includes text excerpted from "Transplant Frequently Asked Questions," Health Resources and Services Administration (HRSA), May 5, 2015.

What Are Blood-Forming Cells?

Blood-forming cells are one of several types of cells in your body that can grow into other types of cells. Blood-forming cells grow into red blood cells, white blood cells, and platelets, all of which are important for your body.

- Red blood cells carry oxygen to all parts of your body.
- White blood cells help your body fight infection.
- Platelets help control bleeding.

A healthy body is always making new blood-forming cells. A person cannot survive for long without healthy blood cells.

Where Do Blood-Forming Cells Used in a Transplant Come From?

The blood-forming cells can come from three sources: bone marrow, peripheral (circulating) blood, and the blood in the umbilical cord and placenta after a baby's birth.

- Bone marrow produces blood-forming cells for the body. Bone marrow is a spongy tissue found inside larger bones. In a surgical procedure, doctors make several small incisions through the skin over the back of the pelvic bone to draw out the marrow.

- Peripheral blood stem cells (PBSC) are blood-forming cells found in the bloodstream. Normally, the bone marrow releases only a small number of blood-forming cells into the bloodstream. To donate PBSC, a donor is given injections of a medication that makes the blood-forming cells move from the bone marrow into the blood. The cells are collected from the blood during an outpatient procedure, similar to plasma or platelet donation.

- Umbilical cord blood is collected from the umbilical cord and placenta after a baby is born. This blood contains a large number of blood-forming cells. (These are not embryonic stem cells.) If the cord blood meets standards for transplant, it is stored at a public cord blood bank for future use.

What Is an Umbilical Cord Blood Unit and How Is It Used in Transplant?

An umbilical cord blood unit is the blood collected from the umbilical cord and placenta after a baby is born. Cord blood is rich in blood-forming cells. (These cells are not embryonic stem cells.) In a cord blood transplant, these healthy cells replace the diseased cells of patients with leukemia, lymphoma, or many other life-threatening diseases.

Cord blood is one of three sources of cells used in transplant; the other two are bone marrow and peripheral blood (circulating blood), which is also called peripheral blood stem cells or PBSC.

When Is a Cord Blood Transplant a Treatment Option?

Like bone marrow, umbilical cord blood is rich in blood-forming cells-cells (The cells in cord blood are not embryonic stem cells.). In a cord blood transplant, these healthy cells replace the diseased cells of patients who have leukemia, lymphoma, or many other life-threatening diseases.

The patient's doctor decides which source of blood-forming cells is best for the patient: cord blood, bone marrow, or PBSC. However, not all transplant centers are able to do cord blood transplants.

The chances of a successful bone marrow or cord blood transplant are better when the blood-forming cells are from a donor who closely matches the patient's tissue type. However, studies suggest that cord blood may not need to match as closely as is required for a marrow donor. Umbilical cord blood may be especially promising for:

- Patients who have difficulty finding a matched marrow donor.

- Patients from diverse heritages who often have an uncommon tissue type.

- Patients who have a life-threatening genetic disorder.

- Patients who need a transplant quickly.

Are the Donors Contacted before the Cord Blood Is Used to Ensure That the Donor Does Not Have Any Conditions, Diseases or Disorders That May Affect Donated Blood Stem Cells?

When a cord blood unit is found to be a potential match for a patient, every effort is made to contact the donor. This is to make sure that the baby's health has not changed since the cord blood donation because some changes could affect the transplant results.

If the Blood Stem Cells Have Already Been Used and the Donor Develops Leukemia (for example), Is There a Way to Notify the Recipient?

Every effort is made to notify the individuals affected if:

- The donor develops health problems that could potentially affect the recipient of the donated unit.

- The recipient develops health problems that could be due to the donated cord blood.

A Donor and Patient Safety Monitoring Committee that is made up of experts in blood stem cell transplant tracks these types of incidents and follows through until they are resolved. This Committee is maintained by one of the Program Contractors.

Deciding Whether to Have a Bone Marrow or Cord Blood Transplant

Is a Bone Marrow or Umbilical Cord Blood Transplant the Right Treatment?

A transplant can help a patient live a longer and healthier life. For many patients, a transplant offers the best or only opportunity for a cure and for survival.

However, there are also risks from a bone marrow or cord blood transplant. Some patients suffer from life-threatening problems as a result of their transplant. These problems can include serious infections and graft-versus-host disease (GVHD), in which the transplanted cells attack the patient's body.

The patient, doctor, and patient's family need to consider many things, including:

- disease

- disease status

- patient's age

- patient's overall health

- availability of a well-matched donor

- other treatment options

A timely referral to a transplant center for consultation can increase a patient's likelihood of a favorable outcome if a transplant is needed.

What Diseases Are Treated Most Often with an Unrelated Bone Marrow or Umbilical Cord Blood Transplant?

Almost three-fourths of transplants using an unrelated marrow donor or cord blood unit are for patients with leukemia or lymphoma.

The specific types of these diseases include:

- Acute lymphoblastic leukemia (ALL)
- Acute myelogenous leukemia (AML)
- Chronic lymphocytic leukemia (CLL)
- Chronic myelogenous leukemia (CML)
- Juvenile myelomonocytic leukemia
- Lymphomas: Hodgkin and non-Hodgkin

Other diseases that may be treated with a transplant include:

- Hemoglobinopathies such as sickle cell anemia and thalassemia
- Inherited immune system disorders, such as severe combined immunodeficiency (SCID) and Wiskott-Aldrich syndrome
- Inherited metabolic disorders, such as Hurler's syndrome and leukodystrophies
- Marrow failure states such as severe aplastic anemia and fanconi anemia
- Myelodysplastic syndromes
- Myeloproliferative disorders
- Plasma disorders such as multiple myeloma

How Many Bone Marrow or Umbilical Cord Blood Transplants Have Been Performed for My Disease?

When considering a bone marrow or cord blood transplant as a treatment option, it may be helpful to view how many other people with your disease received a transplant. However, keep in mind that no two people are exactly alike, and responses to the same treatment can vary greatly.

What Is the Difference between an Autologous and Allogeneic Bone Marrow or Umbilical Cord Blood Transplant?

A transplant may use cells taken from the patient (autologous) or from a volunteer donor (allogeneic).

- An autologous transplant uses the patient's own blood-forming cells that are collected and used later for transplant.

- An allogeneic transplant uses cells from a volunteer marrow donor or cord blood unit. The donor's tissue type must closely match the patient's tissue type. The donor or cord blood unit can be either related or unrelated to the patient. Related donors are usually a brother or sister.

Patients who do not have a closely matched donor in their family may search for an unrelated marrow donor or donated cord blood unit through the registry of the C.W. Bill Young Cell Transplantation Program (also called the Be The Match Registry®).

What Are the Expected Outcomes If I Have a Bone Marrow or Umbilical Cord Blood Transplant?

Survival outcomes data show an estimate of the percentage of people with a certain disease who survive for a specific amount of time. When looking at survival outcomes data, keep in mind that outcomes are affected by:

- Patient factors, such as specific diagnosis, disease status, age, overall health, and previous treatments.

- Donor factors, such as who donated the cells (the patient, a family member, or an unrelated donor), the source of the cells (bone marrow, peripheral blood, or umbilical cord blood) and the level of matching between the patient and the donated cells.

- Number of patients included. Data that include larger number of patients can more accurately predict likely outcomes for other patients.

- When the patients were treated. Treatments can change over time. Data for patients treated five years ago may not be representative of what patients can expect today.

Survival outcomes can help you and your doctor better understand your prognosis and can be helpful in making treatment choices.

- Outcome data can help you and your doctor understand the likely course of your disease (prognosis). The data show how other people with a similar disease responded to different treatments.

- Outcome data cannot predict the outcome of any one person. The data can only report what may happen based on the experiences of other patients.

No two people are exactly alike and responses to the same treatment can vary greatly. To understand how information applies to you, talk to your doctor.

How Does Survival of Patients Receiving a Transplant from an Unrelated Donor Compare to Those from a Related Donor?

Survival is improving. Outcomes of unrelated donor transplants are approaching the rates of related donor transplants. In 2011, overall survival rates at one year were 69 percent (unrelated donor) and 79 percent (related donor).

Unrelated donor transplant outcomes have improved due to a number of factors, including changes in clinical practice and a better understanding of human leukocyte antigen (HLA) typing and matching.

When a sibling donor is unavailable, unrelated donors are a very good alternative.

Is the Patient at Risk of Catching a Disease from an Unrelated Bone Marrow Transplant?

Unrelated donors on the registry of the C.W. Bill Young Cell Transplantation Program (also called The Be The Match Registry®) are carefully screened and tested. These tests significantly reduce the risk—but do not completely eliminate the possibility—that a donor could pass a disease to a patient.

Before they are approved to donate, donors:

- Are tested for infectious diseases such as acquired immunodeficiency syndrome (AIDS) and hepatitis.

- Answer questions about their health history. This helps doctors find risks that the donors may have, such as infectious or hereditary diseases.

- Are checked by doctors for signs of disease.

The National Marrow Donor Program® (NMDP), which operates the registry under Federal contracts, keeps current with diseases and infections transmitted by blood. Sometimes new or rare diseases, such as West Nile virus or severe acute respiratory syndrome (SARS), become public concerns. When this happens, the NMDP uses available methods to watch for these diseases. If a donor shows signs of disease, in some cases he or she will not be allowed to donate. In other cases, where the risk to the patient is considered small, it may be up to the transplant doctor and patient whether or not to use that donor.

Patient and donor safety are top priority for the NMDP. The NMDP Donor and Patient Safety Monitoring Committee helps ensure that the processes and procedures are effective and safe for donors and patients.

Is the Patient at Risk of Catching a Disease from an Unrelated Umbilical Cord Blood Transplant?

Unrelated cord blood units on the registry of the C.W. Bill Young Cell Transplantation Program (also called the Be The Match Registry®) are carefully screened and tested. These tests significantly reduce the risk—but do not completely eliminate the possibility—that the cord blood unit could pass a disease to a patient.

Before a mother donates her baby's umbilical cord blood, she:

- Answers questions about her eligibility to donate.

- Completes health history forms about herself and her family. This information helps doctors determine if the mother is free from diseases that could be transferred to another person through blood-forming cells.

After the cord blood is donated, a sample of the mother's blood is tested for infectious diseases such as acquired immunodeficiency syndrome (AIDS) and hepatitis.

Patient and donor safety are top priority for the National Marrow Donor Program (NMDP). (The NMDP operates the registry under Federal contracts.) The NMDP Donor and Patient Safety Monitoring Committee helps ensure that the processes and procedures are effective and safe for donors and patients.

Chapter 14

Chelation Therapy

Chelation for Coronary Heart Disease[1]

Coronary heart disease is the number-one killer of men and women in the United States. Lifestyle changes (such as quitting smoking), medicines, and medical and surgical procedures are among the mainstays of conventional treatment. Some heart patients also turn to chelation therapy using disodium EDTA (ethylene diamine tetra-acetic acid), a controversial complementary health approach. The use of disodium EDTA for heart disease has not been approved by the U.S. Food and Drug Administration (FDA). Use of this therapy to treat heart disease and other diseases grew, however, in the United States from 2002 to 2007 by nearly 68 percent, to an estimated 111,000 people using it annually.

Chelation is a chemical process in which a substance is used to bind molecules, such as metals or minerals, and hold them tightly so that they can be removed from the body. Chelation has been used to rid the body of excess or toxic metals. It has some uses in conventional medicine, such as treating lead poisoning or iron overload. When used

---

This chapter includes text excerpted from documents published by two public domain sources. Text under headings marked 1 are excerpted from "Chelation for Coronary Heart Disease," National Center for Complementary and Integrative Health (NCCIH), March 25, 2016; text under heading marked 2 is excerpted from "Chelation Therapy Reduces Cardiovascular Events for Older Patients with Diabetes," National Center for Complementary and Integrative Health (NCCIH), January 10, 2014.

as a complementary treatment for heart disease, a healthcare provider typically administers a solution of disodium EDTA, a man-made amino acid, in a series of infusions through the veins. A course of treatment can require 30 or more infusions of several hours each, taken weekly until the maintenance phase. Patients also typically take high-dose pills of vitamins and minerals.

Chelation Therapy Reduces Cardiovascular Events for Older Patients with Diabetes[2]

Chelation treatments reduced cardiovascular events, such as heart attacks, and death in patients with diabetes but not in those who did not have diabetes, according to analyses of data from the National Institutes of Health (NIH)-funded Trial to Assess Chelation Therapy (TACT). However, researchers say more studies are needed before it's known whether this promising finding leads to a treatment option.

Chelation is a chemical process in which a substance is delivered intravenously (through the veins) to bind atoms of metals or minerals, and hold them tightly so that they can be removed from the body. Chelation is conventionally used as a treatment for heavy metal (like lead) poisoning, although some people use chelation as an unapproved and unproven treatment for conditions like heart disease.

Chelation therapy is not approved by the U.S. Food and Drug Administration (FDA) to treat heart disease. However, use of chelation therapy to treat heart disease and other health problems grew in the United States between 2002 and 2007 by nearly 68 percent to 111,000 people, according to the 2008 National Health Statistics Report.

The diabetes subgroup analysis of TACT was published in *Circulation: Cardiovascular Quality and Outcomes* and presented at the American Heart Association's Scientific Sessions 2013. TACT is a study supported by NIH's National Center for Complementary and Alternative Medicine (NCCAM) and National Heart, Lung, and Blood Institute (NHLBI).

TACT's initial report was published in the March 27, 2013, issue of *The Journal of the American Medical Association*. This previous report showed that infusions of a form of chelation therapy using disodium ethylene diamine tetra-acetic acid (EDTA) produced a modest but statistically significant reduction in cardiovascular events in all EDTA-treated participants. However, further examination of the data showed that patients with diabetes were significantly impacted by chelation therapy while patients without diabetes were not.

The patients with diabetes, which made up approximately one third of 1,708 participants, demonstrated a 41 percent overall reduction in the risk of any cardiovascular event; a 40 percent reduction in the risk of death from heart disease nonfatal stroke, or nonfatal heart attack; a 52 percent reduction in recurrent heart attacks; and a 43 percent reduction in death from any cause. In contrast, there was no significant benefit of EDTA treatment in the subgroup of 1,045 participants who did not have diabetes.

"These are striking results that, if supported by future research, could point the way towards new treatments to prevent complications of diabetes," said Gervasio A. Lamas, M.D., the study's principal investigator and chairman of medicine and chief of the Columbia University Division of Cardiology at Mount Sinai Medical Center in Miami Beach.

From 2003 to 2010, 1,708 adults aged 50 and older were enrolled in TACT, of whom 633 had diabetes. Study participants had suffered a heart attack 6 weeks or more before enrollment (on average, the heart attack occurred about 4.5 years earlier). The participants were assigned randomly to receive 40 infusions of disodium EDTA chelation solution or a placebo solution. Patients also were randomly assigned to receive high doses of oral vitamins and minerals or an identical oral placebo. Most participants also took standard medicines for heart attack survivors, such as aspirin, beta blockers, and statins. They were followed for a minimum of 1 year and up to 5 years, with followup ending in October 2011.

TACT was not designed to discover how or why chelation might benefit patients with diabetes.

"Although subgroup analyses of clinical trials do not provide definitive answers, they are very useful in identifying future research questions," said Josephine Briggs, M.D., Director of NCCAM. "The effects seen in this population are large and very intriguing. This analysis suggests strongly that more research is needed to examine possible benefits of chelation in diabetics and the potential mechanisms."

"We share Dr. Briggs's interest in these compelling findings," said Michael Lauer, M.D., Director of the NHLBI's Division of Cardiovascular Sciences. "Additional studies are needed before we can determine the potential place of EDTA chelation therapy, if any, in the treatment of patients with coronary artery disease and diabetes."

Bottom Line[1]

- Overall, TACT showed that infusions of EDTA chelation therapy produced a modest reduction in cardiovascular events in

EDTA-treated participants. However, further examination of the data showed that chelation therapy benefitted only the patients with diabetes.

- Patients with diabetes, who made up approximately one third of the 1,708 TACT participants, had a 41 percent overall reduction in the risk of any cardiovascular event; a 40 percent reduction in the risk of death from heart disease, nonfatal stroke, or nonfatal heart attack; a 52 percent reduction in recurrent heart attacks; and a 43 percent reduction in death from any cause. In contrast, there was no significant benefit of EDTA treatment in participants who didn't have diabetes.

- The TACT study team also looked at the impact of taking high-dose vitamins and minerals in addition to the chelation therapy. They found that chelation plus high-dose vitamins and minerals produced the greatest reduction in risk of cardiovascular events versus placebo.

- Further research is needed to fully understand the TACT results. Since this is the first clinical trial to show a benefit, these results are not, by themselves, sufficient to support the routine use of chelation as a post-heart attack therapy.

Safety[1]

- In the TACT study, which had extensive safety monitoring, 16 percent of people receiving chelation and 15 percent of people receiving the placebo stopped their infusions because of an adverse event. Four of those events were serious; two were in the chelation group (one death) and two were in the placebo group (one death).

- The most common side effect of EDTA chelation is a burning sensation at the site where EDTA is administered. Rare side effects can include fever, headache, nausea, and vomiting. Even more rare are serious and potentially fatal side effects that can include heart failure, a sudden drop in blood pressure, abnormally low calcium levels in the blood (hypocalcemia), permanent kidney damage, and bone marrow depression (blood cell counts fall). Hypocalcemia and death may occur particularly if disodium EDTA is infused too rapidly. Reversible injury to the kidneys, although infrequent, has been reported with EDTA chelation therapy. Other serious side effects can occur if EDTA is not administered by a trained health professional.

- If you're considering chelation therapy, discuss it first with your cardiologist or other healthcare provider for your heart care. Seek out and consider information available from scientific studies on the therapy.

- If you decide to use chelation, choose the practitioner carefully. Do not take over-the-counter products marketed for "chelation" purposes.

- Give all your healthcare providers a full picture of what you do to manage your health. This will help ensure coordinated and safe care.

Part Three

Blood Disorders

Chapter 15

Anemia

Chapter Contents

Section 15.1

Anemia: An Overview

This section includes text excerpted from "Anemia,"
National Heart, Lung, and Blood Institute (NHLBI),
September 15, 2011. Reviewed July 2016.

Anemia is a blood disorder. Blood is a vital liquid that your heart constantly pumps through your veins and arteries and all throughout your body. When something goes wrong in your blood, it can affect your health and quality of life.

Many types of anemia exist, such as iron-deficiency anemia, pernicious anemia, aplastic anemia, and hemolytic anemia. The different types of anemia are linked to various diseases and conditions.

Anemia can affect people of all ages, races, and ethnicities. Some types of anemia are very common, and some are very rare. Some are very mild, and others are severe or even life-threatening if not treated aggressively. The good news is that anemia often can be successfully treated and even prevented.

What Causes Anemia?

Anemia occurs if your body makes too few red blood cells (RBCs), destroys too many RBCs, or loses too many RBCs. RBCs contain hemoglobin, a protein that carries oxygen throughout your body. When you don't have enough RBCs or the amount of hemoglobin in your blood is low, your body doesn't get all the oxygen it needs. As a result, you may feel tired or have other symptoms.

In some types of anemia, such as aplastic anemia, your body also doesn't have enough of other types of blood cells, such as white blood cells (WBCs) and platelets. WBCs help your body's immune system fight infections. Platelets help your blood clot, which helps stop bleeding.

Many diseases, conditions, and other factors can cause anemia. For example, anemia may occur during pregnancy if the body can't meet its increased need for RBCs. Certain autoimmune disorders and other conditions may cause your body to make proteins that destroy your RBCs, which can lead to anemia. Heavy internal or external bleeding—from injuries, for example—may cause anemia because your body loses too many RBCs.

The causes of anemia can be acquired or inherited. "Acquired" means you aren't born with the condition, but you develop it. "Inherited" means your parents passed the gene for the condition on to you. Sometimes the cause of anemia is unknown.

Specific Types of Anemia

- Aplastic Anemia
- Hemolytic Anemia
- Iron-Deficiency Anemia
- Pernicious Anemia

Diagnosing Anemia

People find out they have anemia in a variety of ways. You may have symptoms and go to your doctor, who discovers the anemia through blood tests. Or, your doctor might find out you have anemia as a result of tests done for another reason.

Your doctor will likely ask about your medical and family histories, do a physical exam, and recommend tests or procedures to find out whether you have anemia, what is causing it, and how severe it is.

This information will help your doctor treat the anemia and its underlying cause. Most anemias are treatable, so an accurate diagnosis is important.

Possible Signs and Symptoms of Anemia

- tiredness or weakness
- pale or yellowish skin
- faintness or dizziness
- increased thirst
- sweating
- weak and rapid pulse, rapid breathing
- shortness of breath
- lower leg cramps

- heart-related symptoms (abnormal heart rhythms, heart murmur, enlarged heart, heart failure)

Medical and Family Histories

Your doctor will want to know about your signs and symptoms and how long you've had them. He or she also may ask whether you've had an illness that can cause anemia. You also may be asked about your diet, any medicines or supplements you take, and whether you have a family history of anemia or anemia-related conditions.

Physical Exam

A physical exam can confirm signs and symptoms and provide information about what organs or body systems may be involved. As part of a physical exam, your doctor may check the color of your skin, gums, and nail beds and look for signs of bleeding or infection. He or she may listen to your heart and lungs, feel your abdomen, or do a pelvic or rectal exam to check for internal bleeding.

Tests and Procedures

Your doctor will recommend tests to identify the type of anemia you may have and its severity. Often, the first test is a complete blood count (CBC), which provides useful information about your blood. Depending on the CBC results, your doctor may recommend further tests of your blood or bone marrow (the soft tissue inside bones that makes blood cells).

Treating Anemia

Anemia often is easily treated. The treatment your doctor chooses will depend on the type of anemia you have, its cause, and how severe it is.

The main goals of treatment are to:

- Raise your RBC count or hemoglobin level to improve your blood's ability to carry oxygen

- Treat the underlying condition causing your anemia

- Prevent complications of the anemia, such as heart or nerve damage

- Relieve symptoms and improve your quality of life

If you have a mild or moderate anemia with no symptoms—or if your anemia isn't getting worse—you may not need treatment. Some anemias are treated with dietary changes and nutritional supplements. Other anemias are treated with medicines, procedures, surgery, or blood transfusions (for severe anemia).

Preventing or Controlling Anemia

You can take steps to prevent or control anemia. These actions can give you greater energy and improve your health and quality of life. Here are a few simple things you can do.

Follow a Healthy Diet

Following a healthy diet ensures that you get enough of the nutrients that your body needs to make healthy blood cells. These nutrients include iron, vitamin B12, folate, and vitamin C. These nutrients are found in a variety of foods. Healthy eating also is good for your overall health.

The basics of healthy eating:

- Focus on nutrient-dense foods and beverages—vegetables, fruits, whole grains, fat-free or low-fat dairy products, seafood, lean meats and poultry, eggs, beans and peas, and nuts and seeds.

- Limit your intake of salt, solid fats, added sugars, and refined grains.

- Maintain a healthy weight by balancing the calories you get from foods and beverages with the calories you use through physical activity.

- Follow food safety guidelines when preparing and eating foods to reduce the risk of foodborne illnesses.

Make following a healthy diet a family goal. Infants, young children, and teens grow rapidly. A healthy diet supports growth and development and can help prevent anemia. Have healthy foods at home, and show your children how to make healthy choices when they're away from home.

Also, help your parents or other older relatives enjoy a healthy, nutrient-rich diet. Anemia is common in older adults because of chronic (ongoing) diseases, lack of iron, and poor diet.

Avoid Substances That Can Cause or Trigger Anemia

Contact with chemicals or toxins in the environment can cause some types of anemia. Others types of anemia are triggered by certain foods or cold temperatures. If you have one of these types of anemia, avoid these triggers if you can.

With some types of anemia, you'll want to reduce your chances of getting an infection. To do this, wash your hands often, avoid people who have colds, and stay away from crowds.

Work with Your Doctor

Visit your doctor if you have signs or symptoms of anemia. If you're diagnosed with anemia, follow your doctor's advice about diet, supplements, medicines, and other treatments.

Visit your doctor regularly for checkups and ongoing care, and tell him or her about any new or changing symptoms.

Older children and teens who have severe anemia may have an increased risk of injury or infection. Talk with your doctor about ways to keep them as healthy as possible and whether they need to avoid certain activities.

Girls and women who have heavy menstrual periods may need regular screenings and follow up with their doctors to prevent or control iron-deficiency anemia.

Talk to Your Family

Some types of anemia—such as pernicious anemia, Fanconi anemia, or thalassemia—can be inherited. If you've been diagnosed with one of these kinds of anemia, talk to your family members. Suggest they visit their doctors for a checkup to see whether they also might have anemia.

If you have children or teens who have anemia, talk to them about how they can take an active role in their own care. Encourage them to learn about their condition and make decisions with their doctor. This can help young people feel more in control and have a more positive outlook about their health.

Section 15.2

Anemia of Chronic Disease

This section includes text excerpted from "Anemia of Inflammation
and Chronic Disease," National Institute of Diabetes and
Digestive and Kidney Diseases (NIDDK), September 2013.

What Is Anemia of Inflammation and Chronic Disease (AI/ACD)?

Anemia of inflammation and chronic disease is a type of anemia that commonly occurs with chronic, or long term, illnesses or infections. Cancer and inflammatory disorders, in which abnormal activation of the immune system occurs, can also cause AI/ACD.

AI/ACD is easily confused with iron-deficiency anemia because in both forms of anemia levels of iron circulating in the blood are low. Iron in the body is found both circulating in the blood and stored in body tissues. Circulating iron is necessary for red blood cell production. Low blood iron levels occur in iron-deficiency anemia because levels of the iron stored in the body's tissues are depleted. In AI/ACD, however, iron stores are normal or high. Low blood iron levels occur in AI/ACD, despite normal iron stores, because inflammatory and chronic diseases interfere with the body's ability to use stored iron and absorb iron from the diet. AI/ACD is the second most common form of anemia, after iron-deficiency anemia.

Who Gets AI/ACD?

While AI/ACD can affect people at any age, older adults are especially at risk because they have the highest rates of chronic disease. AI/ACD is also common among hospitalized patients, particularly those with chronic illnesses.

More than 130 million Americans live with at least one chronic illness. Addressing the causes of anemia in people with chronic disease can help improve their health and quality of life.

What Causes AI/ACD?

Anemia of inflammation and chronic disease is caused by red blood cells not functioning normally, so they cannot absorb and use iron efficiently. In addition, the body cannot respond normally to erythropoietin (EPO), a hormone made by the kidneys that stimulates bone marrow to produce red blood cells. Over time, this abnormal functioning causes a lower than normal number of red blood cells in the body.

Some of the chronic diseases that lead to AI/ACD include infectious and inflammatory diseases, kidney disease, and cancer. Certain treatments for chronic diseases may also impair red blood cell production and contribute to AI/ACD.

Infectious and inflammatory diseases. As part of the immune system response that occurs with infectious and inflammatory diseases, cells of the immune system release proteins called cytokines. Cytokines help heal the body and defend it against infection. However, they can also affect normal body functions. In AI/ACD, immune cytokines interfere with the body's ability to absorb and use iron. Cytokines may also interfere with the production and normal activity of EPO.

Infectious diseases that cause AI/ACD include

- tuberculosis, an infection in the lungs

- HIV/AIDS, an infection that destroys the immune system

- endocarditis, an infection in the heart

- osteomyelitis, a bone infection

Sometimes, acute infections—those that develop quickly and may not last long—can also cause AI/ACD.

Inflammatory diseases that can lead to AI/ACD include

- **Rheumatoid arthritis**, which causes pain, swelling, stiffness, and loss of function in the joints.

- **Lupus**, which causes damage to various body tissues, such as the joints, skin, kidneys, heart, lungs, blood vessels, and brain.

- **Diabetes**, in which levels of blood glucose, also called blood sugar, are above normal.

- **Heart failure**, in which the heart cannot pump enough blood to meet the body's needs.

- **Inflammatory bowel disease (IBD)**, diseases that cause inflammation and irritation in the intestines.

IBD, including Crohn's disease, can also cause iron deficiency due to poor absorption of iron by the diseased intestine and bleeding from the gastrointestinal (GI) tract.

Kidney disease. People with kidney disease can develop anemia for several different reasons. Diseased kidneys often fail to make enough EPO. In addition, kidney disease results in abnormal absorption and use of iron, which is typical of AI/ACD. Anemia worsens as kidney disease advances. Therefore, most people with kidney failure have anemia. Kidney failure is described as end-stage kidney disease, sometimes called ESRD, when treated with a kidney transplant or blood-filtering treatments called dialysis.

People with kidney failure can also develop iron deficiency due to blood loss during hemodialysis, a type of dialysis that uses a special filter called a dialyzer to remove wastes from the blood. Low levels of iron and folic acid—another nutrient required for normal red blood cell production—may also contribute to anemia in people with kidney disease.

Cancer. AI/ACD can occur with certain types of cancer, including Hodgkin disease, non-Hodgkin lymphoma, and breast cancer. Like infectious and inflammatory diseases, these types of cancer cause inflammatory cytokines to be released in the body. Anemia can also be made worse by chemotherapy and radiation treatments that damage the bone marrow, and by the cancer's invasion of bone marrow.

What Are the Symptoms of AI/ACD?

Anemia of inflammation and chronic disease typically develops slowly and, because it is usually mild, may cause few or no symptoms. Symptoms of anemia may also be masked by the symptoms of the underlying disease. Sometimes, AI/ACD can cause or contribute to

- fatigue
- weakness
- pale skin
- a fast heartbeat
- shortness of breath
- exercise intolerance

How Is AI/ACD Diagnosed?

To diagnose AI/ACD, a healthcare provider orders a blood test called a complete blood count (CBC). A blood test involves drawing a person's blood at a healthcare provider's office or commercial facility and sending the sample to a lab for analysis. The CBC includes a measurement of a person's hematocrit, the percentage of the blood that consists of red blood cells. The CBC also measures the amount of hemoglobin in the blood and can show whether a person has a lower than normal number of red blood cells.

In addition to measuring hematocrit and hemoglobin, the CBC includes two other measurements to show whether a person has enough iron:

- The ferritin level indicates the amount of iron stored in the body. A ferritin score below 200 nanograms per liter is a sign that a person may have an iron deficiency.

- The transferrin saturation (TSAT) is a score that indicates how much iron is available, or circulating, to make red blood cells. A TSAT score below 20 percent is another sign of iron deficiency.

A CBC result that shows low iron levels in the blood yet normal measures of iron stores in the body is a hallmark of AI/ACD.

How Is AI/ACD Treated?

Anemia of inflammation and chronic disease often is not treated separately from the condition with which it occurs. In general, healthcare providers focus on treating the underlying illness. If this treatment is successful, the anemia usually resolves. For example, antibiotics prescribed for infection and anti-inflammatory medications prescribed for rheumatoid arthritis or IBD can cause AI/ACD to disappear. However, AI/ACD is increasingly being viewed as a medical condition that merits direct treatment.

For people with cancer or kidney disease who have low levels of EPO, a synthetic form of EPO may be prescribed. A healthcare provider usually injects EPO subcutaneously—under the skin—two or three times a week. A person may be taught how to inject the EPO at home. People on hemodialysis who cannot tolerate EPO shots may receive EPO intravenously during hemodialysis.

If iron deficiency has a role in causing AI/ACD, a person may need iron supplements to raise hematocrit to a target level. Iron supplements can be taken by pill, subcutaneously, or intravenously during hemodialysis.

People with kidney disease and AI/ACD may also be advised to take vitamin B12 and folic acid supplements. A person should talk with a healthcare provider before taking any supplements.

Eating, Diet, and Nutrition

People with anemia caused by iron, vitamin B12, or folic acid deficiencies are usually advised to include sources of these nutrients in their diets.

Dietary sources of iron include:

- beans
- breakfast cereals
- chicken
- enriched bread
- spinach
- turkey

Dietary sources of vitamin B12 include:

- beef liver
- breakfast cereals
- chicken
- clams
- fish
- turkey

Dietary sources of folic acid include:

- beans
- breakfast cereals
- chicken
- enriched bread
- rice
- turkey

Section 15.3

Aplastic Anemia and Myelodysplastic Syndromes

This section includes text excerpted from "Aplastic Anemia and Myelodysplastic Syndromes," National Institute of Diabetes and Digestive and Kidney Diseases (NIDDK), February 2014.

What Are Aplastic Anemia and Myelodysplastic Syndromes (MDS)?

Aplastic anemia and myelodysplastic syndromes (MDS) are rare and serious disorders that affect the bone marrow and blood. Bone marrow is the soft, sponge like tissue inside the bones. Bone marrow makes stem cells that develop into one of the three types of blood cells—red blood cells, white blood cells, or platelets. Red blood cells contain hemoglobin, an iron-rich protein that gives blood its red color and carries oxygen from the lungs to all parts of the body. White blood cells help the body fight infections. Platelets are blood cell fragments that stick together to seal small cuts or breaks on blood vessel walls and stop bleeding.

In both disorders, bone marrow does not produce enough healthy red or white blood cells or platelets. Too few functioning red and white blood cells can lead to fatigue and infection. Too few platelets can lead to spontaneous or uncontrolled bleeding.

Anemia most often describes a condition in which the number of red blood cells is less than normal, resulting in less oxygen carried to the body's cells. In aplastic anemia, however, normal production of all blood cells slows or stops. Blood cell production declines because bone marrow stem cells are damaged. The number of stem cells also declines because they are unable to replicate themselves. Although production of mature blood cells is seriously impaired in aplastic anemia, the few blood cells that mature and enter the bloodstream are normal.

In MDS, a shortage of bone marrow stem cells usually does not occur, as it does in aplastic anemia. However, the stem cells are defective and do not mature normally. Progenitor cells and immature blood cells are deformed and fail to develop into healthy, mature red or white blood cells or platelets. These cells often die in the bone marrow. Many of the blood cells that do enter the bloodstream do not survive or function normally. Some forms of MDS are prone to develop into leukemia, an aggressive blood cancer.

Blood Cell Production

All three types of blood cells begin as unspecialized stem cells. Stem cells divide and produce more stem cells or can evolve through a series of stages into mature, specialized blood cells of any type. Early in the maturation process, progenitor cells emerge from stem cells. Unlike stem cells, progenitor cells are committed to develop into only one blood cell type and evolve into mature red or white blood cells or platelets.

Who Has Aplastic Anemia and MDS?

Young adults ages 20 to 25 years and people older than 60 years are most likely to have aplastic anemia. Men and women are equally affected. Most new cases in children are due to inherited bone marrow failure syndromes, caused by abnormal chromosomes. About four out of every 1 million people in the United States get aplastic anemia each year.

MDS affect more than 15,000 people in the United States each year. Researchers consider this number an underestimation resulting from challenges in classifying and reporting the syndromes. MDS are typically diagnosed between the ages of 70 and 80 years.

What Causes Aplastic Anemia and MDS?

Although a cause is not found in most cases of aplastic anemia and MDS, the diseases may be triggered by exposure to

- chemotherapy

- radiation therapy

- high levels of ionizing radiation—the type produced by high-power X-ray machines and in nuclear power plants

- benzene, a chemical used in some manufacturing processes

- toxic chemicals found in some pesticides

- certain viral infections

In most cases of aplastic anemia, these triggers, or other unknown causes, provoke the body's own immune system to destroy the bone marrow stem cells. Certain rare, inherited bone marrow failure syndromes can also lead to aplastic anemia and MDS.

What Are the Symptoms of Aplastic Anemia and MDS?

Symptoms may include

- fatigue
- weakness
- excessive bleeding, such as from external injuries or operations
- pinpoint red spots on the skin caused by bleeding from small blood vessels
- easy bruising
- frequent infections
- fevers
- pale skin
- shortness of breath

Symptoms vary depending on the person and the severity and type of disease. MDS often do not cause symptoms at first. Many of these symptoms also resemble those of other illnesses, making diagnosis difficult.

How Are Aplastic Anemia and MDS Diagnosed?

In addition to a medical history and physical exam, healthcare providers use blood tests, a bone marrow biopsy, and cytogenic analysis to diagnose aplastic anemia or MDS. A healthcare provider may refer a person to a hematologist—a doctor who treats diseases or disorders of the blood. A person also may be referred to an oncologist—a doctor who treats cancer—because aplastic anemia and MDS may be related to bone marrow cancers.

Blood tests. A blood test involves drawing a person's blood at a healthcare provider's office or a commercial facility and sending the sample to a lab for analysis. A complete blood count is usually the first test a healthcare provider uses to detect aplastic anemia or MDS. The test includes measurement of a person's hematocrit, the percentage of the blood that consists of red blood cells. A complete blood count also measures

- the amount of hemoglobin in the blood
- whether a person has a lower-than-normal number of red blood cells
- whether a person has enough iron
- the number of white blood cells and platelets in the blood

Lower-than-normal numbers of one or more blood cell types may suggest aplastic anemia or MDS.

In another test called a peripheral blood smear, the healthcare provider examines a sample of blood with a microscope for unusual changes in the size, shape, and appearance of the blood cells. These cells usually appear normal in aplastic anemia; however, they may be abnormal in MDS.

A healthcare provider also may order blood tests to check for a shortage of folate, vitamin B12, and erythropoietin—a hormone made in the kidneys that stimulates the production of red blood cells.

Bone marrow biopsy. A healthcare provider needs results from a bone marrow biopsy to confirm the diagnosis of aplastic anemia or MDS. A biopsy is a procedure that involves taking a small piece of bone marrow, blood, and a small piece of bone for examination with a microscope. A healthcare provider performs the biopsy during an office visit or in a hospital and uses light sedation and local anesthetic. During the biopsy, the healthcare provider inserts a needle into the hip bone or breastbone. A pathologist—a doctor who specializes in diagnosing diseases—analyzes the bone marrow samples in a lab. The test can show abnormal cells, the number and type of blood progenitor cells, and levels of iron in the bone marrow.

Cytogenic analysis. This test involves sending the person's bone marrow samples from the biopsy to a lab where a pathologist examines them with a microscope to look for abnormal changes in the person's chromosomes.

How Is Aplastic Anemia Treated?

People with mild or moderate aplastic anemia may not need treatment at first. However, people with severe aplastic anemia need immediate medical treatment to prevent or reverse complications from having low blood cell levels. Treatment options, which a healthcare provider may use alone or in combination, include

- blood and bone marrow stem cell transplants, which require chemotherapy and radiation therapy

- medications

- blood transfusions

Treatment options depend on the age and general health of the person and the severity of the disease.

Blood and bone marrow stem cell transplants. Blood and bone marrow stem cell transplants, also called stem cell transplants, replace damaged stem cells in bone marrow with healthy stem cells from a donor's blood or bone marrow and can cure aplastic anemia. Treatment guidelines state that stem cell transplant is the best treatment for people younger than 40 who have an available donor whose blood and bone marrow cells have been tested and found to "match" those of the patient. Stem cell transplants in people older than 40 are possible; however, long-term survival rates are lower. Older adults are generally less able to tolerate the treatments used to prepare the body for transplant and are more likely to develop severe posttransplant complications.

A healthcare provider confirms a matching donor by using a blood test called human leukocyte antigen tissue typing. Human leukocyte antigens are proteins found on the surface of white blood cells.

If healthcare providers do not find a matching donor in a person's family, they will search the National Marrow Donor Program to look for other sources of stem cells for a transplant. Millions of volunteer donors are registered to provide a potential match. Healthcare providers look for

- donors who are a match and not family members

- family members who are close matches, although not exact

- unrelated donors who are close matches, although not exact

- umbilical cord blood that is a match

Umbilical cord blood collected from an umbilical cord and a placenta after a baby is born is frozen and stored at a cord blood bank for future use. Some people donate umbilical cord blood to a public cord blood bank, while others pay to store it at a private bank.

Before the transplant, a healthcare provider uses chemotherapy and sometimes radiation therapy to destroy a person's own damaged bone marrow cells. These therapies also suppress a person's immune system to prevent it from attacking the new stem cells after the transplant.

Chemotherapy and Radiation Therapy

Chemotherapy. Chemotherapy is a treatment that uses medications to stop the growth of immature blood cells, either by killing the cells or stopping them from dividing. A person can take chemotherapy medications by mouth or have them injected into cerebrospinal fluid or a vein, a muscle, an organ, or a body cavity, such as the abdomen. High doses can cause side effects such as nausea, vomiting, diarrhea, and fatigue. Treatment takes place in a hospital or chemotherapy treatment center. People may take oral chemotherapy medications at home. A team of healthcare providers, such as an oncologist and an oncology nurse, cares for people undergoing chemotherapy. A patient does not need anesthesia.

Radiation therapy. Radiation therapy is a treatment that uses external beams of either small doses of radiation over a period of time or a single, precise, high dose of radiation. Treatment takes place in a hospital or radiation treatment center. A team of healthcare providers, including a radiation oncologist—a doctor who specializes in treating tumors or cancer with radiation—cares for people receiving radiation therapy. Most people cannot feel radiation and do not require anesthesia. Side effects may include fatigue and skin sensitivity around the area being treated.

In a hospital, healthcare providers remove stem cells from the donor and freeze them for storage. If the donor stem cells are coming from the blood, the blood is removed from a large vein in the donor's arm or through a central venous catheter, a flexible tube that is placed in a large vein in the neck, chest, or groin area. The blood goes through a machine that removes the stem cells. The blood is then returned to the donor and the healthcare provider stores the collected cells. If the donor stem cells are coming from the bone marrow, the healthcare provider will insert a hollow needle into the donor's pelvis to withdraw the marrow. This procedure occurs in a hospital with local or general anesthesia and is less common.

After receiving chemotherapy or radiation therapy, a person receives the thawed donor stem cells through an intravenous (IV) line, a needle in a vein, or a central venous catheter. The stem cells then travel to the bone marrow where they re-establish and maintain normal blood cell production. The person may be given medication to relax. The transplant will take an hour or longer to complete. The catheter will stay in place for at least 6 months after the transplant, and the person will stay in the hospital from several weeks to months to ensure the transplant is successful. During this time, a person may easily develop an infection due to a weak immune system.

Stem cell transplants carry risks. A person's immune system may attack the donated stem cells, called graft failure. Donated stem cells can attack the recipient's body, called graft-versus-host disease. Both of these complications can be life threatening.

Medications. Healthcare providers often prescribe one or more immunosuppressive medications, which suppress the immune system and reduce damage to bone marrow cells. Medications such as antithymocyte globulin may let the marrow start making blood cells again and reduce or eliminate the need for transfusions. In some people, blood counts return to normal. These medications are the preferred form of treatment for adults with severe aplastic anemia older than 40, younger patients who do not have a matched stem cell donor, and people with aplastic anemia who depend on blood transfusions. Taking these medications alone usually does not result in a cure. Corticosteroids, such as cyclosporine, are often given along with immunosuppressive medications to limit their side effects.

A person also may be given a man-made version of erythropoietin or a growth factor therapy that stimulates white blood cell production.

If infections due to low white blood cell counts occur, a healthcare provider may give the patient medications to kill bacteria, fungi, or viruses.

Healthcare providers often treat people with mild, inherited forms of aplastic anemia with man-made forms of androgens—male sex hormones that stimulate blood production. Androgens can help improve blood counts; however, they are not a cure.

Blood transfusions. A blood transfusion is a procedure in which a person receives healthy blood cells from a donor with the same blood type through an IV line. A healthcare provider performs the procedure during an office visit or in a hospital. The procedure lasts 1 to 4 hours, depending on how much blood the patient needs. Transfusions of red blood cells or platelets can raise blood cell counts and relieve symptoms. Transfusions are not a cure.

Most people with aplastic anemia need repeated transfusions, which can lead to complications. Over time, the body may develop antibodies that damage or destroy donor blood cells. Iron from transfused red blood cells can build up in the body and damage organs unless the healthcare provider prescribes medications called iron chelators to remove extra iron. Healthcare providers avoid giving a transfusion before a blood and bone marrow stem cell transplant because it increases the chances that the transplant will fail.

How Are MDS Treated?

Treatment options for MDS, which a healthcare provider may use alone or in combination, include supportive care, medications, chemotherapy, and blood and bone marrow stem cell transplants. Treatment options depend on the following:

- age and general health of the person
- whether the healthcare provider classifies MDS as a lower-risk or higher-risk disease
- whether the MDS occurred after chemotherapy or radiation therapy for another disease
- whether the MDS has worsened after being treated.

Supportive care. Traditionally the first line of treatment, supportive care aims to manage the symptoms of the disease. This approach may include blood transfusions to help problems caused by low blood cells counts, such as fatigue and infections, and may also include growth factor therapy.

Medications. A healthcare provider may give immunosuppressive medications such as lenalidomide (Revlimid) and antithymocyte globulin with or without cyclosporine to help the bone marrow function more normally. A person may need an iron chelator to treat too much iron in the blood. Some people also may benefit from erythropoietin. A healthcare provider may also give medications to fight infections with bacteria, fungi, or viruses.

Chemotherapy. A healthcare provider may give chemotherapy in an effort to destroy defective blood progenitor cells in severe MDS and let the few remaining normal blood stem cells re-establish normal blood cell production. Chemotherapy medications may include azacitidine (Vidaza), decitabine (Dacogen), or other anticancer medications. This approach is often not effective over the long term. A healthcare provider may also use chemotherapy prior to stem cell transplants.

Blood and bone marrow stem cell transplants. In the past, only a stem cell transplant with a matched sibling donor offered a cure for MDS. However, experts have made much progress with transplants from unrelated matched donors, including unrelated umbilical cord blood transplantation. In the past, healthcare providers did not routinely perform blood and bone marrow stem cell transplants for older adults with MDS. However, healthcare providers who are using newer techniques that use a less toxic pre-transplant regimen are performing successful blood and bone marrow stem cell transplants in this age group.

Eating, Diet, and Nutrition

Eating, diet, and nutrition have not been shown to play a role in preventing or treating aplastic anemia and MDS. However, people with either disorder who receive a stem cell transplant need to eat a healthy diet to help with their recovery. A person also may need to avoid some foods to lower the chances of infection while the immune system is still weak. A healthcare provider will advise a person on which specific foods to eat or avoid and when it is safe to eat in a restaurant. When dining out, stem cell transplant recipients should avoid foods that may be spoiled or not cleaned thoroughly, such as those at buffets or salad bars, to prevent infection.

Some people may not feel hungry, or medication side effects may make eating difficult or painful. Many people also may have nausea, diarrhea, or vomiting. People may need to eat or drink a nutritional supplement in the form of a shake or pudding. Eating foods high in potassium and magnesium will help replace these minerals if they are lost from diarrhea and vomiting. A healthcare provider also may suggest a person eat a diet high in phosphorus and calcium to strengthen and maintain bone health. Eating smaller, more frequent meals can help with nausea. Drinking enough water and other fluids daily is also important.

Stem cell transplant recipients may need to avoid alcohol to prevent reduced liver function. They may also need to avoid sodium, often from salt, to prevent high blood pressure and swelling.

Section 15.4

Fanconi Anemia

This section includes text excerpted from "Fanconi Anemia,"
National Heart, Lung, and Blood Institute (NHLBI),
November 1, 2011. Reviewed July 2016.

What Is Fanconi Anemia?

Fanconi anemia, or FA, is a rare, inherited blood disorder that leads to bone marrow failure. The disorder also is called Fanconi's anemia.

FA prevents your bone marrow from making enough new blood cells for your body to work normally. FA also can cause your bone marrow to make many faulty blood cells. This can lead to serious health problems, such as leukemia (a type of blood cancer).

Although FA is a blood disorder, it also can affect many of your body's organs, tissues, and systems. Children who inherit FA are at higher risk of being born with birth defects. FA also increases the risk of some cancers and other serious health problems.

FA is different from Fanconi syndrome. Fanconi syndrome affects the kidneys. It's a rare and serious condition that mostly affects children.

Children who have Fanconi syndrome pass large amounts of key nutrients and chemicals through their urine. These children may have serious health and developmental problems.

Bone Marrow and Blood

Bone marrow is the spongy tissue inside the large bones of your body. Healthy bone marrow contains stem cells that develop into the three types of blood cells that the body needs:

- Red blood cells, which carry oxygen to all parts of your body. Red blood cells also remove carbon dioxide (a waste product) from your body's cells and carry it to the lungs to be exhaled.

- White blood cells, which help fight infections.

- Platelets, which help your blood clot.

131

It's normal for blood cells to die. The lifespan of red blood cells is about 120 days. White blood cells live less than 1 day. Platelets live about 6 days. As a result, your bone marrow must constantly make new blood cells.

If your bone marrow can't make enough new blood cells to replace the ones that die, serious health problems can occur.

Fanconi Anemia and Your Body

FA is one of many types of anemia. The term "anemia" usually refers to a condition in which the blood has a lower than normal number of red blood cells.

FA is a type of aplastic anemia. In aplastic anemia, the bone marrow stops making or doesn't make enough of all three types of blood cells. Low levels of the three types of blood cells can harm many of the body's organs, tissues, and systems.

With too few red blood cells, your body's tissues won't get enough oxygen to work well. With too few white blood cells, your body may have problems fighting infections. This can make you sick more often and make infections worse. With too few platelets, your blood can't clot normally. As a result, you may have bleeding problems.

What Causes Fanconi Anemia?

FA is an inherited disease. The term "inherited" means that the disease is passed from parents to children through genes. At least 13 faulty genes are associated with FA. FA occurs when both parents pass the same faulty FA gene to their child.

People who have only one faulty FA gene are FA "carriers." Carriers don't have FA, but they can pass the faulty gene to their children.

If both of your parents have a faulty FA gene, you have:

- A 25 percent chance of having FA

- A 25 percent chance of not having FA

- A 50 percent chance of being an FA carrier and passing the gene to any children you have

If only one of your parents has a faulty FA gene, you won't have the disorder. However, you have a 50 percent chance of being an FA carrier and passing the gene to any children you have.

Who Is at Risk for Fanconi Anemia?

FA occurs in all racial and ethnic groups and affects men and women equally.

In the United States, about 1 out of every 181 people is an FA carrier. This carrier rate leads to about 1 in 130,000 people being born with FA.

Two ethnic groups, Ashkenazi Jews and Afrikaners, are more likely than other groups to have FA or be FA carriers.

Ashkenazi Jews are people who are descended from the Jewish population of Eastern Europe. Afrikaners are White natives of South Africa who speak a language called Afrikaans. This ethnic group is descended from early Dutch, French, and German settlers.

In the United States, 1 out of 90 Ashkenazi Jews is an FA carrier, and 1 out of 30,000 is born with FA.

Major Risk Factors

FA is an inherited disease—that is, it's passed from parents to children through genes. At least 13 faulty genes are associated with FA. FA occurs if both parents pass the same faulty FA gene to their child.

Children born into families with histories of FA are at risk of inheriting the disorder. Children whose mothers and fathers both have family histories of FA are at even greater risk. A family history of FA means that it's possible that a parent carries a faulty gene associated with the disorder.

Children whose parents both carry the same faulty gene are at greatest risk of inheriting FA. Even if these children aren't born with FA, they're still at risk of being FA carriers.

Children who have only one parent who carries a faulty FA gene also are at risk of being carriers. However, they're not at risk of having FA.

What Are the Signs and Symptoms of Fanconi Anemia?

Major Signs and Symptoms

Your doctor may suspect you or your child has Fanconi anemia (FA) if you have signs and symptoms of:

- anemia
- bone marrow failure

- birth defects

- developmental or eating problems

FA is an inherited disorder—that is, it's passed from parents to children through genes. If a child has FA, his or her brothers and sisters also should be tested for the disorder.

Anemia

The most common symptom of all types of anemia is fatigue (tiredness). Fatigue occurs because your body doesn't have enough red blood cells to carry oxygen to its various parts. If you have anemia, you may not have the energy to do normal activities.

A low red blood cell count also can cause shortness of breath, dizziness, headaches, coldness in your hands and feet, pale skin, and chest pain.

Bone Marrow Failure

When your bone marrow fails, it can't make enough red blood cells, white blood cells, and platelets. This can cause many problems that have various signs and symptoms.

With too few red blood cells, you can develop anemia. In FA, the size of your red blood cells also can be much larger than normal. This makes it harder for the cells to work well.

With too few white blood cells, you're at risk for infections. Infections also may last longer and be more serious than normal.

With too few platelets, you may bleed and bruise easily, suffer from internal bleeding, or have petechiae. Petechiae are tiny red or purple spots on the skin. Bleeding in small blood vessels just below your skin causes these spots.

In some people who have FA, the bone marrow makes a lot of harmful, immature white blood cells called blasts. Blasts don't work like normal blood cells. As they build up, they prevent the bone marrow from making enough normal blood cells.

A large number of blasts in the bone marrow can lead to a type of blood cancer called acute myeloid leukemia (AML).

Birth Defects

Many birth defects can be signs of FA. These include:

- **Bone or skeletal defects**. FA can cause missing, oddly shaped, or three or more thumbs. Arm bones, hips, legs, hands, and toes

134

may not form fully or normally. People who have FA may have a curved spine, a condition called scoliosis.

- **Eye and ear defects**. The eyes, eyelids, and ears may not have a normal shape. Children who have FA also might be born deaf.

- **Skin discoloration**. This includes coffee-colored areas or odd-looking patches of lighter skin.

- **Kidney problems**. A child who has FA might be born with a missing kidney or kidneys that aren't shaped normally.

- **Congenital heart defects**. The most common congenital heart defect linked to FA is a ventricular septal defect (VSD). A VSD is a hole or defect in the lower part of the wall that separates the heart's left and right chambers.

Developmental Problems

Other signs and symptoms of FA are related to physical and mental development. They include:

- low birth weight
- poor appetite
- delayed growth
- below-average height
- small head size
- mental retardation or learning disabilities

Signs and Symptoms of Fanconi Anemia in Adults

Some signs and symptoms of FA may develop as you or your child gets older. Women who have FA may have some or all of the following:

- Sex organs that are less developed than normal.
- Menstruating later than women who don't have FA.
- Starting menopause earlier than women who don't have FA.
- Problems getting pregnant and carrying a pregnancy to full term.

Men who have FA may have sex organs that are less developed than normal. They also may be less fertile than men who don't have the disease.

How Is Fanconi Anemia Diagnosed?

People who have FA are born with the disorder. They may or may not show signs or symptoms of it at birth. For this reason, FA isn't always diagnosed when a person is born. In fact, most people who have the disorder are diagnosed between the ages of 2 and 15 years.

The tests used to diagnose FA depend on a person's age and symptoms. In all cases, medical and family histories are an important part of diagnosing FA. However, because FA has many of the same signs and symptoms as other diseases, only genetic testing can confirm its diagnosis.

Specialists Involved

A geneticist is a doctor or scientist who studies how genes work and how diseases and traits are passed from parents to children through genes.

Geneticists do genetic testing for FA. They also can provide counseling about how FA is inherited and the types of prenatal (before birth) testing used to diagnose it.

An obstetrician may detect birth defects linked to FA before your child is born. An obstetrician is a doctor who specializes in providing care for pregnant women.

After your child is born, a pediatrician also can help find out whether your child has FA. A pediatrician is a doctor who specializes in treating children and teens.

A hematologist (blood disease specialist) also may help diagnose FA.

Family and Medical Histories

FA is an inherited disease. Some parents are aware that their family has a medical history of FA, even if they don't have the disease.

Other parents, especially if they're FA carriers, may not be aware of a family history of FA. Many parents may not know that FA can be passed from parents to children.

Knowing your family medical history can help your doctor diagnose whether you or your child has FA or another condition with similar symptoms.

If your doctor thinks that you, your siblings, or your children have FA, he or she may ask you detailed questions about:

- Any personal or family history of anemia

- Any surgeries you've had related to the digestive system

- Any personal or family history of immune disorders

- Your appetite, eating habits, and any medicines you take

If you know your family has a history of FA, or if your answers to your doctor's questions suggest a possible diagnosis of FA, your doctor will recommend further testing.

Diagnostic Tests and Procedures

The signs and symptoms of FA aren't unique to the disease. They're also linked to many other diseases and conditions, such as aplastic anemia. For this reason, genetic testing is needed to confirm a diagnosis of FA. Genetic tests for FA include the following.

Chromosome Breakage Test

This is the most common test for FA. It's available only in special laboratories (labs). It shows whether your chromosomes (long chains of genes) break more easily than normal.

Skin cells sometimes are used for the test. Usually, though, a small amount of blood is taken from a vein in your arm using a needle. A technician combines some of the blood cells with certain chemicals.

If you have FA, the chromosomes in your blood sample break and rearrange when mixed with the test chemicals. This doesn't happen in the cells of people who don't have FA.

Cytometric Flow Analysis

Cytometric flow analysis, or CFA, is done in a lab. This test examines how chemicals affect your chromosomes as your cells grow and divide. Skin cells are used for this test.

A technician mixes the skin cells with chemicals that can cause the chromosomes in the cells to act abnormally. If you have FA, your cells are much more sensitive to these chemicals.

The chromosomes in your skin cells will break at a high rate during the test. This doesn't happen in the cells of people who don't have FA.

Mutation Screening

A mutation is an abnormal change in a gene or genes. Geneticists and other specialists can examine your genes, usually using a sample of your skin cells. With special equipment and lab processes, they can look for gene mutations that are linked to FA.

Diagnosing Different Age Groups

Before Birth (Prenatal)

If your family has a history of FA and you get pregnant, your doctor may want to test you or your fetus for FA.

Two tests can be used to diagnose FA in a developing fetus: amniocentesis and chorionic villus sampling (CVS). Both tests are done in a doctor's office or hospital.

Amniocentesis is done 15 to 18 weeks after a pregnant woman's last period. A doctor uses a needle to remove a small amount of fluid from the sac around the fetus. A technician tests chromosomes (chains of genes) from the fluid sample to see whether they have faulty genes associated with FA.

CVS is done 10 to 12 weeks after a pregnant woman's last period. A doctor inserts a thin tube through the vagina and cervix to the placenta (the temporary organ that connects the fetus to the mother).

The doctor removes a tissue sample from the placenta using gentle suction. The tissue sample is sent to a lab to be tested for genetic defects associated with FA.

At Birth

Three out of four people who inherit FA are born with birth defects. If your baby is born with certain birth defects, your doctor may recommend genetic testing to confirm a diagnosis of FA.

Childhood and Later

Some people who have FA are not born with birth defects. Doctors may not diagnose them with the disorder until signs of bone marrow failure or cancer occur. This usually happens within the first 10 years of life.

Signs of bone marrow failure most often begin between the ages of 3 and 12 years, with 7 to 8 years as the most common ages. However, 10 percent of children who have FA aren't diagnosed until after 16 years of age.

If your bone marrow is failing, you may have signs of aplastic anemia. FA is one type of aplastic anemia.

In aplastic anemia, your bone marrow stops making or doesn't make enough of all three types of blood cells: red blood cells, white blood cells, and platelets.

Aplastic anemia can be inherited or acquired after birth through exposure to chemicals, radiation, or medicines.

Doctors diagnose aplastic anemia using:

- Family and medical histories and a physical exam.

- A **complete blood count (CBC)** to check the number, size, and condition of your red blood cells. The CBC also checks numbers of white blood cells and platelets.

- A **reticulocyte count.** This test counts the number of new red blood cells in your blood to see whether your bone marrow is making red blood cells at the proper rate.

- **Bone marrow tests.** For a bone marrow aspiration, a small amount of liquid bone marrow is removed and tested to see whether it's making enough blood cells. For a bone marrow biopsy, a small amount of bone marrow tissue is removed and tested to see whether it's making enough blood cells.

If you or your child is diagnosed with aplastic anemia, your doctor will want to find the cause. If your doctor suspects you have FA, he or she may recommend genetic testing.

How Is Fanconi Anemia Treated?

Doctors decide how to treat Fanconi anemia (FA) based on a person's age and how well the person's bone marrow is making new blood cells.

Goals of Treatment

Long-term treatments for FA can:

- **Cure the anemia**. Damaged bone marrow cells are replaced with healthy ones that can make enough of all three types of blood cells on their own. or

- **Treat the symptoms without curing the cause**. This is done using medicines and other substances that can help your body make more blood cells for a limited time.

Screening and Short-Term Treatment

Even if you or your child has FA, your bone marrow might still be able to make enough new blood cells. If so, your doctor might suggest frequent blood count checks so he or she can watch your condition.

Your doctor will probably want you to have bone marrow tests once a year. He or she also will screen you for any signs of cancer or tumors.

If your blood counts begin to drop sharply and stay low, your bone marrow might be failing. Your doctor may prescribe antibiotics to help your body fight infections. In the short term, he or she also may want to give you blood transfusions to increase your blood cell counts to normal levels.

However, long-term use of blood transfusions can reduce the chance that other treatments will work.

Long-Term Treatment

The four main types of long-term treatment for FA are:

1. blood and marrow stem cell transplant

2. androgen therapy

3. synthetic growth factors

4. gene therapy

Blood and Marrow Stem Cell Transplant

A blood and marrow stem cell transplant is the current standard treatment for patients who have FA that's causing major bone marrow failure. Healthy stem cells from another person, called a donor, are used to replace the faulty cells in your bone marrow.

If you're going to receive stem cells from another person, your doctor will want to find a donor whose stem cells match yours as closely as possible.

Stem cell transplants are most successful in younger people who:

- Have few or no serious health problems.

- Receive stem cells from a brother or sister who is a good donor match.

- Have had few or no previous blood transfusions.

During the transplant, you'll get donated stem cells in a procedure that's like a blood transfusion. Once the new stem cells are in your body, they travel to your bone marrow and begin making new blood cells.

A successful stem cell transplant will allow your body to make enough of all three types of blood cells.

Even if you've had a stem cell transplant to treat FA, you're still at risk for some types of blood cancer and cancerous solid tumors. Your doctor will check your health regularly after the procedure.

Androgen Therapy

Before improvements made stem cell transplants more effective, androgen therapy was the standard treatment for people who had FA. Androgens are man-made male hormones that can help your body make more blood cells for long periods.

Androgens increase your red blood cell and platelet counts. They don't work as well at raising your white blood cell count.

Unlike a stem cell transplant, androgens don't allow your bone marrow to make enough of all three types of blood cells on its own. You may need ongoing treatment with androgens to control the effects of FA.

Also, over time, androgens lose their ability to help your body make more blood cells, which means you'll need other treatments.

Androgen therapy can have serious side effects, such as liver disease. This treatment also can't prevent you from developing leukemia (a type of blood cancer).

Synthetic Growth Factors

Your doctor may choose to treat your FA with growth factors. These are substances found in your body, but they also can be man-made.

Growth factors help your body make more red and white blood cells. Growth factors that help your body make more platelets still are being studied.

More research is needed on growth factor treatment for FA. Early results suggest that growth factors may have fewer and less serious side effects than androgens.

Gene Therapy

Researchers are looking for ways to replace faulty FA genes with normal, healthy genes. They hope these genes will make proteins that can repair and protect your bone marrow cells. Early results of this therapy hold promise, but more research is needed.

Surgery

FA can cause birth defects that affect the arms, thumbs, hips, legs, and other parts of the body. Doctors may recommend surgery to repair some defects.

For example, your child might be born with a ventricular septal defect—a hole or defect in the wall that separates the lower chambers of the heart. His or her doctor may recommend surgery to close the hole so the heart can work properly.

Children who have FA also may need surgery to correct digestive system problems that can harm their nutrition, growth, and survival.

One of the most common problems is an FA-related birth defect in which the trachea (windpipe), which carries air to the lungs, is connected to the esophagus, which carries food to the stomach.

This can cause serious breathing, swallowing, and eating problems and can lead to lung infections. Surgery is needed to separate the two organs and allow normal eating and breathing.

How Can Fanconi Anemia Be Prevented?

You can't prevent FA because it's an inherited disease. If a child gets two copies of the same faulty FA gene, he or she will have the disease.

If you're at high risk for FA and are planning to have children, you may want to consider genetic counseling. A counselor can help you understand your risk of having a child who has FA. He or she also can explain the choices that are available to you.

If you're already pregnant, genetic testing can show whether your child has FA.

In the United States, Ashkenazi Jews (Jews of Eastern European descent) are at higher risk for FA than other ethnic groups. For Ashkenazi Jews, it's recommended that prospective parents get tested for FA-related gene mutations before getting pregnant.

Preventing Complications

If you or your child has FA, you can prevent some health problems related to the disorder. Pneumonia, hepatitis, and chicken pox can occur more often and more severely in people who have FA compared with those who don't. Ask your doctor about vaccines for these conditions.

People who have FA also are at higher risk than other people for some cancers. These cancers include leukemia (a type of blood cancer), myelodysplastic syndrome (abnormal levels of all three types of blood cells), and liver cancer. Screening and early detection can help manage these life-threatening diseases.

Living with Fanconi Anemia

Improvements in blood and marrow stem cell transplants have increased the chances of living longer with FA. Also, researchers are studying new and promising treatments for FA. However, the disorder still presents serious challenges to patients and their families.

What to Expect

FA is a life-threatening illness. If you or your child is diagnosed with FA, you and your family members may feel shock, anger, grief, and depression. If you're the parent or grandparent of a child who has FA, you may blame yourself for causing the disease.

Your doctor will want to test all of your children for FA if one of your children is born with the disorder. If you're diagnosed with FA as an adult, your doctor may suggest testing your brothers and sisters for the disorder.

All of these things can create stress and anxiety for your entire family. Family counseling for FA may give you and other relatives important support, comfort, and advice.

One of the hardest issues to deal with is telling children that they have FA and what effect it will have on their lives.

Most FA support groups believe that parents need to give children information about the disorder in terms they can understand. These groups recommend answering questions honestly and directly, stressing the positive developments in treatment and survival.

If your child becomes upset or begins to act out after learning that he or she has FA, you may want to seek counseling.

Special Concerns and Needs

Many people who have FA survive to adulthood. If you have FA, you'll need ongoing medical care. Your blood counts will need to be checked regularly.

Even if you have a blood and marrow stem cell transplant, you remain at risk for many cancers. You'll need to be screened for cancer more often than people who don't have FA.

If FA has left you with a very low platelet count, your doctor may advise you to avoid contact sports and other activities that can lead to injuries.

If your child has FA, he or she may have problems eating or keeping food down. Your doctor may recommend additional, special feedings to support growth and good health.

Support Groups

You or your family members may find it helpful to know about resources that can give you emotional support and helpful information about FA and its treatments.

Your doctor or hospital social worker may have information about counseling and support services. They also may be able to refer you to support groups that offer help with financial planning (treatment for FA can be costly).

Section 15.5

Biermer Disease (Pernicious Anemia)

This section includes text excerpted from "Biermer's Disease," Genetic and Rare Diseases Information Center (GARD), September 11, 2015.

What Is Biermer Disease?

Biermer disease, also called acquired pernicious anemia, is a condition in which the body is unable to properly utilize vitamin B12. Because vitamin B12 is essential for the formation of red blood cells, this condition is primarily characterized by anemia (too few red blood cells). Affected people may also experience gastrointestinal issues and neurological abnormalities (such as paresthesia, weakness, and clumsiness). Biermer disease and other forms of pernicious anemia are thought to be autoimmune conditions which occur when the body's immune system mistakenly attacks healthy tissue. Treatment generally consists of large doses of vitamin B12, usually as an injection.

What Are the Signs and Symptoms of Biermer Disease?

The Human Phenotype Ontology (HPO) provides the following list of signs and symptoms for Biermer disease.

- Abnormality of the gastric mucosa
- Autoimmunity
- Megaloblastic anemia
- Nausea and vomiting
- Pallor
- Respiratory insufficiency
- Vitamin B12 deficiency
- Arrhythmia

- Decreased antibody level in blood
- Decreased fertility
- Diabetes mellitus
- Glossitis
- Hypoparathyroidism
- Hypopigmented skin patches
- Thyroiditis
- Weight loss
- Xerostomia
- Abdominal pain
- Abnormal renal physiology
- Abnormality of the nose
- Abnormality of the retinal vasculature
- Anorexia
- Congestive heart failure
- Coronary artery disease
- Developmental regression
- Gait disturbance
- Hallucinations
- Hearing abnormality
- Hepatomegaly
- Hypertonia
- Incoordination
- Malabsorption
- Memory impairment
- Migraine
- Neoplasm of the stomach
- Paresthesia
- Recurrent urinary tract infections
- Reduced consciousness/confusion
- Spina bifida
- Splenomegaly

Section 15.6

Hemoglobin E Disease

This section includes text excerpted from "Hemoglobin E Disease," Genetic and Rare Diseases Information Center (GARD), February 21, 2014.

What Is Hemoglobin E Disease?

Hemoglobin E (HbE) disease is an inherited blood disorder characterized by an abnormal form of hemoglobin, called hemoglobin E.

People with this condition have red blood cells that are smaller than normal and have an irregular shape. HbE disease is thought to be a benign condition. It is inherited in an autosomal recessive pattern and is caused by a particular mutation in the *HBB* gene. The mutation that causes hemoglobin E disease has the highest frequency among people of Southeast Asian heritage (Cambodian, Laotian, Vietnamese and Thai). However, it is also found in people of Chinese, Filipino, Asiatic Indian, and Turkish descent.

What Are the Signs and Symptoms of Hemoglobin E Disease?

Affected individuals can develop mild thalassemia in the first few months of life. While mild splenomegaly and/or anemia can occur, it is generally considered a benign condition.

When a person inherits a gene mutation from one of their parents, they are said to be a carrier or have hemoglobin trait. These individuals are typically asymptomatic, although they may have small red blood cells. However, carriers may be at risk to have children with hemoglobin E/ thalassemia (which is similar to thalassemia) or hemoglobin sickle E disease (milder form of sickle cell anemia). Both of these conditions are much more severe than hemoglobin E disease. They are are also inherited in an autosomal recessive fashion.

How Is Hemoglobin E Disease Diagnosed?

Many babies are picked up through state newborn screening programs. A diagnosis is usually made by looking at the red blood cells by doing a Mean Corpuscular Volume (MCV) test, which is commonly part of a Complete Blood Count (CBC) test. More specialized tests, such as a hemoglobin electrophoresis and iron studies might be done. These tests indicate whether a person has different types of hemoglobin. Genetic testing of the *HBB* gene can also be done to confirm a diagnosis.

How Might Hemoglobin E Disease Be Treated?

Treatment is usually not necessary. Folic acid supplements may be prescribed to help the body produce normal red blood cells and improve symptoms of anemia. People with hemoglobin E disease can expect to lead a normal life.

Chapter 16

Hemolytic Anemia

Chapter Contents

Section 16.1

Sickle Cell Disease

This section includes text excerpted from "Sickle Cell
Disease (SCD)," Centers for Disease Control and
Prevention (CDC), September 14, 2015.

Facts about Sickle Cell Disease

Sickle Cell Disease (SCD) is a group of inherited red blood cell
disorders. Healthy red blood cells are round, and they move through
small blood vessels to carry oxygen to all parts of the body. In someone
who has SCD, the red blood cells become hard and sticky and look like
a C-shaped farm tool called a "sickle." The sickle cells die early, which
causes a constant shortage of red blood cells. Also, when they travel
through small blood vessels, they get stuck and clog the blood flow.
This can cause pain and other serious problems such infection, acute
chest syndrome and stroke.

Types of SCD

Following are the most common types of SCD:

HbSS

People who have this form of SCD inherit two sickle cell genes ("S"),
one from each parent. This is commonly called sickle cell anemia and
is usually the most severe form of the disease.

HbSC

People who have this form of SCD inherit a sickle cell gene ("S")
from one parent and from the other parent a gene for an abnormal
hemoglobin called "C." Hemoglobin is a protein that allows red blood
cells to carry oxygen to all parts of the body. This is usually a milder
form of SCD.

HbS Beta Thalassemia

People who have this form of SCD inherit one sickle cell gene ("S") from one parent and one gene for beta thalassemia, another type of anemia, from the other parent. There are two types of beta thalassemia: "0" and "+." Those with HbS beta 0-thalassemia usually have a severe form of SCD. People with HbS beta +-thalassemia tend to have a milder form of SCD.

There also are a few rare types of SCD:

HbSD, HbSE, and HbSO

People who have these forms of SCD inherit one sickle cell gene ("S") and one gene from an abnormal type of hemoglobin ("D," "E," or "O"). Hemoglobin is a protein that allows red blood cells to carry oxygen to all parts of the body. The severity of these rarer types of SCD varies.

Sickle Cell Trait (SCT)

People who inherit one sickle cell gene and one normal gene have sickle cell trait (SCT). People with SCT usually do not have any of the symptoms of sickle cell disease (SCD), but they can pass the trait on to their children.

How Sickle Cell Trait is Inherited

- If both parents have SCT, there is a 50% (or 1 in 2) chance that any child of theirs also will have SCT, if the child inherits the sickle cell gene from one of the parents. Such children will not have symptoms of SCD, but they can pass SCT on to their children.

- If both parents have SCT, there is a 25% (or 1 in 4) chance that any child of theirs will have SCD. There is the same 25% (or 1 in 4) chance that the child will not have SCD or SCT.

Diagnosis

SCT is diagnosed with a simple blood test. People at risk of having SCT can talk with a doctor or health clinic about getting this test.

Complications

Most people with SCT do not have any symptoms of SCD, although— in rare cases—people with SCT might experience complications of SCD, such as pain crises.

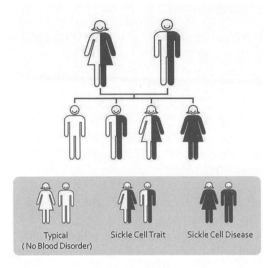

Figure 16.1. *Sickle Cell Inheritance Pattern*

In their extreme form, and in rare cases, the following conditions could be harmful for people with SCT:

- Increased pressure in the atmosphere (which can be experienced, for example, while scuba diving).

- Low oxygen levels in the air (which can be experienced, for example, when mountain climbing, exercising extremely hard in military boot camp, or training for an athletic competition).

- Dehydration (for example, when one has too little water in the body).

- High altitudes (which can be experienced, for example, when flying, mountain climbing, or visiting a city at a high altitude).

More research is needed to find out why some people with SCT have complications and others do not.

SCT and Athletes

Some people with SCT have been shown to be more likely than those without SCT to experience heat stroke and muscle breakdown when doing intense exercise, such as competitive sports or military training under unfavorable temperatures(very high or low) or conditions.

Studies have shown that the chance of this problem can be reduced by avoiding dehydration and getting too hot during training.

People with SCT who participate in competitive or team sports (i.e. student athletes) should be careful when doing training or conditioning activities. To prevent illness it is important to:

- Set your own pace and build your intensity slowly.

- Rest often in between repetitive sets and drills.

- Drink plenty of water before, during and after training and conditioning activities.

- Keep the body temperature cool when exercising in hot and humid temperatures by misting the body with water or going to an air conditioned area during breaks or rest periods.

- Immediately seek medical care when feeling ill.

Cause of SCD

SCD is a genetic condition that is present at birth. It is inherited when a child receives two sickle cell genes—one from each parent.

Diagnosis

SCD is diagnosed with a simple blood test. It most often is found at birth during routine newborn screening tests at the hospital. In addition, SCD can be diagnosed before birth.

Because children with SCD are at an increased risk of infection and other health problems, early diagnosis and treatment are important.

You can call your local sickle cell organization to find out how to get tested.

Complications and Treatments

People with sickle cell disease (SCD) start to have signs of the disease during the first year of life, usually around 5 months of age. Symptoms and complications of SCD are different for each person and can range from mild to severe.

The reason that infants don't show symptoms at birth is because baby or fetal hemoglobin protects the red blood cells from sickling. When the infant is around 4 to 5 months of age, the baby or fetal hemoglobin is replaced by sickle hemoglobin and the cells begin to sickle.

SCD is a disease that worsens over time. Treatments are available that can prevent complications and lengthen the lives of those who have this condition. These treatment options can be different for each person depending on the symptoms and severity.

Hydroxyurea is a medicine that has been shown to decrease several complications of SCD. Stem cell transplants (A stem cell transplant, also called a bone marrow transplant, is a procedure that infuses healthy cells, called stem cells, into the body to replace damaged or diseased bone marrow. Bone marrow is the center of the bone where blood cells are made) from bone marrow or blood of healthy donors are increasingly being used to successfully cure SCD. Complications from hydroxyurea therapy and stem cell transplants are rare but can be serious or life-threatening. People with SCD and their families should ask their doctors about the benefits and risks of each.

Hand-Foot Syndrome

Swelling in the hands and feet usually is the first symptom of SCD. This swelling, often along with a fever, is caused by the sickle cells getting stuck in the blood vessels and blocking the flow of blood in and out of the hands and feet.

Treatment

The most common treatments for swelling in the hands and the feet are pain medicine and an increase in fluids, such as water.

Pain "Episode" or "Crisis"

Pain is the most common complication of SCD, and the top reason that people with SCD go to the emergency room or hospital. When sickle cells travel through small blood vessels, they can get stuck and clog the blood flow. This causes pain that can start suddenly, be mild to severe, and can last for any length of time.

Prevention

There are simple steps that people with SCD can take to help prevent and reduce the number of pain crises:

- Drink plenty of water.

- Try not to get too hot or too cold.

- Try to avoid places or situations that expose you to high altitudes (for example, flying, mountain climbing, or cities with a high altitude).

- Try to avoid places or situations that expose you to low oxygen levels (for example, mountain climbing or exercising extremely hard, such as in military boot camp or when training for an athletic competition).

- Adults with severe SCD can take a medicine called hydroxyurea to help reduce the number of pain crises.

- People taking hydroxyurea are checked often by a doctor to prevent complications including an increased risk of infections.

- New research has shown that babies and children with SCD also benefit from hydroxurea therapy.

Treatment

Most pain related to SCD can be treated with over the counter pain medications such as ibuprofen and aspirin. Some people who have severe pain are given opioid (i.e. morphine) medications daily, along with additional pain medication. Some people may be admitted to the hospital for intense treatment.

Anemia

Anemia is a very common complication of SCD. With SCD, the red blood cells die early. This means there are not enough healthy red blood cells to carry oxygen throughout the body. When this happens, a person might have:

- tiredness

- irritability

- dizziness and lightheadedness

- a fast heart rate

- difficulty breathing

- pale skin color

- jaundice (yellow color to the skin and whites of the eyes)

- slow growth

- delayed puberty

Treatment

Blood transfusions are used to treat severe anemia. A sudden worsening of anemia resulting from infection or enlargement of the spleen is a common reason for a transfusion. Multiple blood transfusions, however, might cause health problems because of the iron content of blood. Iron overload, called hemosiderosis, can damage liver, heart, pancreas and other organs, leading to diseases such as diabetes mellitus. Iron chelation therapy should be started in patients with SCD receiving regular blood transfusions to reduce excess iron levels.

Infection

People with SCD, especially infants and children, are more at risk for infections, especially those due to bacteria with capsules because of damage to the spleen. Pneumonia is a leading cause of death in infants and young children with SCD.

Prevention

Vaccines can protect against harmful infections.

- Washing your hands is one of the best ways to help prevent getting an infection. People with SCD, their family, and other caretakers should wash their hands with soap and clean water many times each day.

- Because bacteria in some foods can be especially harmful to children with SCD, food should be prepared safely.

- Vaccines can protect against harmful infections. Children with SCD should get all regular childhood vaccines, plus a few extra. Adults should have the flu vaccine every year, as well as the pneumococcal vaccine and any others recommended by a doctor.

- Take penicillin (or other antibiotic prescribed by a doctor) every day until at least 5 years of age.

Treatment

Infections are treated with antibiotic medicines and sometimes blood transfusions. At the first sign of an infection, such as a fever, it is important to see a doctor right away as this may represent a medical emergency for people with SCD. Early treatment of infection can help prevent problems.

Acute Chest Syndrome

This can be life-threatening and should be treated in a hospital. Symptoms and signs are similar to pneumonia. Signs and symptoms include chest pain, coughing, difficulty breathing, and fever.

Prevention

Adults with severe SCD can take a medicine called hydroxyurea to help prevent acute chest syndrome. People taking hydroxyurea are monitored closely with regular blood testing and dose adjustments to prevent complications.

A person who is on bed rest or has recently had surgery can use an incentive spirometer, also called "blow bottle," to help prevent acute chest syndrome.

Treatment

Depending on the cause, treatment might include oxygen, medicine to treat an infection, medicine to open up airways to improve air, and blood transfusions.

Splenic Sequestration

This can be life-threatening and should be treated in a hospital. It happens when a large number of sickle cells get trapped in the spleen and cause it to suddenly get large. Symptoms include sudden weakness, pale lips, fast breathing, extreme thirst, abdominal (belly) pain on the left side of body, and fast heartbeat.

Parents of a child with SCD should learn how to feel and measure the size of their child's spleen and seek help if the spleen is enlarged.

Prevention

For those who have had a very severe, life-threatening episode of splenic sequestration or who have had many episodes in the past, it might be necessary to have regular blood transfusions or the spleen can be removed (called splenectomy) to stop it from happening again.

Treatment

Treatment typically is a blood transfusion. This should be done in consultation with a blood specialist as patients sometimes become overloaded with fluid when the blood is released from the spleen. Removal of blood may be necessary to prevent this from happening.

Vision Loss

Vision loss, including blindness, can occur when blood vessels in the eye become blocked with sickle cells and the retina (the thin layer of tissue inside the back of the eye) gets damaged. Some patients develop extra blood vessels in the eye from the lack of oxygen.

Prevention

People with sickle cell disease should have their eyes checked every year to look for damage to the retina. If possible, this should be done by an eye doctor who specializes in diseases of the retina.

Treatment

If the retina is damaged by excessive blood vessel growth, laser treatment often can prevent further vision loss.

Leg Ulcers

This usually occurs on the lower part of the leg. They happen more often in males than in females and usually appear from 10 through 50 years of age. A combination of factors cause ulcer formation, including trauma, infection, inflammation, and interruption of the circulation in the smallest blood vessels of the leg.

Treatment

Leg ulcers can be treated with medicated creams and ointments. Leg ulcers can be painful, and patients can be given strong pain medicine. Management of leg ulcers could also include the use of cultured skin grafts. This treatment is provided in specialized centers. Bed rest and keeping the leg (or legs) raised to reduce swelling is helpful, although not always possible.

Stroke

A stroke can happen if sickle cells get stuck in a blood vessel and clog blood flow to the brain. About 10% of children with SCD will have a symptomatic stroke. Stroke can cause learning problems and lifelong disabilities.

Prevention

Children who are at risk for stroke can be identified using a special type of exam called, transcranial Doppler ultrasound (TCD). If the child is found to have an abnormal TCD, a doctor might recommend frequent blood transfusions to help prevent a stroke. People who have frequent blood transfusions must be watched closely because there are serious side effects. For example, too much iron can build up in the body, causing life-threatening damage to the organs.

Deep Vein Thrombosis (DVT) and Pulmonary Embolism (PE)

Sickling of red cells can increase blood coagulation and induce an increased risk of blood clot in a deep vein (DVT), or in the lung (PE) if the blood clot moves from the deep veins. People with SCD have a high chance of developing DVT or PE. DVT and PE can cause serious illness, disability and, in some cases, death.

Prevention and Treatment

Medication is used to prevent and treat DVT and PE. PE requires immediate medical attention.

Other Possible Complications

- Damage to body organs (like the liver, heart, or kidneys), tissues, or bones because not enough blood is flowing to the affected area(s).

- Malnutrition and growth retardation among adolescents can cause a delayed onset of puberty and, in males, infertility.

- Gallstones.

- Painful erection of the penis, called priapism, can last less than 2 hours or more than 4 hours. If it lasts more than 4 hours, the person should get urgent medical help. It can lead to impotence.

- A very rare form of kidney cancer (renal medullary carcinoma) has been associated with sickle cell trait.

Cure

The only cure for SCD is bone marrow or stem cell transplant.

Bone marrow is a soft, fatty tissue inside the center of the bones where blood cells are made. A bone marrow or stem cell transplant is a procedure that takes healthy cells that form blood from one person—the donor—and puts them into someone whose bone marrow is not working properly.

Bone marrow or stem cell transplants are very risky, and can have serious side effects, including death. For the transplant to work, the bone marrow must be a close match. Usually, the best donor is a brother or sister. Bone marrow or stem cell transplants are used only in cases of severe SCD for children who have minimal organ damage from the disease.

Section 16.2

Thalassemia

This section includes text excerpted from "Thalassemia," Centers for Disease Control and Prevention (CDC), May 24, 2016.

Facts about Thalassemia

Thalassemia is an inherited (i.e., passed from parents to children through genes) blood disorder caused when the body doesn't make enough of a protein called hemoglobin, an important part of red blood cells. When there isn't enough hemoglobin, the body's red blood cells don't function properly and they last shorter periods of time, so there are fewer healthy red blood cells traveling in the bloodstream.

Red blood cells carry oxygen to all the cells of the body. Oxygen is a sort of food that cells use to function. When there are not enough healthy red blood cells, there is also not enough oxygen delivered to all the other cells of the body, which may cause a person to feel tired, weak or short of breath. This is a condition called anemia. People with thalassemia may have mild or severe anemia. Severe anemia can damage organs and lead to death.

What Are the Different Types of Thalassemia?

When we talk about different "types" of thalassemia, we might be talking about one of two things: the specific part of hemoglobin that is affected (usually either "alpha" or "beta"), or the severity of thalassemia, which is noted by words like trait, carrier, intermedia, or major.

Hemoglobin, which carries oxygen to all cells in the body, is made of two different parts, called alpha and beta. When thalassemia is called "alpha" or "beta," this refers to the part of hemoglobin that isn't being made. If either the alpha or beta part is not made, there aren't enough building blocks to make normal amounts of hemoglobin. Low alpha is called alpha thalassemia. Low beta is called beta thalassemia.

When the words "trait," "minor," "intermedia," or "major" are used, these words describe how severe the thalassemia is. A person who has thalassemia trait may not have any symptoms at all or may have only mild anemia, while a person with thalassemia major may have severe symptoms and may need regular blood transfusions.

In the same way that traits for hair color and body structure are passed down from parents to children, thalassemia traits are passed from parents to children. The type of thalassemia that a person has depends on how many and what type of traits for thalassemia a person has inherited, or received from their parents. For instance, if a person receives a beta thalassemia trait from his father and another from his mother, he will have beta thalassemia major. If a person received an alpha thalassemia trait from her mother and the normal alpha parts from her father, she would have alpha thalassemia trait (also called alpha thalassemia minor). Having a thalassemia trait means that you may not have any symptoms, but you might pass that trait on to your children and increase their risk for having thalassemia.

Sometimes, thalassemias have other names, like Constant Spring, Cooley Anemia, or hemoglobin Bart hydrops fetalis. These names are specific to certain thalassemias—for instance, Cooley Anemia is the same thing as beta thalassemia major.

How Do I Know If I Have Thalassemia?

People with moderate and severe forms of thalassemia usually find out about their condition in childhood, since they have symptoms of severe anemia early in life. People with less severe forms of thalassemia may only find out because they are having symptoms of anemia, or maybe because a doctor finds anemia on a routine blood test or a test done for another reason.

Because thalassemias are inherited, the condition sometimes runs in families. Some people find out about their thalassemia because they have relatives with a similar condition.

People who have family members from certain parts of the world have a higher risk for having thalassemia. Traits for thalassemia are more common in people from Mediterranean countries, like Greece and Turkey, and in people from Asia, Africa, and the Middle East. If you have anemia and you also have family members from these areas, your doctor might test your blood further to find out if you have thalassemia.

How Can I Prevent Thalassemia?

Because thalassemia is passed from parents to children, it is very hard to prevent. However, if you or your partner knows of family members with thalassemia, or if you both have family members from places in the world where thalassemia is common, you can speak to a genetic counselor to determine what your risk would be of passing thalassemia to your children.

Complications and Treatment

If I Have Thalassemia, How Does It Affect My Body?

Since your body has fewer red blood cells when you have thalassemia, you may have symptoms of a low blood count, or anemia. When you have anemia, you might feel tired or weak. You might also experience:

- dizziness
- shortness of breath
- a fast heart beat
- headache
- leg cramps
- difficulty concentrating
- pale skin

Your body will try very hard to make more red blood cells. The main place where blood cells are made is the bone marrow, the dark spongy part in the middle of bones. Because your bone marrow may be working harder than normal, it might grow bigger. This causes your bones to expand, and may stretch your bones and make them thinner and more easily broken.

Another place where blood is made is an organ called the spleen. It sits on the left side of your abdomen, just under your lower ribs. The spleen has many other jobs. Two of the major ones are filtering the blood and monitoring the blood for certain infections. When it finds these infections, it can start the process of fighting them. When you have thalassemia, the spleen can get very big as it tries to make blood cells. Because it is working so hard on this job, it can't work as hard to filter blood or monitor for and fight infections. Because of this, people with thalassemia are said to be "immunocompromised," which means that some of the body's defenses against infection aren't working. When you are immunocompromised, it is easier for you to get infections and you sometimes need extra protection, like flu shots and other vaccines.

How Is Thalassemia Treated?

The type of treatment a person receives depends on how severe the thalassemia is. The more severe the thalassemia, the less hemoglobin the body has, and the more severe the anemia may be.

One way to treat anemia is to provide the body with more red blood cells to carry oxygen. This can be done through a blood transfusion, a safe, common procedure in which you receive blood through a small plastic tube inserted into one of your blood vessels. Some people with thalassemia—usually with thalassemia major—need regular blood transfusions because their body makes such low amounts of hemoglobin. People with thalassemia intermedia (not as severe as major, but not as mild as trait) may need blood transfusions sometimes, such as when they have an infection or an illness. People with thalassemia minor or trait usually do not need blood transfusions because they either do not have anemia or have only a mild anemia.

Many times people with thalassemia are prescribed a supplemental B vitamin, known as folic acid, to help treat anemia. Folic acid can help red blood cells develop. Treatment with folic acid is usually done in addition to other therapies.

How Do Blood Transfusions Affect My Body?

People who receive a lot of blood transfusions are at risk for iron overload. Red blood cells contain a lot of iron, and over time, the iron from all of the transfusions can build up in the body. When it builds up, the iron collects in places like the heart, liver, and brain, and can make it hard for these organs to work properly. To prevent iron overload, people with thalassemia may need chelation therapy, which is when doctors give a medicine—either a pill or a shot under the skin—to remove excess iron before it builds up in the organs.

Every time a person gets a blood transfusion, their risk for a problem called "alloimmunization" goes up. Alloimmunization happens when a person's body reacts to blood from a transfusion because it is seen as harmful by their immune system, and tries to destroy it. Persons with alloimmunization can still receive blood transfusions, but the blood they receive has to be checked and compared to their own blood to make sure that it won't be destroyed by their immune system. This takes time and can mean that persons with alloimmunization have to wait longer for blood, or may have a harder time finding blood that won't be destroyed by their body.

Another concern for people who receive a lot of blood transfusions is the safety of the blood they receive. Some infections, like hepatitis, can be carried in blood. In the United States, the blood supply is screened and monitored for safety, and the risk of getting an infection from a blood transfusion is very low. Nevertheless, there is still a very small risk of getting an infection through a blood transfusion.

Section 16.3

Hereditary Spherocytosis

This section includes text excerpted from "Hereditary Spherocytosis," Genetic and Rare Diseases Information Center (GARD), September 11, 2015.

What Is Hereditary Spherocytosis?

Hereditary spherocytosis is a condition characterized by hemolytic anemia (when red blood cells are destroyed earlier than normal). Signs and symptoms can range from mild to severe and may include pale skin, fatigue, anemia, jaundice, gallstones, and/or enlargement of the spleen. Some people with a severe form may have short stature, delayed sexual development, and skeletal abnormalities. The condition is caused by mutations in any of several genes, such as the *ANK1, EPB42, SLC4A1, SPTA1*, and *SPTB* genes. It is most commonly inherited in an autosomal dominant manner, but may be inherited in an autosomal recessive manner. There are different types of hereditary spherocytosis, which are distinguished by severity and genetic cause. Depending on severity, treatment may involve splenectomy, red cell transfusions, folic acid supplementation, and/or cholecystectomy.

What Are the Signs and Symptoms of Hereditary Spherocytosis?

- Autosomal dominant inheritance
- Cholelithiasis
- Hemolytic anemia
- Hyperbilirubinemia
- Jaundice
- Reticulocytosis
- Spherocytosis
- Splenomegaly

What Causes Hereditary Spherocytosis?

Hereditary spherocytosis may be caused by changes (mutations) in any of several genes. These genes give the body instructions to make proteins that exist on the membranes of red blood cells. These proteins carry molecules in and out of cells, keep cell structure, and attach to other proteins. Some increase the flexibility of cells so they can easily travel from larger blood vessels to smaller, narrow blood vessels.

The gene mutations that cause hereditary spherocytosis cause red blood cells to have an abnormal, spherical shape with decreased flexibility. The misshapen red blood cells are called spherocytes. The spherocytes are taken out of circulation and sent to the spleen to be destroyed (hemolysis). This results in a shortage of red blood cells in the blood, and too many in the spleen.

About half of all cases of hereditary spherocytosis are due to mutations in the *ANK1* gene. Other genes associated with the condition include the *EPB42, SLC4A1, SPTA1,* and *SPTB* genes.

How Is Hereditary Spherocytosis Inherited?

About 75% of cases of hereditary spherocytosis are inherited in an autosomal dominant manner. This means that having a change (mutation) in only one copy of the responsible gene in each cell is enough to cause features of the condition. In some cases, an affected person inherits the mutated gene from an affected parent. In other cases, the mutation occurs for the first time in a person with no family history of the condition. This is called a de novo mutation. When a person with a mutation that causes an autosomal dominant condition has children, each child has a 50% (1 in 2) chance to inherit that mutation.

Less commonly, hereditary spherocytosis is inherited in an autosomal recessive manner.This means that to be affected, a person must have a mutation in both copies of the responsible gene in each cell. Affected people inherit one mutated copy of the gene from each parent, who is referred to as a carrier. Carriers of an autosomal recessive condition typically do not have any signs or symptoms (they are unaffected). When 2 carriers of an autosomal recessive condition have children, each child has a:

- 25% (1 in 4) chance to be affected

- 50% (1 in 2) chance to be an unaffected carrier like each parent

- 25% chance to be unaffected and not be a carrier

In some of the cases that result from new mutations in people with no family history of the condition, the inheritance pattern may be unclear.

What Is the Long-Term Outlook for People with Hereditary Spherocytosis?

Overall, the long-term outlook (prognosis) for people with hereditary spherocytosis (HS) is usually good with treatment. However, it may depend on the severity of the condition in each person. HS is often classified as being mild, moderate or severe. People with very mild HS may not have any signs or symptoms unless an environmental "trigger" causes symptom onset. In many cases, no specific therapy is needed other than monitoring for anemia and watching for signs and symptoms. Moderately and severely affected people are likely to benefit from splenectomy. Most people who undergo splenectomy are able to maintain a normal hemoglobin level. However, people with severe HS may remain anemic post-splenectomy, and may need blood transfusions during an infection.

Information about life expectancy in the medical literature appears to be limited. However, we are not aware of reports that state that life expectancy is known to be significantly shortened in people without other medical problems who are managed appropriately. In all people who undergo splenectomy, there is a lifelong, increased risk of developing a life-threatening infection (sepsis). Although most septic episodes have been observed in children whose spleens were removed in the first years of life, older children and adults also are susceptible. Fortunately, taking certain precautions can reduce this risk and can prevent minor infections from becoming life-threatening.

Section 16.4

Iron-Deficiency Anemia

This section includes text excerpted from "Iron-Deficiency Anemia," National Heart, Lung, and Blood Institute (NHLBI), March 26, 2014.

What Is Iron-Deficiency Anemia?

Iron-deficiency anemia is a common, easily treated condition that occurs if you don't have enough iron in your body. Low iron levels usually are due to blood loss, poor diet, or an inability to absorb enough iron from food.

What Causes Iron-Deficiency Anemia?

Not having enough iron in your body causes iron-deficiency anemia. Lack of iron usually is due to blood loss, poor diet, or an inability to absorb enough iron from food.

Blood Loss

When you lose blood, you lose iron. If you don't have enough iron stored in your body to make up for the lost iron, you'll develop iron-deficiency anemia.

In women, long or heavy menstrual periods or bleeding fibroids in the uterus may cause low iron levels. Blood loss that occurs during childbirth is another cause of low iron levels in women.

Internal bleeding (bleeding inside the body) also may lead to iron-deficiency anemia. This type of blood loss isn't always obvious, and it may occur slowly. Some causes of internal bleeding are:

- A bleeding ulcer, colon polyp, or colon cancer.

- Regular use of aspirin or other pain medicines, such as non-steroidal anti-inflammatory drugs (for example, ibuprofen and naproxen).

- Urinary tract bleeding.

Blood loss from severe injuries, surgery, or frequent blood drawings also can cause iron-deficiency anemia.

Poor Diet

The best sources of iron are meat, poultry, fish, and iron-fortified foods (foods that have iron added). If you don't eat these foods regularly, or if you don't take an iron supplement, you're more likely to develop iron-deficiency anemia.

Vegetarian diets can provide enough iron if you eat the right foods. For example, good nonmeat sources of iron include iron-fortified breads and cereals, beans, tofu, dried fruits, and spinach and other dark green leafy vegetables.

During some stages of life, such as pregnancy and childhood, it may be hard to get enough iron in your diet. This is because your need for iron increases during these times of growth and development.

Inability to Absorb Enough Iron

Even if you have enough iron in your diet, your body may not be able to absorb it. This can happen if you have intestinal surgery (such as gastric bypass) or a disease of the intestine (such as Crohn disease or celiac disease).

Prescription medicines that reduce acid in the stomach also can interfere with iron absorption.

Who Is at Risk for Iron-Deficiency Anemia?

Infants and Young Children

Infants and young children need a lot of iron to grow and develop. The iron that full-term infants have stored in their bodies is used up in the first 4 to 6 months of life.

Premature and low-birth-weight babies (weighing less than 5.5 pounds) are at even greater risk for iron-deficiency anemia. These babies don't have as much iron stored in their bodies as larger, full-term infants.

Iron-fortified baby food or iron supplements, when used properly, can help prevent iron-deficiency anemia in infants and young children. Talk with your child's doctor about your child's diet.

Young children who drink a lot of cow's milk may be at risk for iron-deficiency anemia. Milk is low in iron, and too much milk may take the place of iron-rich foods in the diet. Too much milk also may prevent children's bodies from absorbing iron from other foods.

Children who have lead in their blood also may be at risk for iron-deficiency anemia. Lead can interfere with the body's ability to make hemoglobin. Lead may get into the body from breathing in lead dust, eating lead in paint or soil, or drinking water that contains lead.

Teens

Teens are at risk for iron-deficiency anemia if they're underweight or have chronic (ongoing) illnesses. Teenage girls who have heavy periods also are at increased risk for the condition.

Women

Women of childbearing age are at higher risk for iron-deficiency anemia because of blood loss during their monthly periods. About 1 in 5 women of childbearing age has iron-deficiency anemia.

Pregnant women also are at higher risk for the condition because they need twice as much iron as usual. The extra iron is needed for increased blood volume and for the fetus' growth.

About half of all pregnant women develop iron-deficiency anemia. The condition can increase a pregnant woman's risk for a premature or low-birth-weight baby.

Adults Who Have Internal Bleeding

Adults who have internal bleeding, such as intestinal bleeding, can develop iron-deficiency anemia due to blood loss. Certain conditions, such as colon cancer and bleeding ulcers, can cause blood loss. Some medicines, such as aspirin, also can cause internal bleeding.

Other At-Risk Groups

People who get kidney dialysis treatment may develop iron-deficiency anemia. This is because blood is lost during dialysis. Also, the kidneys are no longer able to make enough of a hormone that the body needs to produce red blood cells.

People who have gastric bypass surgery also may develop iron-deficiency anemia. This type of surgery can prevent the body from absorbing enough iron.

Certain eating patterns or habits may put you at higher risk for iron-deficiency anemia. This can happen if you:

- Follow a diet that excludes meat and fish, which are the best sources of iron. However, vegetarian diets can provide enough iron if you eat the right foods.

- Eat poorly because of money, social, health, or other problems.

- Follow a very low-fat diet over a long time. Some higher fat foods, like meat, are the best sources of iron.

- Follow a high-fiber diet. Large amounts of fiber can slow the absorption of iron.

What Are the Signs and Symptoms of Iron-Deficiency Anemia?

The signs and symptoms of iron-deficiency anemia depend on its severity. Mild to moderate iron-deficiency anemia may have no signs or symptoms.

When signs and symptoms do occur, they can range from mild to severe. Many of the signs and symptoms of iron-deficiency anemia apply to all types of anemia.

Signs and Symptoms of Anemia

The most common symptom of all types of anemia is fatigue (tiredness). Fatigue occurs because your body doesn't have enough red blood cells to carry oxygen to its many parts.

Also, the red blood cells your body makes have less hemoglobin than normal. Hemoglobin is an iron-rich protein in red blood cells. It helps red blood cells carry oxygen from the lungs to the rest of the body.

Anemia also can cause shortness of breath, dizziness, headache, coldness in your hands and feet, pale skin, chest pain, weakness, and fatigue (tiredness).

If you don't have enough hemoglobin-carrying red blood cells, your heart has to work harder to move oxygen-rich blood through your body. This can lead to irregular heartbeats called arrhythmias, a heart murmur, an enlarged heart, or even heart failure.

In infants and young children, signs of anemia include poor appetite, slowed growth and development, and behavioral problems.

Signs and Symptoms of Iron Deficiency

Signs and symptoms of iron deficiency may include brittle nails, swelling or soreness of the tongue, cracks in the sides of the mouth, an enlarged spleen, and frequent infections.

People who have iron-deficiency anemia may have an unusual craving for nonfood items, such as ice, dirt, paint, or starch. This craving is called pica.

Some people who have iron-deficiency anemia develop restless legs syndrome (RLS). RLS is a disorder that causes a strong urge to move the legs. This urge to move often occurs with strange and unpleasant feelings in the legs. People who have RLS often have a hard time sleeping.

Iron-deficiency anemia can put children at greater risk for lead poisoning and infections.

Some signs and symptoms of iron-deficiency anemia are related to the condition's causes. For example, a sign of intestinal bleeding is bright red blood in the stools or black, tarry-looking stools.

Very heavy menstrual bleeding, long periods, or other vaginal bleeding may suggest that a woman is at risk for iron-deficiency anemia.

How Is Iron-Deficiency Anemia Diagnosed?

Your doctor will diagnose iron-deficiency anemia based on your medical history, a physical exam, and the results from tests and procedures.

Once your doctor knows the cause and severity of the condition, he or she can create a treatment plan for you.

Mild to moderate iron-deficiency anemia may have no signs or symptoms. Thus, you may not know you have it unless your doctor discovers it from a screening test or while checking for other problems.

Specialists Involved

Primary care doctors often diagnose and treat iron-deficiency anemia. These doctors include pediatricians, family doctors, gynecologists/obstetricians, and internal medicine specialists.

A hematologist (a blood disease specialist), a gastroenterologist (a digestive system specialist), and other specialists also may help treat iron-deficiency anemia.

Medical History

Your doctor will ask about your signs and symptoms and any past problems you've had with anemia or low iron. He or she also may ask about your diet and whether you're taking any medicines.

If you're a woman, your doctor may ask whether you might be pregnant.

Physical Exam

Your doctor will do a physical exam to look for signs of iron-deficiency anemia. He or she may:

- Look at your skin, gums, and nail beds to see whether they're pale.

- Listen to your heart for rapid or irregular heartbeats.

- Listen to your lungs for rapid or uneven breathing.

- Feel your abdomen to check the size of your liver and spleen.

- Do a pelvic and rectal exam to check for internal bleeding.

Diagnostic Tests and Procedures

Many tests and procedures are used to diagnose iron-deficiency anemia. They can help confirm a diagnosis, look for a cause, and find out how severe the condition is.

Complete Blood Count

Often, the first test used to diagnose anemia is a complete blood count (CBC). The CBC measures many parts of your blood.

This test checks your hemoglobin and hematocrit levels. Hemoglobin is an iron-rich protein in red blood cells that carries oxygen to the body. Hematocrit is a measure of how much space red blood cells take up in your blood. A low level of hemoglobin or hematocrit is a sign of anemia.

The normal range of these levels varies in certain racial and ethnic populations. Your doctor can explain your test results to you.

The CBC also checks the number of red blood cells, white blood cells, and platelets in your blood. Abnormal results may be a sign of infection, a blood disorder, or another condition.

Finally, the CBC looks at mean corpuscular volume (MCV). MCV is a measure of the average size of your red blood cells. The results may be a clue as to the cause of your anemia. In iron-deficiency anemia, for example, red blood cells usually are smaller than normal.

Other Blood Tests

If the CBC results confirm you have anemia, you may need other blood tests to find out what's causing the condition, how severe it is, and the best way to treat it.

Reticulocyte count. This test measures the number of reticulocytes in your blood. Reticulocytes are young, immature red blood cells. Over time, reticulocytes become mature red blood cells that carry oxygen throughout your body.

A reticulocyte count shows whether your bone marrow is making red blood cells at the correct rate.

Peripheral smear. For this test, a sample of your blood is examined under a microscope. If you have iron-deficiency anemia, your red blood cells will look smaller and paler than normal.

Tests to measure iron levels. These tests can show how much iron has been used from your body's stored iron. Tests to measure iron levels include:

- Serum iron. This test measures the amount of iron in your blood. The level of iron in your blood may be normal even if the total amount of iron in your body is low. For this reason, other iron tests also are done.

- Serum ferritin. Ferritin is a protein that helps store iron in your body. A measure of this protein helps your doctor find out how much of your body's stored iron has been used.

- Transferrin level, or total iron-binding capacity. Transferrin is a protein that carries iron in your blood. Total iron-binding capacity measures how much of the transferrin in your blood isn't carrying iron. If you have iron-deficiency anemia, you'll have a high level of transferrin that has no iron.

Other tests. Your doctor also may recommend tests to check your hormone levels, especially your thyroid hormone. You also may have a blood test for a chemical called erythrocyte protoporphyrin. This chemical is a building block for hemoglobin.

Children also may be tested for the level of lead in their blood. Lead can make it hard for the body to produce hemoglobin.

Tests and Procedures for Gastrointestinal Blood Loss

To check whether internal bleeding is causing your iron-deficiency anemia, your doctor may suggest a fecal occult blood test. This test looks for blood in the stools and can detect bleeding in the intestines.

If the test finds blood, you may have other tests and procedures to find the exact spot of the bleeding. These tests and procedures may look for bleeding in the stomach, upper intestines, colon, or pelvic organs.

How Is Iron-Deficiency Anemia Treated?

Treatment for iron-deficiency anemia will depend on its cause and severity. Treatments may include dietary changes and supplements, medicines, and surgery.

Severe iron-deficiency anemia may require a blood transfusion, iron injections, or intravenous (IV) iron therapy. Treatment may need to be done in a hospital.

The goals of treating iron-deficiency anemia are to treat its underlying cause and restore normal levels of red blood cells, hemoglobin, and iron.

Dietary Changes and Supplements

Iron

You may need iron supplements to build up your iron levels as quickly as possible. Iron supplements can correct low iron levels within months. Supplements come in pill form or in drops for children.

Large amounts of iron can be harmful, so take iron supplements only as your doctor prescribes. Keep iron supplements out of reach from children. This will prevent them from taking an overdose of iron.

Iron supplements can cause side effects, such as dark stools, stomach irritation, and heartburn. Iron also can cause constipation, so your doctor may suggest that you use a stool softener.

Your doctor may advise you to eat more foods that are rich in iron. The best source of iron is red meat, especially beef and liver. Chicken, turkey, pork, fish, and shellfish also are good sources of iron.

The body tends to absorb iron from meat better than iron from nonmeat foods. However, some nonmeat foods also can help you raise your iron levels. Examples of nonmeat foods that are good sources of iron include:

- iron-fortified breads and cereals
- peas; lentils; white, red, and baked beans; soybeans; and chickpeas
- tofu
- dried fruits, such as prunes, raisins, and apricots
- spinach and other dark green leafy vegetables
- prune juice

The Nutrition Facts labels on packaged foods will show how much iron the items contain. The amount is given as a percentage of the total amount of iron you need every day.

Vitamin C

Vitamin C helps the body absorb iron. Good sources of vitamin C are vegetables and fruits, especially citrus fruits. Citrus fruits include oranges, grapefruits, tangerines, and similar fruits. Fresh and frozen fruits, vegetables, and juices usually have more vitamin C than canned ones.

If you're taking medicines, ask your doctor or pharmacist whether you can eat grapefruit or drink grapefruit juice. Grapefruit can affect the strength of a few medicines and how well they work.

Other fruits rich in vitamin C include kiwi fruit, strawberries, and cantaloupes.

Vegetables rich in vitamin C include broccoli, peppers, Brussels sprouts, tomatoes, cabbage, potatoes, and leafy green vegetables like turnip greens and spinach.

Treatment To Stop Bleeding

If blood loss is causing iron-deficiency anemia, treatment will depend on the cause of the bleeding. For example, if you have a bleeding ulcer, your doctor may prescribe antibiotics and other medicines to treat the ulcer.

If a polyp or cancerous tumor in your intestine is causing bleeding, you may need surgery to remove the growth.

If you have heavy menstrual flow, your doctor may prescribe birth control pills to help reduce your monthly blood flow. In some cases, surgery may be advised.

Treatments for Severe Iron-Deficiency Anemia

Blood Transfusion

If your iron-deficiency anemia is severe, you may get a transfusion of red blood cells. A blood transfusion is a safe, common procedure in which blood is given to you through an IV line in one of your blood vessels. A transfusion requires careful matching of donated blood with the recipient's blood.

A transfusion of red blood cells will treat your anemia right away. The red blood cells also give a source of iron that your body can reuse. However, a blood transfusion is only a short-term treatment. Your doctor will need to find and treat the cause of your anemia.

Blood transfusions are usually reserved for people whose anemia puts them at a higher risk for heart problems or other severe health issues.

Iron Therapy

If you have severe anemia, your doctor may recommend iron therapy. For this treatment, iron is injected into a muscle or an IV line in one of your blood vessels.

IV iron therapy presents some safety concerns. It must be done in a hospital or clinic by experienced staff. Iron therapy usually is given to people who need iron long-term but can't take iron supplements by mouth. This therapy also is given to people who need immediate treatment for iron-deficiency anemia.

How Can Iron-Deficiency Anemia Be Prevented?

Eating a well-balanced diet that includes iron-rich foods may help you prevent iron-deficiency anemia.

Taking iron supplements also may lower your risk for the condition if you're not able to get enough iron from food. Large amounts of iron can be harmful, so take iron supplements only as your doctor prescribes.

Infants and young children and women are the two groups at highest risk for iron-deficiency anemia. Special measures can help prevent the condition in these groups.

Infants and Young Children

A baby's diet can affect his or her risk for iron-deficiency anemia. For example, cow's milk is low in iron. For this and other reasons, cow's milk isn't recommended for babies in their first year. After the first year, you may need to limit the amount of cow's milk your baby drinks.

Also, babies need more iron as they grow and begin to eat solid foods. Talk with your child's doctor about a healthy diet and food choices that will help your child get enough iron.

Your child's doctor may recommend iron drops. However, giving a child too much iron can be harmful. Follow the doctor's instructions and keep iron supplements and vitamins away from children. Asking for child-proof packages for supplements can help prevent overdosing in children.

Because recent research supports concerns that iron deficiency during infancy and childhood can have long-lasting, negative effects on brain health, the American Academy of Pediatrics recommends testing all infants for anemia at 1 year of age.

Women and Girls

Women of childbearing age may be tested for iron-deficiency anemia, especially if they have:

- A history of iron-deficiency anemia.

- Heavy blood loss during their monthly periods.

- Other risk factors for iron-deficiency anemia.

The Centers for Disease Control and Prevention (CDC) has developed guidelines for who should be screened for iron deficiency, and how often:

- Girls aged 12 to 18 and women of childbearing age who are not pregnant: Every 5 to 10 years.

- Women who have risk factors for iron deficiency: Once a year.

- Pregnant women: At the first prenatal visit.

For pregnant women, medical care during pregnancy usually includes screening for anemia. Also, your doctor may prescribe iron supplements or advise you to eat more iron-rich foods. This not only will help you avoid iron-deficiency anemia, but also may lower your risk of having a low-birth-weight baby.

Living with Iron-Deficiency Anemia

If you have iron-deficiency anemia, get ongoing care to make sure your iron levels are improving. At your checkups, your doctor may change your medicines or supplements. He or she also may suggest ways to improve your diet.

Take iron supplements only with your doctor's approval, and only as he or she prescribes. It's possible to have too much iron in your body (a condition called iron overload). Too much iron in your body can damage your organs.

You may have fatigue (tiredness) and other symptoms of iron-deficiency anemia until your iron levels return to normal, which can take months. Tell your doctor if you have any new symptoms or if your symptoms get worse.

Chapter 17

Hemochromatosis

What Is Hemochromatosis?

Hemochromatosis is the most common form of iron overload disease. Too much iron in the body causes hemochromatosis. Iron is important because it is part of hemoglobin, a molecule in the blood that transports oxygen from the lungs to all body tissues. However, too much iron in the body leads to iron overload—a buildup of extra iron that, without treatment, can damage organs such as the liver, heart, and pancreas; endocrine glands; and joints.

The three types of hemochromatosis are primary hemochromatosis, also called hereditary hemochromatosis; secondary hemochromatosis; and neonatal hemochromatosis.

What Causes Hemochromatosis?

Primary Hemochromatosis

Inherited genetic defects cause primary hemochromatosis, and mutations in the *HFE* gene are associated with up to 90 percent of cases. The HFE gene helps regulate the amount of iron absorbed from food. The two known mutations of *HFE* are C282Y and H63D. C282Y defects are the most common cause of primary hemochromatosis.

This chapter includes text excerpted from "Hemochromatosis," National Institute of Diabetes and Digestive and Kidney Diseases (NIDDK), March 2014.

People inherit two copies of the *HFE* gene—one copy from each parent. Most people who inherit two copies of the *HFE* gene with the *C282Y* defect will have higher-than-average iron absorption. However, not all of these people will develop health problems associated with hemochromatosis. One recent study found that 31 percent of people with two copies of the *C282Y* defect developed health problems by their early fifties. Men who develop health problems from *HFE* defects typically develop them after age 40. Women who develop health problems from *HFE* defects typically develop them after menopause.

People who inherit two *H63D* defects or one *C282Y* and one *H63D* defect may have higher-than-average iron absorption. However, they are unlikely to develop iron overload and organ damage.

Rare defects in other genes may also cause primary hemochromatosis. Mutations in the hemojuvelin or hepcidin genes cause juvenile hemochromatosis, a type of primary hemochromatosis. People with juvenile hemochromatosis typically develop severe iron overload and liver and heart damage between ages 15 and 30.

Secondary Hemochromatosis

Hemochromatosis that is not inherited is called secondary hemochromatosis. The most common cause of secondary hemochromatosis is frequent blood transfusions in people with severe anemia. Anemia is a condition in which red blood cells are fewer or smaller than normal, which means they carry less oxygen to the body's cells. Types of anemia that may require frequent blood transfusions include

- congenital, or inherited, anemias such as sickle cell disease, thalassemia, and Fanconi syndrome

- severe acquired anemias, which are not inherited, such as aplastic anemia and autoimmune hemolytic anemia

Liver diseases—such as alcoholic liver disease, nonalcoholic steatohepatitis, and chronic hepatitis C infection—may cause mild iron overload. However, this iron overload causes much less liver damage than the underlying liver disease causes.

Neonatal Hemochromatosis

Neonatal hemochromatosis is a rare disease characterized by liver failure and death in fetuses and newborns. Researchers are studying the causes of neonatal hemochromatosis and believe more than one factor may lead to the disease.

Experts previously considered neonatal hemochromatosis a type of primary hemochromatosis. However, recent studies suggest genetic defects that increase iron absorption do not cause this disease. Instead, the mother's immune system may produce antibodies—proteins made by the immune system to protect the body from foreign substances such as bacteria or viruses—that damage the liver of the fetus. Women who have had one child with neonatal hemochromatosis are at risk for having more children with the disease. Treating these women during pregnancy with intravenous (IV) immunoglobulin—a solution of antibodies from healthy people—can prevent fetal liver damage.

Researchers supported by the National Institute of Diabetes and Digestive and Kidney Diseases (NIDDK) recently found that a combination of exchange transfusion—removing blood and replacing it with donor blood—and IV immunoglobulin is an effective treatment for babies born with neonatal hemochromatosis.

Who Is More Likely to Develop Hemochromatosis?

Primary hemochromatosis mainly affects Caucasians of Northern European descent. This disease is one of the most common genetic disorders in the United States. About four to five out of every 1,000 Caucasians carry two copies of the *C282Y* mutation of the *HFE* gene and are susceptible to developing hemochromatosis. About one out of every 10 Caucasians carries one copy of *C282Y*.

Hemochromatosis is extremely rare in African Americans, Asian Americans, Hispanics/Latinos, and American Indians. *HFE* mutations are usually not the cause of hemochromatosis in these populations.

Both men and women can inherit the gene defects for hemochromatosis; however, not all will develop the symptoms of hemochromatosis. Men usually develop symptoms at a younger age than women. Women lose blood—which contains iron—regularly during menstruation; therefore, women with the gene defects that cause hemochromatosis may not develop iron overload and related symptoms and complications until after menopause.

What Are the Symptoms of Hemochromatosis?

A person with hemochromatosis may notice one or more of the following symptoms:

- joint pain
- fatigue, or feeling tired

179

- unexplained weight loss

- abnormal bronze or gray skin color

- abdominal pain

- loss of sex drive

Not everyone with hemochromatosis will develop these symptoms.

What Are the Complications of Hemochromatosis?

Without treatment, iron may build up in the organs and cause complications, including

- cirrhosis, or scarring of liver tissue

- diabetes

- irregular heart rhythms or weakening of the heart muscle

- arthritis

- erectile dysfunction

The complication most often associated with hemochromatosis is liver damage. Iron buildup in the liver causes cirrhosis, which increases the chance of developing liver cancer.

For some people, complications may be the first sign of hemochromatosis. However, not everyone with hemochromatosis will develop complications.

How Is Hemochromatosis Diagnosed?

Healthcare providers use medical and family history, a physical exam, and routine blood tests to diagnose hemochromatosis or other conditions that could cause the same symptoms or complications.

- **Medical and family history.** Taking a medical and family history is one of the first things a healthcare provider may do to help diagnose hemochromatosis. The healthcare provider will look for clues that may indicate hemochromatosis, such as a family history of arthritis or unexplained liver disease.

- **Physical exam.** After taking a medical history, a healthcare provider will perform a physical exam, which may help diagnose hemochromatosis.

- **Blood tests.** A blood test involves drawing blood at a healthcare provider's office or a commercial facility and sending the sample to a lab for analysis. Blood tests can determine whether the amount of iron stored in the body is higher than normal:

  - The **transferrin saturation test** shows how much iron is bound to the protein that carries iron in the blood. Transferrin saturation values above or equal to 45 percent are considered abnormal.

  - The **serum ferritin test** detects the amount of ferritin—a protein that stores iron—in the blood. Levels above 300 μg/L in men and 200 μg/L in women are considered abnormal. Levels above 1,000 μg/L in men or women indicate a high chance of iron overload and organ damage.

  If either test shows higher-than-average levels of iron in the body, healthcare providers can order a special blood test that can detect two copies of the *C282Y* mutation to confirm the diagnosis. If the mutation is not present, healthcare providers will look for other causes.

- **Liver biopsy.** Healthcare providers may perform a liver biopsy, a procedure that involves taking a piece of liver tissue for examination with a microscope for signs of damage or disease. The healthcare provider may ask the patient to temporarily stop taking certain medications before the liver biopsy. The healthcare provider may ask the patient to fast for 8 hours before the procedure.

Hemochromatosis is rare, and healthcare providers may not think to test for this disease. Thus, the disease is often not diagnosed or treated. The initial symptoms can be diverse, vague, and similar to the symptoms of many other diseases. Healthcare providers may focus on the symptoms and complications caused by hemochromatosis rather than on the underlying iron overload. However, if a healthcare provider diagnoses and treats the iron overload caused by hemochromatosis before organ damage has occurred, a person can live a normal, healthy life.

Who Should Be Tested for Hemochromatosis?

Experts recommend testing for hemochromatosis in people who have symptoms, complications, or a family history of the disease.

Some researchers have suggested widespread screening for the *C282Y* mutation in the general population. However, screening is not cost-effective. Although the *C282Y* mutation occurs quite frequently, the disease caused by the mutation is rare, and many people with two copies of the mutation never develop iron overload or organ damage.

Researchers and public health officials suggest the following:

- Siblings of people who have hemochromatosis should have their blood tested to see if they have the *C282Y* mutation.

- Parents, children, and other close relatives of people who have hemochromatosis should consider being tested.

- Healthcare providers should consider testing people who have severe and continuing fatigue, unexplained cirrhosis, joint pain or arthritis, heart problems, erectile dysfunction, or diabetes because these health issues may result from hemochromatosis.

How Is Hemochromatosis Treated?

Healthcare providers treat hemochromatosis by drawing blood. This process is called phlebotomy. Phlebotomy rids the body of extra iron. This treatment is simple, inexpensive, and safe.

Based on the severity of the iron overload, a patient will have phlebotomy to remove a pint of blood once or twice a week for several months to a year, and occasionally longer. Healthcare providers will test serum ferritin levels periodically to monitor iron levels. The goal is to bring serum ferritin levels to the low end of the average range and keep them there. Depending on the lab, the level is 25 to 50 μg/L.

After phlebotomy reduces serum ferritin levels to the desired level, patients may need maintenance phlebotomy treatment every few months. Some patients may need phlebotomies more often. Serum ferritin tests every 6 months or once a year will help determine how often a patient should have blood drawn. Many blood donation centers provide free phlebotomy treatment for people with hemochromatosis.

Treating hemochromatosis before organs are damaged can prevent complications such as cirrhosis, heart problems, arthritis, and diabetes. Treatment cannot cure these conditions in patients who already have them at diagnosis. However, treatment will help most of these conditions improve. The treatment's effectiveness depends on the degree of organ damage. For example, treating hemochromatosis can stop the progression of liver damage in its early stages and lead to a normal life expectancy. However, if a patient develops cirrhosis, his or her chance of developing liver cancer increases, even with phlebotomy treatment. Arthritis usually does not improve even after phlebotomy removes extra iron.

Eating, Diet, and Nutrition

Iron is an essential nutrient found in many foods. Healthy people usually absorb less than 10 percent of iron in the food they eat. People with hemochromatosis absorb up to 30 percent of that iron. People with hemochromatosis can help prevent iron overload by

- eating only moderate amounts of iron-rich foods, such as red meat and organ meat.

- avoiding supplements that contain iron.

- avoiding supplements that contain vitamin C, which increases iron absorption.

People with hemochromatosis can take steps to help prevent liver damage, including

- limiting the amount of alcoholic beverages they drink because alcohol increases their chance of cirrhosis and liver cancer.

- avoiding alcoholic beverages entirely if they already have cirrhosis.

Chapter 18

Leukemia

Chapter Contents

Section 18.1

Adult Acute Lymphoblastic Leukemia

This section includes text excerpted from "Adult Acute Lymphoblastic
Leukemia Treatment (PDQ®)—Patient Version," National Cancer
Institute (NCI), February 5, 2016.

Adult acute lymphoblastic leukemia (ALL; also called acute lymphocytic leukemia) is a cancer of the blood and bone marrow. This type
of cancer usually gets worse quickly if it is not treated.

Leukemia May Affect Red Blood Cells, White Blood Cells, and Platelets

Normally, the bone marrow makes blood stem cells (immature
cells) that become mature blood cells over time. A blood stem cell may
become a myeloid stem cell or a lymphoid stem cell.

A myeloid stem cell becomes one of three types of mature blood cells:

- Red blood cells that carry oxygen and other substances to all tissues of the body.

- Platelets that form blood clots to stop bleeding.

- Granulocytes (white blood cells) that fight infection and disease.

A lymphoid stem cell becomes a lymphoblast cell and then one of
three types of lymphocytes (white blood cells):

- B lymphocytes that make antibodies to help fight infection.

- T lymphocytes that help B lymphocytes make the antibodies
  that help fight infection.

- Natural killer cells that attack cancer cells and viruses.

In ALL, too many stem cells become lymphoblasts, B lymphocytes,
or T lymphocytes. These cells are also called leukemia cells. These leukemia cells are not able to fight infection very well. Also, as the number
of leukemia cells increases in the blood and bone marrow, there is less
room for healthy white blood cells, red blood cells, and platelets. This

may cause infection, anemia, and easy bleeding. The cancer can also spread to the central nervous system (brain and spinal cord).

Previous Chemotherapy and Exposure to Radiation May Increase the Risk of Developing ALL

Anything that increases your risk of getting a disease is called a risk factor. Having a risk factor does not mean that you will get cancer; not having risk factors doesn't mean that you will not get cancer. Talk with your doctor if you think you may be at risk. Possible risk factors for ALL include the following:

- being male
- being white
- being older than 70
- past treatment with chemotherapy or radiation therapy
- being exposed to high levels of radiation in the environment (such as nuclear radiation)
- having certain genetic disorders, such as Down syndrome

Signs and Symptoms of Adult ALL Include Fever, Feeling Tired, and Easy Bruising or Bleeding.

The early signs and symptoms of ALL may be like the flu or other common diseases. Check with your doctor if you have any of the following:

- weakness or feeling tired
- fever or night sweats
- easy bruising or bleeding
- petechiae (flat, pinpoint spots under the skin, caused by bleeding)
- shortness of breath
- weight loss or loss of appetite
- pain in the bones or stomach
- pain or feeling of fullness below the ribs
- painless lumps in the neck, underarm, stomach, or groin
- having many infections

These and other signs and symptoms may be caused by adult acute lymphoblastic leukemia or by other conditions.

Tests That Examine the Blood and Bone Marrow Are Used to Detect (Find) and Diagnose Adult ALL

The following tests and procedures may be used:

- **Physical exam and history:** An exam of the body to check general signs of health, including checking for signs of disease, such as infection or anything else that seems unusual. A history of the patient's health habits and past illnesses and treatments will also be taken.

- **Complete blood count (CBC) with differential:** A procedure in which a sample of blood is drawn and checked for the following:

  - The number of red blood cells and platelets.

  - The number and type of white blood cells.

  - The amount of hemoglobin (the protein that carries oxygen) in the red blood cells.

  - The portion of the blood sample made up of red blood cells.

- **Blood chemistry studies:** A procedure in which a blood sample is checked to measure the amounts of certain substances released into the blood by organs and tissues in the body. An unusual (higher or lower than normal) amount of a substance can be a sign of disease.

- **Peripheral blood smear:** A procedure in which a sample of blood is checked for blast cells, the number and kinds of white blood cells, the number of platelets, and changes in the shape of blood cells.

- **Bone marrow aspiration and biopsy:** The removal of bone marrow, blood, and a small piece of bone by inserting a hollow needle into the hipbone or breastbone. A pathologist views the bone marrow, blood, and bone under a microscope to look for abnormal cells.

The following tests may be done on the samples of blood or bone marrow tissue that are removed:

- **Cytogenetic analysis:** A laboratory test in which the cells in a sample of blood or bone marrow are looked at under a microscope to find out if there are certain changes in the chromosomes of lymphocytes. For example, in Philadelphia chromosome –positive ALL, part of one chromosome switches places with part of another chromosome. This is called the "Philadelphia chromosome."

- **Immunophenotyping:** A process used to identify cells, based on the types of antigens or markers on the surface of the cell. This process is used to diagnose the subtype of ALL by comparing the cancer cells to normal cells of the immune system. For example, a cytochemistry study may test the cells in a sample of tissue using chemicals (dyes) to look for certain changes in the sample. A chemical may cause a color change in one type of leukemia cell but not in another type of leukemia cell.

Certain Factors Affect Prognosis (Chance of Recovery) and Treatment Options

The prognosis (chance of recovery) and treatment options depend on the following:

- The age of the patient.

- Whether the cancer has spread to the brain or spinal cord.

- Whether there are certain changes in the genes, including the Philadelphia chromosome.

- Whether the cancer has been treated before or has recurred (come back).

Section 18.2

Childhood Acute Lymphoblastic Leukemia

This section includes text excerpted from "Childhood Acute
Lymphoblastic Leukemia Treatment (PDQ®)—Patient Version,"
National Cancer Institute (NCI), April 1, 2016.

Childhood acute lymphoblastic leukemia (also called ALL or acute
lymphocytic leukemia) is a cancer of the blood and bone marrow. This
type of cancer usually gets worse quickly if it is not treated.

ALL is the most common type of cancer in children.

Leukemia May Affect Red Blood Cells, White Blood Cells, and Platelets

In a child with ALL, too many stem cells become lymphoblasts,
B lymphocytes, or T lymphocytes. These cells are cancer (leukemia)
cells. The leukemia cells do not work like normal lymphocytes and are
not able to fight infection very well. Also, as the number of leukemia
cells increases in the blood and bone marrow, there is less room for
healthy white blood cells, red blood cells, and platelets. This may lead
to infection, anemia, and easy bleeding.

Past Treatment for Cancer and Certain Genetic Conditions Affect the Risk of Having Childhood ALL

Possible risk factors for ALL include the following:

- being exposed to X-rays before birth

- being exposed to radiation

- past treatment with chemotherapy

- having certain changes in the chromosomes or genes

- having certain genetic conditions, such as:

  - Down syndrome

  - neurofibromatosis type 1 (NF1)

- Shwachman syndrome
- Bloom syndrome
- ataxia-telangiectasia

Signs of Childhood ALL Include Fever and Bruising

These and other signs and symptoms may be caused by childhood ALL or by other conditions. Check with your child's doctor if your child has any of the following:

- fever
- easy bruising or bleeding
- petechiae (flat, pinpoint, dark-red spots under the skin caused by bleeding)
- bone or joint pain
- painless lumps in the neck, underarm, stomach, or groin
- pain or feeling of fullness below the ribs
- weakness, feeling tired, or looking pale
- loss of appetite

Tests That Examine the Blood and Bone Marrow Are Used to Detect (Find) and Diagnose Childhood ALL

The following tests and procedures may be used to diagnose childhood ALL and find out if leukemia cells have spread to other parts of the body such as the brain or testicles:

- physical exam and history
- complete blood count (CBC) with differential
- blood chemistry studies
- bone marrow aspiration and biopsy

The following tests may be done on the tissue that is removed:

- **Cytogenetic analysis:** A laboratory test in which the cells in a sample of blood or bone marrow are viewed under a microscope to look for certain changes in the chromosomes of lymphocytes. For example, in Philadelphia chromosome–positive ALL, part of one chromosome switches places with part of another chromosome. This is called the "Philadelphia chromosome."

- **Immunophenotyping:** A laboratory test in which the antigens or markers on the surface of a blood or bone marrow cell are checked to see if they are lymphocytes or myeloid cells. If the cells are malignant lymphocytes (cancer) they are checked to see if they are B lymphocytes or T lymphocytes.

- **Lumbar puncture:** A procedure used to collect a sample of cerebrospinal fluid (CSF) from the spinal column. This is done by placing a needle between two bones in the spine and into the CSF around the spinal cord and removing a sample of the fluid. The sample of CSF is checked under a microscope for signs that leukemia cells have spread to the brain and spinal cord. This procedure is also called an LP or spinal tap.

- **Chest X-ray:** An X-ray of the organs and bones inside the chest. An X-ray is a type of energy beam that can go through the body and onto film, making a picture of areas inside the body. The chest X-ray is done to see if leukemia cells have formed a mass in the middle of the chest.

- **Testicular biopsy:** The removal of cells or tissues from the testicles so they can be viewed under a microscope by a pathologist to check for signs of cancer. This procedure is done only if there seems to be anything unusual about the testicles during the physical exam.

Certain Factors Affect Prognosis (Chance of Recovery) and Treatment Options

The prognosis (chance of recovery) depends on:

- Age at diagnosis, gender, and race.

- The number of white blood cells in the blood at diagnosis.

- Whether the leukemia cells began from B lymphocytes or T lymphocytes.

- Whether there are certain changes in the chromosomes or genes of the lymphocytes with cancer.

- Whether the child has Down syndrome.

- Whether leukemia cells are found in the cerebrospinal fluid.

- Weight at diagnosis and during treatment.

- How quickly and how low the leukemia cell count drops after the first or second phase of treatment.

Treatment options depend on:

- Whether the leukemia cells began from B lymphocytes or T lymphocytes.

- Whether the child has standard-risk or high-risk ALL.

- The age of the child at diagnosis.

- Whether there are certain changes in the chromosomes of lymphocytes, such as the Philadelphia chromosome.

- How quickly and how low the leukemia cell count drops after initial treatment.

For leukemia that relapses (comes back) after initial treatment, the prognosis and treatment options depend partly on the following:

- How long it is between diagnosis and when the leukemia comes back after initial treatment.

- Whether the leukemia comes back in the bone marrow or in other parts of the body.

Section 18.3

Adult Acute Myeloid Leukemia

This section includes text excerpted from "Adult Acute Myeloid Leukemia Treatment (PDQ®)—Patient Version," National Cancer Institute (NCI), September 17, 2015.

Adult acute myeloid leukemia (AML) is a cancer of the blood and bone marrow. This type of cancer usually gets worse quickly if it is not treated. It is the most common type of acute leukemia in adults. AML is also called acute myelogenous leukemia, acute myeloblastic leukemia, acute granulocytic leukemia, and acute nonlymphocytic leukemia.

Leukemia May Affect Red Blood Cells, White Blood Cells, and Platelets

In AML, the myeloid stem cells usually become a type of immature white blood cell called myeloblasts (or myeloid blasts). The myeloblasts in AML are abnormal and do not become healthy white blood cells. Sometimes in AML, too many stem cells become abnormal red blood cells or platelets. These abnormal white blood cells, red blood cells, or platelets are also called leukemia cells or blasts. Leukemia cells can build up in the bone marrow and blood so there is less room for healthy white blood cells, red blood cells, and platelets. When this happens, infection, anemia, or easy bleeding may occur. The leukemia cells can spread outside the blood to other parts of the body, including the central nervous system (brain and spinal cord), skin, and gums.

There Are Different Subtypes of AML

Most AML subtypes are based on how mature (developed) the cancer cells are at the time of diagnosis and how different they are from normal cells.

Acute promyelocytic leukemia (APL) is a subtype of AML that occurs when parts of two genes stick together. APL usually occurs in middle-aged adults. Signs of APL may include both bleeding and forming blood clots.

Smoking, Previous Chemotherapy Treatment, and Exposure to Radiation May Affect the Risk of Adult AML

Anything that increases your risk of getting a disease is called a risk factor. Having a risk factor does not mean that you will get cancer; not having risk factors doesn't mean that you will not get cancer. Talk with your doctor if you think you may be at risk. Possible risk factors for AML include the following:

- being male
- smoking, especially after age 60
- having had treatment with chemotherapy or radiation therapy in the past
- having had treatment for childhood acute lymphoblastic leukemia (ALL) in the past
- being exposed to radiation from an atomic bomb or to the chemical benzene

- having a history of a blood disorder such as myelodysplastic syndrome

Signs and Symptoms of Adult AML Include Fever, Feeling Tired, and Easy Bruising or Bleeding

The early signs and symptoms of AML may be like those caused by the flu or other common diseases. Check with your doctor if you have any of the following:

- fever
- shortness of breath
- easy bruising or bleeding
- petechiae (flat, pinpoint spots under the skin caused by bleeding)
- weakness or feeling tired
- weight loss or loss of appetite

Tests That Examine the Blood and Bone Marrow Are Used to Detect (Find) and Diagnose Adult AML

The following tests and procedures may be used:

- physical exam and history
- complete blood count (CBC)
- peripheral blood smear
- bone marrow aspiration and biopsy
- cytogenetic analysis
- immunophenotyping
- reverse transcription–polymerase chain reaction test (RT–PCR)

Certain Factors Affect Prognosis (Chance of Recovery) and Treatment Options

The prognosis (chance of recovery) and treatment options depend on:

- the age of the patient
- the subtype of AML

- whether the patient received chemotherapy in the past to treat a different cancer

- whether there is a history of a blood disorder such as myelodysplastic syndrome

- whether the cancer has spread to the central nervous system

- whether the cancer has been treated before or recurred (come back)

It is important that acute leukemia be treated right away.

Section 18.4

Childhood Acute Myeloid Leukemia

This section includes text excerpted from "Childhood Acute Myeloid Leukemia/Other Myeloid Malignancies Treatment (PDQ®)—Patient Version," National Cancer Institute (NCI), February 5, 2016.

Childhood acute myeloid leukemia (AML) is a cancer of the blood and bone marrow. AML is also called acute myelogenous leukemia, acute myeloblastic leukemia, acute granulocytic leukemia, and acute nonlymphocytic leukemia. Cancers that are acute usually get worse quickly if they are not treated. Cancers that are chronic usually get worse slowly.

Leukemia and Other Diseases of the Blood and Bone Marrow May Affect Red Blood Cells, White Blood Cells, and Platelets

In AML, the myeloid stem cells usually become a type of immature white blood cell called myeloblasts (or myeloid blasts). The myeloblasts, or leukemia cells, in AML are abnormal and do not become healthy white blood cells. The leukemia cells can build up in the blood and bone marrow so there is less room for healthy white blood cells, red blood cells, and platelets. When this happens, infection, anemia, or easy bleeding may occur. The leukemia cells can spread outside the blood to other parts of the body, including the central nervous system (brain and spinal cord), skin, and gums. Sometimes leukemia cells form a solid tumor called a granulocytic sarcoma or chloroma.

There are subtypes of AML based on the type of blood cell that is affected. The treatment of AML is different when it is a subtype called acute promyelocytic leukemia (APL) or when the child has Down syndrome.

Other Myeloid Diseases Can Affect the Blood and Bone Marrow

Chronic Myelogenous Leukemia

In chronic myelogenous leukemia (CML), too many bone marrow stem cells become a type of white blood cell called granulocytes. Some of these bone marrow stem cells never become mature white blood cells. These are called blasts. Over time, the granulocytes and blasts crowd out the red blood cells and platelets in the bone marrow. CML is rare in children.

Juvenile Myelomonocytic Leukemia

Juvenile myelomonocytic leukemia (JMML) is a rare childhood cancer that occurs more often in children around the age of 2 years and is more common in boys. In JMML, too many bone marrow stem cells become 2 types of white blood cells called myelocytes and monocytes. Some of these bone marrow stem cells never become mature white blood cells. These immature cells, called blasts, are unable to do their usual work. Over time, the myelocytes, monocytes, and blasts crowd out the red blood cells and platelets in the bone marrow. When this happens, infection, anemia, or easy bleeding may occur.

Myelodysplastic Syndromes

Myelodysplastic syndromes (MDS) occur less often in children than in adults. In MDS, the bone marrow makes too few red blood cells, white blood cells, and platelets. These blood cells may not mature and enter the blood. The treatment for MDS depends on how low the numbers of red blood cells, white blood cells, or platelets are. Over time, MDS may become AML.

Transient myeloproliferative disorder (TMD) is a type of MDS. This disorder of the bone marrow can develop in newborns who have Down syndrome. It usually goes away on its own within the first 3 weeks of life. Infants who have Down syndrome and TMD have an increased chance of developing AML before the age of 3 years.

AML or MDS May Occur after Treatment with Certain Anticancer Drugs and/or Radiation Therapy

Cancer treatment with certain anticancer drugs and/or radiation therapy may cause therapy-related AML (t-AML) or therapy-related MDS (t-MDS). The risk of these therapy-related myeloid diseases depends on the total dose of the anticancer drugs used and the radiation dose and treatment field. Some patients also have an inherited risk for t-AML and t-MDS. These therapy-related diseases usually occur within 7 years after treatment, but are rare in children.

The Risk Factors for Childhood AML, Childhood CML, JMML, and MDS Are Similar

Anything that increases your risk of getting a disease is called a risk factor. Having a risk factor does not mean that you will get cancer; not having risk factors doesn't mean that you will not get cancer. Talk with your child's doctor if you think your child may be at risk. These and other factors may increase the risk of childhood AML, childhood CML, JMML, and MDS:

- having a brother or sister, especially a twin, with leukemia
- being Hispanic
- being exposed to cigarette smoke or alcohol before birth
- having a personal history of aplastic anemia
- having a personal or family history of MDS
- having a family history of AML
- past treatment with chemotherapy or radiation therapy
- being exposed to ionizing radiation or chemicals such as benzene
- having certain genetic disorders, such as:
    - Down syndrome
    - Fanconi anemia
    - neurofibromatosis type 1
    - Noonan syndrome
    - Shwachman-Diamond syndrome

Signs and Symptoms of Childhood AML, Childhood CML, JMML, or MDS Include Fever, Feeling Tired, and Easy Bleeding or Bruising

These and other signs and symptoms may be caused by childhood AML, childhood CML, JMML, or MDS or by other conditions. Check with a doctor if your child has any of the following:

- fever with or without an infection
- night sweats
- shortness of breath
- weakness or feeling tired
- easy bruising or bleeding
- petechiae (flat, pinpoint spots under the skin caused by bleeding)
- pain in the bones or joints
- pain or feeling of fullness below the ribs
- painless lumps in the neck, underarm, stomach, groin, or other parts of the body. In childhood AML, these lumps, called leukemia cutis, may be blue or purple
- painless lumps that are sometimes around the eyes. These lumps, called chloromas, are sometimes seen in childhood AML and may be blue-green
- an eczema-like skin rash

The signs and symptoms of TMD may include the following:

- swelling all over the body
- shortness of breath
- trouble breathing
- weakness or feeling tired
- pain below the ribs

Tests That Examine the Blood and Bone Marrow Are Used to Detect (Find) and Diagnose Childhood AML, Childhood CML, JMML, and MDS

The following tests and procedures may be used:

- physical exam and history

- complete blood count (CBC) with differential
- peripheral blood smear
- blood chemistry studies
- chest X-ray
- biopsy:
  - bone marrow aspiration and biopsy
  - tumor biopsy
  - lymph node biopsy
- cytogenetic analysis
- reverse transcription–polymerase chain reaction (RT–PCR) test
- immunophenotyping
- molecular testing
- lumbar puncture

Certain Factors Affect Prognosis (Chance of Recovery) and Treatment Options

The prognosis (chance of recovery) and treatment options for childhood AML depend on the following:

- The age of the child when the cancer is diagnosed.
- The race or ethnic group of the child.
- Whether the child is greatly overweight.
- Number of white blood cells in the blood at diagnosis.
- Whether the AML occurred after previous cancer treatment.
- The subtype of AML.
- Whether there are certain chromosome or gene changes in the leukemia cells.
- Whether the child has Down syndrome. Most children with AML and Down syndrome can be cured of their leukemia.
- Whether the leukemia is in the central nervous system (brain and spinal cord).
- How quickly the leukemia responds to treatment.

- Whether the AML is newly diagnosed (untreated) or has recurred (come back) after being treated.

- The length of time since treatment ended, for AML that has recurred.

The prognosis and treatment options for childhood CML depend on how long it has been since the patient was diagnosed and how many blast cells are in the blood.

The prognosis (chance of recovery) and treatment options for JMML depend on the following:

- The age of the child when the cancer is diagnosed.

- The type of gene affected and the number of genes that have changes.

- How many red blood cells, white blood cells, or platelets are in the blood.

- Whether the JMML is newly diagnosed (untreated) or has recurred after treatment.

The prognosis (chance of recovery) and treatment options for MDS depend on the following:

- Whether the MDS was caused by previous cancer treatment.

- How low the numbers of red blood cells, white blood cells, or platelets are.

- Whether the MDS is newly diagnosed (untreated) or has recurred after treatment.

Section 18.5

Chronic Lymphocytic Leukemia

This section includes text excerpted from "Chronic Lymphocytic Leukemia Treatment (PDQ®)—Patient Version," National Cancer Institute (NCI), October 23, 2015.

Chronic lymphocytic leukemia (also called CLL) is a blood and bone marrow disease that usually gets worse slowly. CLL is one of the most common types of leukemia in adults. It often occurs during or after middle age; it rarely occurs in children.

Leukemia May Affect Red Blood Cells, White Blood Cells, and Platelets

In CLL, too many blood stem cells become abnormal lymphocytes and do not become healthy white blood cells. The abnormal lymphocytes may also be called leukemia cells. The lymphocytes are not able to fight infection very well. Also, as the number of lymphocytes increases in the blood and bone marrow, there is less room for healthy white blood cells, red blood cells, and platelets. This may cause infection, anemia, and easy bleeding.

Older Age Can Affect the Risk of Developing Chronic Lymphocytic Leukemia

Anything that increases your risk of getting a disease is called a risk factor. Having a risk factor does not mean that you will get cancer; not having risk factors doesn't mean that you will not get cancer. Talk with your doctor if you think you may be at risk. Risk factors for CLL include the following:

- Being middle-aged or older, male, or white.

- A family history of CLL or cancer of the lymph system.

- Having relatives who are Russian Jews or Eastern European Jews.

Signs and Symptoms of Chronic Lymphocytic Leukemia Include Swollen Lymph Nodes and Tiredness

Usually CLL does not cause any signs or symptoms and is found during a routine blood test. Signs and symptoms may be caused by CLL or by other conditions. Check with your doctor if you have any of the following:

- painless swelling of the lymph nodes in the neck, underarm, stomach, or groin
- feeling very tired
- pain or fullness below the ribs
- fever and infection
- weight loss for no known reason

Tests That Examine the Blood, Bone Marrow, and Lymph Nodes Are Used to Detect (Find) and Diagnose Chronic Lymphocytic Leukemia

The following tests and procedures may be used:

- physical exam and history
- complete blood count (CBC) with differential
- immunophenotyping
- FISH (fluorescence in situ hybridization)
- flow cytometry
- *IgVH* gene mutation test
- bone marrow aspiration and biopsy

Certain Factors Affect Treatment Options and Prognosis (Chance of Recovery)

Treatment options depend on:

- the stage of the disease
- red blood cell, white blood cell, and platelet blood counts
- whether there are signs or symptoms, such as fever, chills, or weight loss

- whether the liver, spleen, or lymph nodes are larger than normal

- the response to initial treatment

- whether the CLL has recurred (come back)

The prognosis (chance of recovery) depends on:

- whether there is a change in the DNA and the type of change, if there is one

- whether lymphocytes are spread throughout the bone marrow

- the stage of the disease

- whether the CLL gets better with treatment or has recurred (come back)

- whether the CLL progresses to lymphoma or prolymphocytic leukemia

- the patient's general health

Section 18.6

Chronic Myelogenous Leukemia

This section includes text excerpted from "Chronic Myelogenous Leukemia Treatment (PDQ®)—Patient Version," National Cancer Institute (NCI), September 21, 2015.

Chronic myelogenous leukemia (also called CML or chronic granulocytic leukemia) is a slowly progressing blood and bone marrow disease that usually occurs during or after middle age, and rarely occurs in children.

Leukemia May Affect Red Blood Cells, White Blood Cells, and Platelets

In CML, too many blood stem cells become a type of white blood cell called granulocytes. These granulocytes are abnormal and do not become healthy white blood cells. They are also called leukemia cells. The leukemia cells can build up in the blood and bone marrow so there is less room for healthy white blood cells, red blood cells, and platelets. When this happens, infection, anemia, or easy bleeding may occur.

Signs and Symptoms of Chronic Myelogenous Leukemia Include Fever, Night Sweats, and Tiredness

These and other signs and symptoms may be caused by CML or by other conditions. Check with your doctor if you have any of the following:

- feeling very tired
- weight loss for no known reason
- night sweats
- fever
- pain or a feeling of fullness below the ribs on the left side

Sometimes CML does not cause any symptoms at all.

Most People with CML Have a Gene Mutation (Change) Called the Philadelphia Chromosome

Every cell in the body contains DNA (genetic material) that determines how the cell looks and acts. DNA is contained inside chromosomes. In CML, part of the DNA from one chromosome moves to another chromosome. This change is called the " Philadelphia chromosome." It results in the bone marrow making an enzyme, called tyrosine kinase, that causes too many stem cells to become white blood cells (granulocytes or blasts).

The Philadelphia chromosome is not passed from parent to child.

Tests That Examine the Blood and Bone Marrow Are Used to Detect (Find) and Diagnose Chronic Myelogenous Leukemia

The following tests and procedures may be used:

- physical exam and history
- complete blood count (CBC) with differential

- blood chemistry studies

- bone marrow aspiration and biopsy

Certain Factors Affect Prognosis (Chance of Recovery) and Treatment Options

The prognosis (chance of recovery) and treatment options depend on the following:

- the patient's age

- the phase of CML

- the amount of blasts in the blood or bone marrow

- the size of the spleen at diagnosis

- the patient's general health

Section 18.7

Hairy Cell Leukemia

This section includes text excerpted from "Hairy Cell Leukemia Treatment (PDQ®)—Patient Version," National Cancer Institute (NCI), April 6, 2016.

Hairy cell leukemia is a cancer of the blood and bone marrow. This rare type of leukemia gets worse slowly or does not get worse at all. The disease is called hairy cell leukemia because the leukemia cells look "hairy" when viewed under a microscope.

Leukemia May Affect Red Blood Cells, White Blood Cells, and Platelets

In hairy cell leukemia, too many blood stem cells become lymphocytes. These lymphocytes are abnormal and do not become healthy white blood cells. They are also called leukemia cells. The leukemia cells can build up in the blood and bone marrow so there is less room for healthy white blood cells, red blood cells, and platelets. This may cause infection, anemia, and easy bleeding. Some of the leukemia cells may collect in the spleen and cause it to swell.

Gender and Age May Affect the Risk of Hairy Cell Leukemia

The cause of hairy cell leukemia is unknown. It occurs more often in older men.

Signs and Symptoms of Hairy Cell Leukemia Include Infections, Tiredness, and Pain below the Ribs

These and other signs and symptoms may be caused by hairy cell leukemia or by other conditions. Check with your doctor if you have any of the following:

- weakness or feeling tired
- fever or frequent infections
- easy bruising or bleeding
- shortness of breath
- weight loss for no known reason
- pain or a feeling of fullness below the ribs
- painless lumps in the neck, underarm, stomach, or groin

Tests That Examine the Blood and Bone Marrow Are Used to Detect (Find) and Diagnose Hairy Cell Leukemia

The following tests and procedures may be used:

- physical exam and history
- complete blood count (CBC)
- peripheral blood smear
- blood chemistry studies
- bone marrow aspiration and biopsy
- immunophenotyping
- flow cytometry

- cytogenetic analysis
- CT scan (CAT scan)

Certain Factors Affect Treatment Options and Prognosis (Chance of Recovery)

The treatment options may depend on the following:

- The number of hairy (leukemia) cells and healthy blood cells in the blood and bone marrow.
- Whether the spleen is swollen.
- Whether there are signs or symptoms of leukemia, such as infection.
- Whether the leukemia has recurred (come back) after previous treatment.

The prognosis (chance of recovery) depends on the following:

- Whether the hairy cell leukemia does not grow or grows so slowly it does not need treatment.
- Whether the hairy cell leukemia responds to treatment.

Treatment often results in a long-lasting remission (a period during which some or all of the signs and symptoms of the leukemia are gone). If the leukemia returns after it has been in remission, retreatment often causes another remission.

Chapter 19

Lymphoma

Chapter Contents

Section 19.1

AIDS-Related Lymphoma

This section includes text excerpted from "AIDS-Related Lymphoma
Treatment (PDQ®)—Patient Version," National Cancer Institute
(NCI), September 17, 2015.

AIDS is caused by the human immunodeficiency virus (HIV), which
attacks and weakens the body's immune system. The immune system
is then unable to fight infection and disease. People with HIV disease
have an increased risk of infection and lymphoma or other types of
cancer. A person with HIV disease who develops certain types of infections or cancer is then diagnosed with AIDS. Sometimes, people are
diagnosed with AIDS and AIDS-related lymphoma at the same time.

AIDS-related lymphoma is a type of cancer that affects the lymph
system, which is part of the body's immune system. The immune system protects the body from foreign substances, infection, and diseases.
The lymph system is made up of the following:

- **Lymph:** Colorless, watery fluid that carries white blood cells
  called lymphocytes through the lymph system. Lymphocytes
  protect the body against infections and the growth of tumors.

- **Lymph vessels:** A network of thin tubes that collect lymph
  from different parts of the body and return it to the bloodstream.

- **Lymph nodes:** Small, bean-shaped structures that filter lymph
  and store white blood cells that help fight infection and disease.
  Lymph nodes are located along the network of lymph vessels
  found throughout the body. Clusters of lymph nodes are found in
  the neck, underarm, abdomen, pelvis, and groin.

- **Spleen:** An organ that makes lymphocytes, filters the blood,
  stores blood cells, and destroys old blood cells. The spleen is on
  the left side of the abdomen near the stomach.

- **Thymus:** An organ in which lymphocytes grow and multiply.
  The thymus is in the chest behind the breastbone.

- **Tonsils:** Two small masses of lymph tissue at the back of the
  throat. The tonsils make lymphocytes.

- **Bone marrow:** The soft, spongy tissue in the center of large bones. Bone marrow makes white blood cells, red blood cells, and platelets.

Lymph tissue is also found in other parts of the body such as the brain, stomach, thyroid gland, and skin.

Sometimes AIDS-related lymphoma occurs outside the lymph nodes in the bone marrow, liver, meninges (thin membranes that cover the brain) and gastrointestinal tract. Less often, it may occur in the anus, heart, bile duct, gingiva, and muscles.

There Are Many Different Types of Lymphoma

Lymphomas are divided into two general types:

1. Hodgkin lymphoma

2. Non-Hodgkin lymphoma

Both Hodgkin lymphoma and non-Hodgkin lymphoma may occur in patients with AIDS, but non-Hodgkin lymphoma is more common. When a person with AIDS has non-Hodgkin lymphoma, it is called AIDS-related lymphoma. When AIDS-related lymphoma occurs in the central nervous system (CNS), it is called AIDS-related primary CNS lymphoma.

Non-Hodgkin lymphomas are grouped by the way their cells look under a microscope. They may be indolent (slow-growing) or aggressive (fast-growing). AIDS-related lymphomas are aggressive. There are two main types of AIDS-related non-Hodgkin lymphoma:

1. Diffuse large B-cell lymphoma (including B-cell immunoblastic lymphoma)

2. Burkitt or Burkitt-like lymphoma

Signs of AIDS-Related Lymphoma Include Weight Loss, Fever, and Night Sweats

These and other signs and symptoms may be caused by AIDS-related lymphoma or by other conditions. Check with your doctor if you have any of the following:

- weight loss or fever for no known reason

- night sweats

- painless, swollen lymph nodes in the neck, chest, underarm, or groin

- a feeling of fullness below the ribs

Tests That Examine the Lymph System and Other Parts of the Body Are Used to Help Detect (Find) and Diagnose AIDS-Related Lymphoma

The following tests and procedures may be used:

- **Physical exam and history:** An exam of the body to check general signs of health, including checking for signs of disease, such as lumps or anything else that seems unusual. A history of the patient's health habits and past illnesses and treatments will also be taken.

- Complete blood count (CBC): A procedure in which a sample of blood is drawn and checked for the following:

  - The number of red blood cells, white blood cells, and platelets.

  - The amount of hemoglobin (the protein that carries oxygen) in the red blood cells.

  - The portion of the sample made up of red blood cells.

- **HIV test**: A test to measure the level of HIV antibodies in a sample of blood. Antibodies are made by the body when it is invaded by a foreign substance. A high level of HIV antibodies may mean the body has been infected with HIV.

- **Lymph node biopsy:** The removal of all or part of a lymph node. A pathologist views the tissue under a microscope to look for cancer cells. One of the following types of biopsies may be done:

  - **Excisional biopsy:** The removal of an entire lymph node.

  - **Incisional biopsy:** The removal of part of a lymph node.

  - **Core biopsy**: The removal of tissue from a lymph node using a wide needle.

- **Fine-needle aspiration (FNA) biopsy:** The removal of tissue from a lymph node using a thin needle.

- **Bone marrow aspiration and biopsy:** The removal of bone marrow and a small piece of bone by inserting a hollow needle into the hipbone or breastbone. A pathologist views the bone marrow and bone under a microscope to look for signs of cancer.

- **Chest X-ray:** An X-ray of the organs and bones inside the chest. An X-ray is a type of energy beam that can go through the body and onto film, making a picture of areas inside the body.

Certain Factors Affect Prognosis (Chance of Recovery) and Treatment Options

The prognosis (chance of recovery) and treatment options depend on the following:

- The stage of the cancer.

- The age of the patient.

- The number of CD4 lymphocytes (a type of white blood cell) in the blood.

- The number of places in the body lymphoma is found outside the lymph system.

- Whether the patient has a history of intravenous (IV) drug use.

- The patient's ability to carry out regular daily activities.

Section 19.2

Adult Hodgkin Lymphoma

This section includes text excerpted from "Adult Hodgkin Lymphoma Treatment (PDQ®)—Patient Version," National Cancer Institute (NCI), October 27, 2015.

Adult Hodgkin lymphoma is a type of cancer that develops in the lymph system, part of the body's immune system. The immune system protects the body from foreign substances, infection, and diseases.

Lymphomas are divided into two general types: Hodgkin lymphoma and non-Hodgkin lymphoma. This section is about the treatment of adult Hodgkin lymphoma.

Hodgkin lymphoma can occur in both adults and children. Treatment for adults is different than treatment for children. Hodgkin lymphoma may also occur in patients who have acquired immunodeficiency syndrome (AIDS); these patients require special treatment.

Hodgkin lymphoma in pregnant women is the same as the disease in nonpregnant women of childbearing age. However, treatment is different for pregnant women. This section includes information about treating Hodgkin lymphoma during pregnancy.

There Are Two Main Types of Hodgkin Lymphoma: Classical and Nodular Lymphocyte-Predominant

Most Hodgkin lymphomas are the classical type. The classical type is broken down into the following four subtypes:

1. nodular sclerosing Hodgkin lymphoma

2. mixed cellularity Hodgkin lymphoma

3. lymphocyte depletion Hodgkin lymphoma

4. lymphocyte-rich classical Hodgkin lymphoma

Age, Gender, and Epstein-Barr Infection Can Affect the Risk of Adult Hodgkin Lymphoma

Risk factors for adult Hodgkin lymphoma include the following:

- being in young or late adulthood

- being male

- being infected with the Epstein-Barr virus

- having a first-degree relative (parent, brother, or sister) with Hodgkin lymphoma

Pregnancy is not a risk factor for Hodgkin lymphoma.

Signs of Adult Hodgkin Lymphoma Include Swollen Lymph Nodes, Fever, Night Sweats, and Weight Loss

These and other signs and symptoms may be caused by adult Hodgkin lymphoma or by other conditions. Check with your doctor if any of the following do not go away:

- painless, swollen lymph nodes in the neck, underarm, or groin
- fever for no known reason
- drenching night sweats
- weight loss for no known reason
- itchy skin
- feeling very tired

Tests That Examine the Lymph Nodes Are Used to Detect (Find) and Diagnose Adult Hodgkin Lymphoma

The following tests and procedures may be used:

- Physical exam and history
- Complete blood count (CBC)
- Blood chemistry studies
- Sedimentation rate
- Lymph node biopsy
  - Excisional biopsy
  - Incisional biopsy
  - Core biopsy

Certain Factors Affect Prognosis (Chance of Recovery) and Treatment Options

The prognosis (chance of recovery) and treatment options depend on the following:

- the patient's signs and symptoms
- the stage of the cancer
- the type of Hodgkin lymphoma
- blood test results
- the patient's age, gender, and general health
- whether the cancer is recurrent or progressive

For Hodgkin lymphoma during pregnancy, treatment options also depend on:

- the wishes of the patient

- the age of the fetus

Adult Hodgkin lymphoma can usually be cured if found and treated early.

Section 19.3

Adult Non-Hodgkin Lymphoma

This section includes text excerpted from "Adult Non-Hodgkin Lymphoma Treatment (PDQ®)—Patient Version," National Cancer Institute (NCI), March 3, 2016.

Non-Hodgkin lymphoma is a type of cancer that forms in the lymph system, which is part of the body's immune system. The immune system protects the body from foreign substances, infection, and diseases. The lymph system is made up of the following:

- **Lymph:** Colorless, watery fluid that carries white blood cells called lymphocytes through the lymph system. Lymphocytes protect the body against infection and the growth of tumors. There are three types of lymphocytes:

- B lymphocytes that make antibodies to help fight infection. Also called B cells. Most types of non-Hodgkin lymphoma begin in B lymphocytes.

  - T lymphocytes that help B lymphocytes make the antibodies that help fight infection. Also called T cells.

  - Natural killer cells that attack cancer cells and viruses. Also called NK cells.

Non-Hodgkin lymphoma can begin in B lymphocytes, T lymphocytes, or natural killer cells. Lymphocytes can also be found in the blood and also collect in the lymph nodes, spleen, and thymus.

Non-Hodgkin lymphoma during pregnancy is rare. Non-Hodgkin lymphoma in pregnant women is the same as the disease in nonpregnant women of childbearing age. However, treatment is different for pregnant women.

Non-Hodgkin lymphoma can occur in both adults and children. Treatment for adults is different than treatment for children.

Non-Hodgkin Lymphoma Can Be Indolent or Aggressive

Non-Hodgkin lymphoma grows and spreads at different rates and can be indolent or aggressive. Indolent lymphoma tends to grow and spread slowly, and has few signs and symptoms. Aggressive lymphoma grows and spreads quickly, and has signs and symptoms that can be severe. The treatments for indolent and aggressive lymphoma are different.

This section is about the following types of non-Hodgkin lymphoma:

Indolent Non-Hodgkin Lymphomas

Follicular lymphoma. Follicular lymphoma is the most common type of indolent non-Hodgkin lymphoma. It is a very slow-growing type of non-Hodgkin lymphoma that begins in B lymphocytes. It affects the lymph nodes and may spread to the bone marrow or spleen. Most patients with follicular lymphoma are age 50 years and older when they are diagnosed. Follicular lymphoma may go away without treatment. The patient is closely watched for signs or symptoms that the disease has come back. Treatment is needed if signs or symptoms occur after the cancer disappeared or after initial cancer treatment. Sometimes follicular lymphoma can become a more aggressive type of lymphoma, such as diffuse large B-cell lymphoma.

Lymphoplasmacytic lymphoma. In most cases of lymphoplasmacytic lymphoma, B lymphocytes that are turning into plasma cells make large amounts of a protein called monoclonal immunoglobulin M (IgM) antibody. High levels of IgM antibody in the blood cause the blood plasma to thicken. This may cause signs or symptoms such as trouble seeing or hearing, heart problems, shortness of breath, headache, dizziness, and numbness or tingling of the hands and feet. Sometimes there are no signs or symptoms of lymphoplasmacytic lymphoma. It may be found when a blood test is done for another reason. Lymphoplasmacytic lymphoma often spreads to the bone marrow, lymph nodes, and spleen. It is also called Waldenström's macroglobulinemia.

Marginal zone lymphoma. This type of non-Hodgkin lymphoma begins in B lymphocytes in a part of lymph tissue called the marginal zone. There are five different types of marginal zone lymphoma. They are grouped by the type of tissue where the lymphoma formed:

1. **Monocytoid B cell lymphoma.** Monocytoid B-cell lymphoma forms in lymph nodes. This type of non-Hodgkin lymphoma is rare. It is also called nodal marginal zone lymphoma.

2. **Gastric mucosa-associated lymphoid tissue (MALT) lymphoma.** Gastric MALT lymphoma usually begins in the stomach. This type of marginal zone lymphoma forms in cells in the mucosa that help make antibodies. Patients with gastric MALT lymphoma may also have *Helicobacter* gastritis or an autoimmune disease, such as Hashimoto thyroiditis or Sjögren syndrome.

3. **Extragastric MALT lymphoma.** Extragastric MALT lymphoma begins outside of the stomach in almost every part of the body including other parts of the gastrointestinal tract, salivary glands, thyroid, lung, skin, and around the eye. This type of marginal zone lymphoma forms in cells in the mucosa that help make antibodies. Extragastric MALT lymphoma may come back many years after treatment.

4. **Mediterranean abdominal lymphoma.** This is a type of MALT lymphoma that occurs in young adults in eastern Mediterranean countries. It often forms in the abdomen and patients may also be infected with bacteria called *Campylobacter jejuni*. This type of lymphoma is also called immunoproliferative small intestinal disease.

5. **Splenic marginal zone lymphoma.** This type of marginal zone lymphoma begins in the spleen and may spread to the peripheral blood and bone marrow. The most common sign of this type of splenic marginal zone lymphoma is a spleen that is larger than normal.

Primary cutaneous anaplastic large cell lymphoma. This type of non-Hodgkin lymphoma is in the skin only. It can be a benign (not cancer) nodule that may go away on its own or it can spread to many places on the skin and need treatment.

Aggressive Non-Hodgkin Lymphomas

Diffuse large B-cell lymphoma. Diffuse large B-cell lymphoma is the most common type of non-Hodgkin lymphoma. It grows quickly in the lymph nodes and often the spleen, liver, bone marrow, or other organs are also affected. Signs and symptoms of diffuse large B-cell lymphoma may include fever, recurring night sweats, and weight loss. These are also called B symptoms.

Primary mediastinal large B-cell lymphoma is a type of diffuse large B-cell lymphoma.

- Primary mediastinal large B-cell lymphoma. This type of non-Hodgkin lymphoma is marked by the overgrowth of fibrous (scar-like) lymph tissue. A tumor most often forms behind the breastbone. It may press on the airways and cause coughing and trouble breathing. Most patients with primary mediastinal large B-cell lymphoma are women who are age 30 to 40 years.

Follicular large cell lymphoma, stage III. Follicular large cell lymphoma, stage III, is a very rare type of non-Hodgkin lymphoma. It is more like diffuse large B-cell lymphoma than other types of follicular lymphoma.

Anaplastic large cell lymphoma. Anaplastic large cell lymphoma is a type of non-Hodgkin lymphoma that usually begins in T lymphocytes. The cancer cells also have a marker called CD30 on the surface of the cell.

There are two types of anaplastic large cell lymphoma:

1. **Cutaneous anaplastic large cell lymphoma.** This type of anaplastic large cell lymphoma mostly affects the skin, but other parts of the body may also be affected. Signs of cutaneous anaplastic large cell lymphoma include one or more bumps or ulcers on the skin.

2. **Systemic anaplastic large cell lymphoma.** This type of anaplastic large cell lymphoma begins in the lymph nodes and may affect other parts of the body. Patients may have a lot of anaplastic lymphoma kinase (ALK) protein inside the lymphoma cells. These patients have a better prognosis than patients who do not have extra ALK protein. Systemic anaplastic large cell lymphoma is more common in children than adults.

Extranodal NK-/T-cell lymphoma. Extranodal NK-/T-cell lymphoma usually begins in the area around the nose. It may also affect the paranasal sinus (hollow spaces in the bones around the nose), roof of the mouth, trachea, skin, stomach, and intestines. Most cases of extranodal NK-/T-cell lymphoma have Epstein-Barr virus in the tumor cells. Sometimes hemophagocytic syndrome occurs (a serious condition in which there are too many active histiocytes and T cells that cause severe inflammation in the body). Treatment to suppress the immune system is needed. This type of non-Hodgkin lymphoma is not common in the United States.

Lymphomatoid granulomatosis. Lymphomatoid granulomatosis mostly affects the lungs. It may also affect the paranasal sinuses (hollow spaces in the bones around the nose), skin, kidneys, and central nervous system. In lymphomatoid granulomatosis, cancer invades the blood vessels and kills tissue. Because the cancer may spread to the brain, intrathecal chemotherapy or radiation therapy to the brain is given.

Angioimmunoblastic T-cell lymphoma. This type of non-Hodgkin lymphoma begins in T cells. Swollen lymph nodes are a common sign. Other signs may include a skin rash, fever, weight loss, or night sweats. There may also be high levels of gamma globulin (antibodies) in the blood. Patients may also have opportunistic infections because their immune systems are weakened.

Peripheral T-cell lymphoma. Peripheral T-cell lymphoma begins in mature T lymphocytes. This type of T lymphocyte matures in the thymus gland and travels to other lymphatic sites in the body such as the lymph nodes, bone marrow, and spleen. There are three subtypes of peripheral T-cell lymphoma:

- Hepatosplenic T-cell lymphoma. This is an uncommon type of peripheral T-cell lymphoma that occurs mostly in young men. It begins in the liver and spleen and the cancer cells also have a T-cell receptor called gamma/delta on the surface of the cell.

- Subcutaneous panniculitis-like T-cell lymphoma. Subcutaneous panniculitis-like T-cell lymphoma begins in the skin or mucosa. It may occur with hemophagocytic syndrome (a serious condition in which there are too many active histiocytes and T cells that cause severe inflammation in the body). Treatment to suppress the immune system is needed.

- Enteropathy-type intestinal T-cell lymphoma. This type of peripheral T-cell lymphoma occurs in the small bowel of patients with untreated celiac disease (an immune response to gluten that causes malnutrition). Patients who are diagnosed with celiac disease in childhood and stay on a gluten-free diet rarely develop enteropathy-type intestinal T-cell lymphoma.

Intravascular large B-cell lymphoma. This type of non-Hodgkin lymphoma affects blood vessels, especially the small blood vessels in the brain, kidney, lung, and skin. Signs and symptoms of intravascular large B-cell lymphoma are caused by blocked blood vessels. It is also called intravascular lymphomatosis.

Burkitt lymphoma. Burkitt lymphoma is a type of B-cell non-Hodgkin lymphoma that grows and spreads very quickly. It may affect the jaw, bones of the face, bowel, kidneys, ovaries, or other organs. There are three main types of Burkitt lymphoma (endemic, sporadic, and immunodeficiency related). Endemic Burkitt lymphoma commonly occurs in Africa and is linked to the Epstein-Barr virus, and sporadic Burkitt lymphoma occurs throughout the world. Immunodeficiency-related Burkitt lymphoma is most often seen in patients who have AIDS. Burkitt lymphoma may spread to the brain and spinal cord and treatment to prevent its spread may be given. Burkitt lymphoma occurs most often in children and young adults. Burkitt lymphoma is also called diffuse small noncleaved-cell lymphoma.

Lymphoblastic lymphoma. Lymphoblastic lymphoma may begin in T cells or B cells, but it usually begins in T cells. In this type of non-Hodgkin lymphoma, there are too many lymphoblasts (immature white blood cells) in the lymph nodes and the thymus gland. These lymphoblasts may spread to other places in the body, such as the bone marrow, brain, and spinal cord. Lymphoblastic lymphoma is most common in teenagers and young adults. It is a lot like acute lymphoblastic leukemia (lymphoblasts are mostly found in the bone marrow and blood).

Adult T-cell leukemia/lymphoma. Adult T-cell leukemia/lymphoma is caused by the human T-cell leukemia virus type 1 (HTLV-1). Signs include bone and skin lesions, high blood calcium levels, and lymph nodes, spleen, and liver that are larger than normal.

Mantle cell lymphoma. Mantle cell lymphoma is a type of B-cell non-Hodgkin lymphoma that usually occurs in middle-aged or older adults. It begins in the lymph nodes and spreads to the spleen, bone marrow, blood, and sometimes the esophagus, stomach, and intestines. Patients with mantle cell lymphoma have too much of a protein called cyclin-D1 or a certain gene change in the lymphoma cells. In some patients who do not have signs or symptoms of lymphoma delaying the start of treatment does not affect the prognosis.

Posttransplantation lymphoproliferative disorder. This disease occurs in patients who have had a heart, lung, liver, kidney, or pancreas transplant and need lifelong immunosuppressive therapy. Most posttransplant lymphoproliferative disorders affect the B cells and have Epstein-Barr virus in the cells. Lymphoproliferative disorders are often treated like cancer.

True histiocytic lymphoma. This is a rare, very aggressive type of lymphoma. It is not known whether it begins in B cells or T cells. It does not respond well to treatment with standard chemotherapy.

Primary effusion lymphoma. Primary effusion lymphoma begins in B cells that are found in an area where there is a large build-up of fluid, such as the areas between the lining of the lung and chest wall (pleural effusion), the sac around the heart and the heart (pericardial effusion), or in the abdominal cavity. There is usually no tumor that can be seen. This type of lymphoma often occurs in patients who have AIDS.

Plasmablastic lymphoma. Plasmablastic lymphoma is a type of large B-cell non-Hodgkin lymphoma that is very aggressive. It is most often seen in patients with HIV infection.

Age, Gender, and a Weakened Immune System Can Affect the Risk of Adult Non-Hodgkin Lymphoma

These and other risk factors may increase the risk of certain types of adult non-Hodgkin lymphoma:

- Being older, male, or white.

- Having one of the following medical conditions:

    - An inherited immune disorder (such as hypogammaglobulin-emia or Wiskott-Aldrich syndrome).

    - An autoimmune disease (such as rheumatoid arthritis, psoriasis, or Sjögren syndrome).

    - HIV/AIDS.

    - Human T-lymphotrophic virus type I or Epstein-Barr virus infection.

    - Helicobacter pylori infection.

- Taking immunosuppressant drugs after an organ transplant.

Signs and Symptoms of Adult Non-Hodgkin Lymphoma Include Swelling in the Lymph Nodes, Fever, Night Sweats, Weight Loss, and Fatigue

These signs and symptoms may be caused by adult non-Hodgkin lymphoma or by other conditions. Check with your doctor if you have any of the following:

- swelling in the lymph nodes in the neck, underarm, groin, or stomach

- fever for no known reason

- recurring night sweats

- feeling very tired

- weight loss for no known reason

- skin rash or itchy skin

- pain in the chest, abdomen, or bones for no known reason

When fever, night sweats, and weight loss occur together, this group of symptoms is called B symptoms.

Other signs and symptoms of adult non-Hodgkin lymphoma may occur and depend on the following:

- where the cancer forms in the body

- the size of the tumor

- how fast the tumor grows

Tests That Examine the Body and Lymph System Are Used to Help Detect (Find) and Diagnose Adult Non-Hodgkin Lymphoma

The following tests and procedures may be used:

- Physical exam and history

- Flow cytometry

- Bone marrow aspiration and biopsy

- Lymph node biopsy

- Excisional biopsy

- Incisional biopsy

- Core biopsy

- Fine-needle aspiration (FNA) biopsy

- Laparoscopy

- Laparotomy

If cancer is found, the following tests may be done to study the cancer cells:

- Immunohistochemistry

- Cytogenetic analysis

- FISH (fluorescence in situ hybridization)

- Immunophenotyping

Other tests and procedures may be done depending on the signs and symptoms seen and where the cancer forms in the body.

Certain Factors Affect Prognosis (Chance of Recovery) and Treatment Options

The prognosis (chance of recovery) and treatment options depend on the following:

- The stage of the cancer.

- The type of non-Hodgkin lymphoma.

- The amount of lactate dehydrogenase (LDH) in the blood.

- Whether there are certain changes in the genes.

- The patient's age and general health.

- Whether the lymphoma has just been diagnosed or has recurred (come back).

For non-Hodgkin lymphoma during pregnancy, the treatment options also depend on:

- The wishes of the patient.

- Which trimester of pregnancy the patient is in.

- Whether the baby can be delivered early.

Some types of non-Hodgkin lymphoma spread more quickly than others do. Most non-Hodgkin lymphomas that occur during pregnancy are aggressive. Delaying treatment of aggressive lymphoma until after the baby is born may lessen the mother's chance of survival. Immediate treatment is often recommended, even during pregnancy.

Section 19.4

Childhood Hodgkin Lymphoma

This section includes text excerpted from "Childhood Hodgkin Lymphoma Treatment (PDQ®)—Patient Version," National Cancer Institute (NCI), December 16, 2015.

Childhood Hodgkin lymphoma is a type of cancer that develops in the lymph system, which is part of the body's immune system. The immune system protects the body from foreign substances, infection, and diseases.

There are two general types of lymphoma: Hodgkin lymphoma and non-Hodgkin lymphoma.

Hodgkin lymphoma often occurs in adolescents 15 to 19 years of age. The treatment for children and adolescents is different than treatment for adults.

There Are Two Types of Childhood Hodgkin Lymphoma

The two types of childhood Hodgkin lymphoma are:

1. Classical Hodgkin lymphoma

2. Nodular lymphocyte-predominant Hodgkin lymphoma

Classical Hodgkin lymphoma is divided into four subtypes, based on how the cancer cells look under a microscope:

1. Lymphocyte-rich classical Hodgkin lymphoma

2. Nodular sclerosis Hodgkin lymphoma

3. Mixed cellularity Hodgkin lymphoma

4. Lymphocyte-depleted Hodgkin lymphoma

Epstein-Barr Virus Infection Increases the Risk of Childhood Hodgkin Lymphoma

Anything that increases your risk of getting a disease is called a risk factor. Having a risk factor does not mean that you will get cancer;

not having risk factors doesn't mean that you will not get cancer. Talk with your child's doctor if you think your child may be at risk.

Risk factors for childhood Hodgkin lymphoma include the following:

- Being infected with the Epstein-Barr virus.
- Being infected with the human immunodeficiency virus (HIV).
- Having certain diseases of the immune system.
- Having a personal history of mononucleosis ("mono").
- Having a parent or sibling with a personal history of Hodgkin lymphoma.

Being exposed to common infections in early childhood may decrease the risk of Hodgkin lymphoma in children because of the effect it has on the immune system.

Signs of Childhood Hodgkin Lymphoma Include Swollen Lymph Nodes, Fever, Night Sweats, and Weight Loss

These and other signs and symptoms may be caused by childhood Hodgkin lymphoma or by other conditions. Check with your child's doctor if your child has any of the following:

- painless, swollen lymph nodes near the collarbone or in the neck, chest, underarm, or groin
- fever for no known reason
- weight loss for no known reason
- night sweats
- fatigue
- anorexia
- itchy skin
- pain in the lymph nodes after drinking alcohol

Fever, weight loss, and night sweats are called B symptoms.

Tests That Examine the Lymph System Are Used to Detect (Find) and Diagnose Childhood Hodgkin Lymphoma

The following tests and procedures may be used:

- Physical exam and history

- CT scan (CAT scan)
- PET scan (positron emission tomography scan)
- Chest X-ray
- Complete blood count (CBC)
- Blood chemistry studies
- Sedimentation rate
- Lymph node biopsy
  - Excisional biopsy
  - Incisional biopsy
  - Core biopsy
  - Fine-needle aspiration (FNA) biopsy

Certain Factors Affect Prognosis (Chance of Recovery) and Treatment Options

The prognosis (chance of recovery) and treatment options depend on the following:

- The stage of the cancer.
- The size of the tumor.
- Whether there are B symptoms at diagnosis.
- The type of Hodgkin lymphoma.
- Certain features of the cancer cells.
- Whether there are too many white blood cells or too few red blood cells at the time of diagnosis.
- How well the tumor responds to initial treatment with chemotherapy.
- Whether the cancer is newly diagnosed or has recurred (come back).

The treatment options also depend on:

- The child's age and gender.
- The risk of long-term side effects.

Most children and adolescents with newly diagnosed Hodgkin lymphoma can be cured.

Section 19.5

Childhood Non-Hodgkin Lymphoma

This section includes text excerpted from "Childhood Non-Hodgkin Lymphoma Treatment (PDQ®)—Patient Version," National Cancer Institute (NCI), April 7, 2016.

Childhood non-Hodgkin lymphoma is a type of cancer that forms in the lymph system, which is part of the body's immune system. The immune system protects the body from foreign substances, infection, and diseases.

Non-Hodgkin lymphoma can begin in B lymphocytes, T lymphocytes, or natural killer cells. Lymphocytes can also be found in the blood and collect in the lymph nodes, spleen, and thymus.

The Main Types of Lymphoma Are Hodgkin Lymphoma and Non-Hodgkin Lymphoma

Lymphomas are divided into two general types: Hodgkin lymphoma and non-Hodgkin lymphoma. This summary is about the treatment of childhood non-Hodgkin lymphoma.

There Are Three Major Types of Childhood Non-Hodgkin Lymphoma

The type of lymphoma is determined by how the cells look under a microscope. The three major types of childhood non-Hodgkin lymphoma are:

Mature B-cell non-Hodgkin lymphoma

Mature B-cell non-Hodgkin lymphomas include:

- **Burkitt and Burkitt-like lymphoma/leukemia:** Burkitt lymphoma and Burkitt leukemia are different forms of the same disease. Burkitt lymphoma/leukemia is an aggressive (fast-growing) disorder of B lymphocytes that is most common in children and young adults. It may form in the abdomen, Waldeyer's

228

ring, testicles, bone, bone marrow, skin, or central nervous system (CNS). Burkitt leukemia may start in the lymph nodes as Burkitt lymphoma and then spread to the blood and bone marrow, or it may start in the blood and bone marrow without forming in the lymph nodes first.

Both Burkitt leukemia and Burkitt lymphoma have been linked to infection with the Epstein-Barr virus (EBV), although EBV infection is more likely to occur in patients in Africa than in the United States. Burkitt and Burkitt-like lymphoma/leukemia are diagnosed when a sample of tissue is checked and a certain change to the *c*-myc gene is found.

- **Diffuse large B-cell lymphoma:** Diffuse large B-cell lymphoma is the most common type of non-Hodgkin lymphoma. It is a type of B-cell non-Hodgkin lymphoma that grows quickly in the lymph nodes. The spleen, liver, bone marrow, or other organs are also often affected. Diffuse large B-cell lymphoma occurs more often in adolescents than in children.

- **Primary mediastinal B-cell lymphoma:** A type of lymphoma that develops from B cells in the mediastinum (the area behind the breastbone). It may spread to nearby organs including the lungs and the sac around the heart. It may also spread to lymph nodes and distant organs including the kidneys. In children and adolescents, primary mediastinal B-cell lymphoma occurs more often in older adolescents.

Lymphoblastic lymphoma

Lymphoblastic lymphoma is a type of lymphoma that mainly affects T-cell lymphocytes. It usually forms in the mediastinum (the area behind the breastbone). This causes trouble breathing, wheezing, trouble swallowing, or swelling of the head and neck. It may spread to lymph nodes, bone, bone marrow, skin, the CNS, abdominal organs, and other areas. Lymphoblastic lymphoma is a lot like acute lymphoblastic leukemia (ALL).

Anaplastic large cell lymphoma

Anaplastic large cell lymphoma is a type of lymphoma that mainly affects T-cell lymphocytes. It usually forms in the lymph nodes, skin, or bone, and sometimes forms in the gastrointestinal tract, lung, tissue that covers the lungs, and muscle. Patients with anaplastic large cell lymphoma have a receptor, called CD30, on the surface of their T cells. In many children, anaplastic large cell lymphoma is marked by changes in the *ALK* gene that makes a protein called anaplastic lymphoma kinase. A pathologist checks for these cell and gene changes to help diagnose anaplastic large cell lymphoma.

Some Types of Non-Hodgkin Lymphoma Are Rare in Children

- **Pediatric follicular lymphoma:** In children, follicular lymphoma occurs mainly in males. It is more likely to be found in one area and does not spread to other places in the body. It usually forms in the tonsils and lymph nodes in the neck, but may also form in the testicles, kidney, gastrointestinal tract, and salivary gland.

- **Marginal zone lymphoma:** Marginal zone lymphoma is a type of lymphoma that tends to grow and spread slowly and is usually found at an early stage. It may be found in the lymph nodes or in areas outside the lymph nodes. Marginal zone lymphoma found outside the lymph nodes in children is called mucosa-associated lymphoid tissue (MALT) lymphoma and may be linked to *Helicobacter pylori* infection of the gastrointestinal tract and *Chlamydophila psittaci* infection of the conjunctival membrane which lines the eye.

- **Primary central nervous system (CNS) lymphoma:** Primary CNS lymphoma is extremely rare in children.

- **Peripheral T-cell lymphoma:** Peripheral T-cell lymphoma is an aggressive (fast-growing) non-Hodgkin lymphoma that begins in mature T lymphocytes. The T lymphocytes mature in the thymus gland and travel to other parts of the lymph system, such as the lymph nodes, bone marrow, and spleen.

- **Cutaneous T-cell lymphoma:** Cutaneous T-cell lymphoma begins in the skin and can cause the skin to thicken or form a tumor. It is very rare in children, but is more common in adolescents and young adults. There are different types of cutaneous T-cell lymphoma, such as cutaneous anaplastic large cell lymphoma, subcutaneous panniculitis-like T-cell lymphoma, gamma-delta T-cell lymphoma, and mycosis fungoides. Mycosis fungoides rarely occurs in children and adolescents.

Past Treatment for Cancer and Having a Weakened Immune System Affect the Risk of Having Childhood Non-Hodgkin Lymphoma

Anything that increases your risk of getting a disease is called a risk factor. Having a risk factor does not mean that you will get cancer; not having risk factors doesn't mean that you will not get cancer. Talk with your child's doctor if you think your child may be at risk.

Possible risk factors for childhood non-Hodgkin lymphoma include the following:

- Past treatment for cancer.

- Being infected with the Epstein-Barr virus or human immuno-deficiency virus (HIV).

- Having a weakened immune system after a transplant or from medicines given after a transplant.

- Having certain inherited diseases of the immune system.

If lymphoma or lymphoproliferative disease is linked to a weak-ened immune system from certain inherited diseases, HIV infection, a transplant or medicines given after a transplant, the condition is called lymphoproliferative disease associated with immunodeficiency. The different types of lymphoproliferative disease associated with immunodeficiency include:

Lymphoproliferative disease associated with primary immunodeficiency.

- HIV-associated non-Hodgkin lymphoma.

- Post-transplant lymphoproliferative disease.

- Signs of childhood non-Hodgkin lymphoma include breathing problems and swollen lymph nodes.

Signs of Childhood Non-Hodgkin Lymphoma Include Breathing Problems and Swollen Lymph Nodes

These and other signs may be caused by childhood non-Hodgkin lymphoma or by other conditions. Check with a doctor if your child has any of the following:

- trouble breathing

- wheezing

- coughing

- high-pitched breathing sounds

- swelling of the head, neck, upper body, or arms

- trouble swallowing

- painless swelling of the lymph nodes in the neck, underarm, stomach, or groin

- painless lump or swelling in a testicle

- fever for no known reason

- weight loss for no known reason

- night sweats

Tests That Examine the Body and Lymph System Are Used to Detect (Find) and Diagnose Childhood Non-Hodgkin Lymphoma

The following tests and procedures may be used:

- Physical exam and history

- Blood chemistry studies

- Liver function tests

- CT scan (CAT scan)

- PET scan (positron emission tomography scan)

- MRI (magnetic resonance imaging)

- Lumbar puncture

- Chest X-ray

- Ultrasound exam

A Biopsy Is Done to Diagnose Childhood Non-Hodgkin Lymphoma

Cells and tissues are removed during a biopsy so they can be viewed under a microscope by a pathologist to check for signs of cancer. Because treatment depends on the type of non-Hodgkin lymphoma, biopsy samples should be checked by a pathologist who has experience in diagnosing childhood non-Hodgkin lymphoma.

One of the following types of biopsies may be done:

- Excisional biopsy
- Incisional biopsy
- Core biopsy
- Fine-needle aspiration (FNA) biopsy

The procedure used to remove the sample of tissue depends on where the tumor is in the body:

- Bone marrow aspiration and biopsy
- Mediastinoscopy
- Anterior mediastinotomy
- Thoracentesis

If cancer is found, the following tests may be done to study the cancer cells:

- Immunohistochemistry
- Flow cytometry
- Cytogenetic analysis
- FISH (fluorescence in situ hybridization)
- Immunophenotyping

Certain Factors Affect Prognosis (Chance of Recovery) and Treatment Options

The prognosis (chance of recovery) and treatment options depend on:

- the type of lymphoma
- where the tumor is in the body when the tumor is diagnosed
- the stage of the cancer
- whether there are certain changes in the chromosomes
- the type of initial treatment
- whether the lymphoma responded to initial treatment
- the patient's age and general health

A Biopsy Is Done to Diagnose Childhood Non-Hodgkin Lymphoma

Section 19.6

Mycosis Fungoides and the Sézary Syndrome

This section includes text excerpted from "Mycosis Fungoides and the Sézary Syndrome Treatment (PDQ®)—Patient Version," National Cancer Institute (NCI), February 5, 2016.

Normally, the bone marrow makes blood stem cells (immature cells) that become mature blood stem cells over time. A blood stem cell may become a myeloid stem cell or a lymphoid stem cell. A myeloid stem cell becomes a red blood cell, white blood cell, or platelet. A lymphoid stem cell becomes a lymphoblast and then one of three types of lymphocytes (white blood cells):

- B-cell lymphocytes that make antibodies to help fight infection.

- T-cell lymphocytes that help B-lymphocytes make the antibodies that help fight infection.

- Natural killer cells that attack cancer cells and viruses.

In mycosis fungoides, T-cell lymphocytes become cancerous and affect the skin. In the Sézary syndrome, cancerous T-cell lymphocytes affect the skin and are in the blood.

Mycosis Fungoides and the Sézary Syndrome Are Types of Cutaneous T-Cell Lymphoma

Mycosis fungoides and the Sézary syndrome are the two most common types of cutaneous T-cell lymphoma (a type of non-Hodgkin lymphoma).

A Sign of Mycosis Fungoides Is a Red Rash on the Skin

Mycosis fungoides may go through the following phases:

- **Premycotic phase:** A scaly, red rash in areas of the body that usually are not exposed to the sun. This rash does not cause symptoms and may last for months or years. It is hard to diagnose the rash as mycosis fungoides during this phase.

- **Patch phase:** Thin, reddened, eczema-like rash.
- **Plaque phase:** Small raised bumps (papules) or hardened lesions on the skin, which may be reddened.
- **Tumor phase:** Tumors form on the skin. These tumors may develop ulcers and the skin may get infected.

Check with your doctor if you have any of these signs.

In the Sézary Syndrome, Cancerous T-Cells Are Found in the Blood

Also, skin all over the body is reddened, itchy, peeling, and painful. There may also be patches, plaques, or tumors on the skin. It is not known if the Sézary syndrome is an advanced form of mycosis fungoides or a separate disease.

Tests That Examine the Skin and Blood Are Used to Detect (Find) and Diagnose Mycosis Fungoides and the Sézary Syndrome

The following tests and procedures may be used:

- Physical exam and history
- Complete blood count with differential
- Peripheral blood smear
- Skin biopsy
- Immunophenotyping
- T-cell receptor (TCR) gene rearrangement test
- Flow cytometry

Certain Factors Affect Prognosis (Chance of Recovery) and Treatment Options

The prognosis (chance of recovery) and treatment options depend on the following:

- The stage of the cancer.
- The type of lesion (patches, plaques, or tumors).

Mycosis fungoides and the Sézary syndrome are hard to cure. Treatment is usually palliative, to relieve symptoms and improve the quality of life. Patients with early stage disease may live many years.

Section 19.7

Primary CNS Lymphoma

This section includes text excerpted from "Primary
CNS Lymphoma Treatment (PDQ®)—Patient Version,"
National Cancer Institute (NCI), September 21, 2015.

Lymphoma is a disease in which malignant (cancer) cells form in the lymph system. The lymph system is part of the immune system and is made up of the lymph, lymph vessels, lymph nodes, spleen, thymus, tonsils, and bone marrow. Lymphocytes (carried in the lymph) travel in and out of the central nervous system (CNS). It is thought that some of these lymphocytes become malignant and cause lymphoma to form in the CNS. Primary CNS lymphoma can start in the brain, spinal cord, or meninges (the layers that form the outer covering of the brain). Because the eye is so close to the brain, primary CNS lymphoma can also start in the eye (called ocular lymphoma).

Having a Weakened Immune System May Increase the Risk of Developing Primary CNS Lymphoma

Primary CNS lymphoma may occur in patients who have acquired immunodeficiency syndrome (AIDS) or other disorders of the immune system or who have had a kidney transplant.

Tests That Examine the Eyes, Brain, and Spinal Cord Are Used to Detect (Find) and Diagnose Primary CNS Lymphoma

The following tests and procedures may be used:

• Physical exam and history

- Neurological exam
- Slit-lamp eye exam
- MRI (magnetic resonance imaging)
- PET scan (positron emission tomography scan)
- Lumbar puncture
- Stereotactic biopsy

The following tests may be done on the samples of tissue that are removed:

- Flow cytometry
- Immunohistochemistry
- Cytogenetic analysis
- Complete blood count (CBC) with differential
- Blood chemistry studies

Certain Factors Affect Prognosis (Chance of Recovery) and Treatment Options

The prognosis (chance of recovery) depends on the following:

- The patient's age and general health.
- The level of certain substances in the blood and cerebrospinal fluid (CSF).
- Where the tumor is in the central nervous system.
- Whether the patient has AIDS.

Treatment options depend on the following:

- The stage of the cancer.
- Where the tumor is in the central nervous system.
- The patient's age and general health.
- Whether the cancer has just been diagnosed or has recurred (come back).

Treatment of primary CNS lymphoma works best when the tumor has not spread outside the cerebrum (the largest part of the brain) and the patient is younger than 60 years, able to carry out most daily activities, and does not have AIDS or other diseases that weaken the immune system.

Section 19.8

Waldenström's Macroglobulinemia

This section includes text excerpted from "Waldenstrom Macroglobulinemia," Genetic and Rare Diseases Information Center (GARD), October 1, 2013.

What Is Waldenström's Macroglobulinemia?

Waldenström's macroglobulinemia is a chronic, slow-growing lymphoproliferative disorder. It usually affects older adults and is primarily found in the bone marrow, although lymph nodes and the spleen may be involved. Affected individuals have a high level of an antibody called immunoglobulin M (IgM) in their blood, which can cause thickening of the blood (hyperviscosity). Although some individuals initially do not have symptoms and are diagnosed from routine blood work, common symptoms may include weakness, appetite loss and weight loss. Other symptoms may include peripheral neuropathy, fever, Raynaud's phenomenon, and mental status changes. Hyperviscosity of the blood may cause nosebleeds, headaches, dizziness, and blurring or loss of vision. The cause of the condition is not known but environmental, genetic, and viral factors have been suggested. There have been some reports of familial cases suggesting a genetic predisposition. Treatment is often reserved for those with symptoms and may include various medications including corticosteroids, alkylating agents, biologic response modifiers and purine analogues.

What Are the Signs and Symptoms of Waldenström's Macroglobulinemia?

The Human Phenotype Ontology (HPO) provides the following list of signs and symptoms for Waldenström's macroglobulinemia.

- Leukemia

- Lymphoma

- Autosomal dominant inheritance

- Impaired lymphocyte transformation with phytohemagglutinin

- Polyclonal elevation of IgM

- Polyneuropathy

- Waldenström's macroglobulinemia

How Might Waldenström's Macroglobulinemia Be Treated?

For individuals who do not have any symptoms, doctors may decide to "watch and wait" and not treat the disease right away. This can last many years for some individuals. For individuals requiring treatment, the type and severity of symptoms present, aggressiveness of the disease, and age all play a role in the type of therapy chosen.

Some affected individuals have a procedure called plasmapheresis, to reverse or prevent the symptoms associated with the thickening of the blood (hyperviscosity). This involves removing the blood, passing it through a machine that removes the part of the blood with the IgM antibody, and returning the blood to the body. This may be combined with other treatments such as various types of chemotherapy. Many different drugs can be used to manage this condition, both alone and/or in various combinations.

For many individuals, there is a delayed response to treatment and the best response sometimes occurs several months after the treatment ends. Although the condition is not curable, many individuals do have a long-term response to treatment. Those who relapse after treatment or do not respond to initial treatment may consider secondary therapies. There are also several new drugs and drug combinations that are being studied in clinical trials.

Chapter 20

Myeloproliferative Disorders

Chapter Contents

Section 20.1

Myelodysplastic Syndromes

This section includes text excerpted from "Myelodysplastic
Syndromes Treatment (PDQ®)—Patient Version," National
Cancer Institute (NCI), August 12, 2015.

Myelodysplastic Syndromes Are a Group of Cancers in Which Immature Blood Cells in the Bone Marrow Do Not Mature or Become Healthy Blood Cells

In a healthy person, the bone marrow makes blood stem cells
(immature cells) that become mature blood cells over time.

In a patient with a myelodysplastic syndrome, the blood stem cells
(immature cells) do not become mature red blood cells, white blood
cells, or platelets in the bone marrow. These immature blood cells,
called blasts, do not work the way they should and either die in the
bone marrow or soon after they go into the blood. This leaves less room
for healthy white blood cells, red blood cells, and platelets to form in
the bone marrow. When there are fewer healthy blood cells, infection,
anemia, or easy bleeding may occur.

The Different Types of Myelodysplastic Syndromes Are Diagnosed Based on Certain Changes in the Blood Cells and Bone Marrow

- **Refractory anemia:** There are too few red blood cells in the
  blood and the patient has anemia. The number of white blood
  cells and platelets is normal.

- **Refractory anemia with ring sideroblasts:** There are too
  few red blood cells in the blood and the patient has anemia. The
  red blood cells have too much iron inside the cell. The number of
  white blood cells and platelets is normal.

- **Refractory anemia with excess blasts:** There are too few red
  blood cells in the blood and the patient has anemia. Five percent
  to 19% of the cells in the bone marrow are blasts. There also

may be changes to the white blood cells and platelets. Refractory anemia with excess blasts may progress to acute myeloid leukemia (AML).

- **Refractory cytopenia with multilineage dysplasia:** There are too few of at least two types of blood cells (red blood cells, platelets, or white blood cells). Less than 5% of the cells in the bone marrow are blasts and less than 1% of the cells in the blood are blasts. If red blood cells are affected, they may have extra iron. Refractory cytopenia may progress to acute myeloid leukemia (AML).

- **Refractory cytopenia with unilineage dysplasia:** There are too few of one type of blood cell (red blood cells, platelets, or white blood cells). There are changes in 10% or more of two other types of blood cells. Less than 5% of the cells in the bone marrow are blasts and less than 1% of the cells in the blood are blasts.

- **Unclassifiable myelodysplastic syndrome:** The numbers of blasts in the bone marrow and blood are normal, and the disease is not one of the other myelodysplastic syndromes.

- **Myelodysplastic syndrome associated with an isolated del(5q) chromosome abnormality:** There are too few red blood cells in the blood and the patient has anemia. Less than 5% of the cells in the bone marrow and blood are blasts. There is a specific change in the chromosome.

Age and past Treatment with Chemotherapy or Radiation Therapy Affect the Risk of a Myelodysplastic Syndrome

Risk factors for myelodysplastic syndromes include the following:

- Past treatment with chemotherapy or radiation therapy for cancer.

- Being exposed to certain chemicals, including tobacco smoke, pesticides, fertilizers, and solvents such as benzene.

- Being exposed to heavy metals, such as mercury or lead.

The cause of myelodysplastic syndromes in most patients is not known.

Signs and Symptoms of a Myelodysplastic Syndrome Include Shortness of Breath and Feeling Tired

Myelodysplastic syndromes often do not cause early signs or symptoms. They may be found during a routine blood test. Signs and symptoms may be caused by myelodysplastic syndromes or by other conditions. Check with your doctor if you have any of the following:

- shortness of breath
- weakness or feeling tired
- having skin that is paler than usual
- easy bruising or bleeding
- petechiae (flat, pinpoint spots under the skin caused by bleeding)

Tests That Examine the Blood and Bone Marrow Are Used to Detect (Find) and Diagnose Myelodysplastic Syndromes

The following tests and procedures may be used:

- Physical exam and history
- Complete blood count (CBC) with differential
- Peripheral blood smear
- Cytogenetic analysis
- Blood chemistry studies
- Bone marrow aspiration and biopsy

The following tests may be done on the sample of tissue that is removed:

- Immunocytochemistry
- Immunophenotyping
- Flow cytometry
- FISH (fluorescence in situ hybridization)

Certain Factors Affect Prognosis and Treatment Options

The prognosis (chance of recovery) and treatment options depend on the following:

- The number of blast cells in the bone marrow.

- Whether one or more types of blood cells are affected.

- Whether the patient has signs or symptoms of anemia, bleeding, or infection.

- Whether the patient has a low or high risk of leukemia.

- Certain changes in the chromosomes.

- Whether the myelodysplastic syndrome occurred after chemo-therapy or radiation therapy for cancer.

- The age and general health of the patient.

Section 20.2

Myeloproliferative Neoplasms

This section includes text excerpted from "Chronic Myeloproliferative Neoplasms Treatment (PDQ®)—Patient Version," National Cancer Institute (NCI), April 7, 2016.

Myeloproliferative Neoplasms Are a Group of Diseases in Which the Bone Marrow Makes Too Many Red Blood Cells, White Blood Cells, or Platelets

Normally, the bone marrow makes blood stem cells (immature cells) that become mature blood cells over time.

In myeloproliferative neoplasms, too many blood stem cells become one or more types of blood cells. The neoplasms usually get worse slowly as the number of extra blood cells increases.

There Are 6 Types of Chronic Myeloproliferative Neoplasms

The type of myeloproliferative neoplasm is based on whether too many red blood cells, white blood cells, or platelets are being made. Sometimes the body will make too many of more than one type of blood cell, but usually one type of blood cell is affected more than the others are. Chronic myeloproliferative neoplasms include the following 6 types:

- chronic myelogenous leukemia
- polycythemia vera
- primary myelofibrosis (also called chronic idiopathic myelofibrosis)
- essential thrombocythemia
- chronic neutrophilic leukemia
- chronic eosinophilic leukemia

Chronic myeloproliferative neoplasms sometimes become acute leukemia, in which too many abnormal white blood cells are made.

Tests That Examine the Blood and Bone Marrow Are Used to Detect (Find) and Diagnose Chronic Myeloproliferative Neoplasms

The following tests and procedures may be used:

- Physical exam and history
- Complete blood count (CBC) with differential
- Peripheral blood smear
- Blood chemistry studies
- Bone marrow aspiration and biopsy
- Cytogenetic analysis
- Gene mutation test

Section 20.3

Primary Myelofibrosis

This section includes text excerpted from "Primary Myelofibrosis," Genetic Home Reference (GHR), July 19, 2016.

What Is Primary Myelofibrosis?

Primary myelofibrosis is a condition characterized by the buildup of scar tissue (fibrosis) in the bone marrow, the tissue that produces blood cells. Because of the fibrosis, the bone marrow is unable to make enough normal blood cells. The shortage of blood cells causes many of the signs and symptoms of primary myelofibrosis.

Initially, most people with primary myelofibrosis have no signs or symptoms. Eventually, fibrosis can lead to a reduction in the number of red blood cells, white blood cells, and platelets. A shortage of red blood cells (anemia) often causes extreme tiredness (fatigue) or shortness of breath. A loss of white blood cells can lead to an increased number of infections, and a reduction of platelets can cause easy bleeding or bruising.

Because blood cell formation (hematopoiesis) in the bone marrow is disrupted, other organs such as the spleen or liver may begin to produce blood cells. This process, called extramedullary hematopoiesis, often leads to an enlarged spleen (splenomegaly) or an enlarged liver (hepatomegaly). People with splenomegaly may feel pain or fullness in the abdomen, especially below the ribs on the left side. Other common signs and symptoms of primary myelofibrosis include fever, night sweats, and bone pain.

Primary myelofibrosis is most commonly diagnosed in people aged 50 to 80 but can occur at any age.

Frequency

Primary myelofibrosis is a rare condition that affects approximately 1 in 500,000 people worldwide.

Genetic Changes

Mutations in the *JAK2*, *MPL*, *CALR*, and *TET2* genes are associated with most cases of primary myelofibrosis. The *JAK2* and *MPL* genes provide instructions for making proteins that promote the growth and division (proliferation) of blood cells. The *CALR* gene provides instructions for making a protein with multiple functions, including ensuring the proper folding of newly formed proteins and maintaining the correct levels of stored calcium in cells. The *TET2* gene provides instructions for making a protein whose function is unknown.

The proteins produced from the *JAK2* and *MPL* genes are both part of a signaling pathway called the JAK/STAT pathway, which transmits chemical signals from outside the cell to the cell's nucleus. The protein produced from the *MPL* gene, called thrombopoietin receptor, turns on (activates) the pathway, and the *JAK2* protein transmits signals after activation. Through the JAK/STAT pathway, these two proteins promote the proliferation of blood cells, particularly a type of blood cell known as a megakaryocyte.

Mutations in either the *JAK2* gene or the *MPL* gene that are associated with primary myelofibrosis lead to overactivation of the JAK/STAT pathway. The abnormal activation of JAK/STAT signaling leads to overproduction of abnormal megakaryocytes, and these megakaryocytes stimulate another type of cell to release collagen. Collagen is a protein that normally provides structural support for the cells in the bone marrow. However, in primary myelofibrosis, the excess collagen forms scar tissue in the bone marrow.

Although mutations in the *CALR* gene and the *TET2* gene are relatively common in primary myelofibrosis, it is unclear how these mutations are involved in the development of the condition.

Some people with primary myelofibrosis do not have a mutation in any of the known genes associated with this condition. Researchers are working to identify other genes that may be involved in the condition.

Inheritance Pattern

This condition is generally not inherited but arises from gene mutations that occur in early blood-forming cells after conception. These alterations are called somatic mutations.

Section 20.4

Polycythemia Vera

This section includes text excerpted from "Polycythemia Vera," National Heart, Lung, and Blood Institute (NHLBI), March 1, 2011. Reviewed July 2016.

What Is Polycythemia Vera?

Polycythemia vera, or PV, is a rare blood disease in which your body makes too many red blood cells.

The extra red blood cells make your blood thicker than normal. As a result, blood clots can form more easily. These clots can block blood flow through your arteries and veins, which can cause a heart attack or stroke.

Thicker blood also doesn't flow as quickly to your body as normal blood. Slowed blood flow prevents your organs from getting enough oxygen, which can cause serious problems, such as angina and heart failure. (Angina is chest pain or discomfort.)

Other Names for Polycythemia Vera

- Cryptogenic polycythemia
- Erythremia
- Erythrocytosis megalosplenica
- Myelopathic polycythemia
- Myeloproliferative disorder
- Osler disease
- Polycythemia rubra vera
- Polycythemia with chronic cyanosis
- Primary polycythemia
- Splenomegalic polycythemia
- Vaquez disease

What Causes Polycythemia Vera?

Primary Polycythemia

PV also is known as primary polycythemia. A mutation, or change, in the body's *JAK2* gene is the main cause of PV. The *JAK2* gene makes a protein that helps the body produce blood cells.

What causes the change in the *JAK2* gene isn't known. PV generally isn't inherited—that is, passed from parents to children through genes. However, in some families, the *JAK2* gene may have a tendency to mutate. Other, unknown genetic factors also may play a role in causing PV.

Secondary Polycythemia

Another type of polycythemia, called secondary polycythemia, isn't related to the *JAK2* gene. Long-term exposure to low oxygen levels causes secondary polycythemia.

A lack of oxygen over a long period can cause your body to make more of the hormone erythropoietin (EPO). High levels of EPO can prompt your body to make more red blood cells than normal. This leads to thicker blood, as seen in PV.

People who have severe heart or lung disease may develop secondary polycythemia. People who smoke, spend long hours at high altitudes, or are exposed to high levels of carbon monoxide where they work or live also are at risk.

For example, working in an underground parking garage or living in a home with a poorly vented fireplace or furnace can raise your risk for secondary polycythemia.

Rarely, tumors can make and release EPO, or certain blood problems can cause the body to make more EPO.

Sometimes doctors can cure secondary polycythemia—it depends on whether the underlying cause can be stopped, controlled, or cured.

Who Is at Risk for Polycythemia Vera?

PV is a rare blood disease. The disease affects people of all ages, but it's most common in adults who are older than 60. PV is rare in children and young adults. Men are at slightly higher risk for PV than women.

What Are the Signs and Symptoms of Polycythemia Vera?

PV develops slowly. The disease may not cause signs or symptoms for years.

When signs and symptoms are present, they're the result of the thick blood that occurs with PV. This thickness slows the flow of oxygen-rich blood to all parts of your body. Without enough oxygen, many parts of your body won't work normally.

The signs and symptoms of PV include:

- headaches, dizziness, and weakness

- shortness of breath and problems breathing while lying down

- feelings of pressure or fullness on the left side of the abdomen due to an enlarged spleen (an organ in the abdomen)

- double or blurred vision and blind spots

- itching all over (especially after a warm bath), reddened face, and a burning feeling on your skin (especially your hands and feet)

- bleeding from your gums and heavy bleeding from small cuts

- unexplained weight loss

- fatigue (tiredness)

- excessive sweating

- very painful swelling in a single joint, usually the big toe (called gouty arthritis)

In rare cases, people who have PV may have pain in their bones.

Polycythemia Vera Complications

If you have PV, the thickness of your blood and the slowed blood flow can cause serious health problems.

Blood clots are the most serious complication of PV. Blood clots can cause a heart attack or stroke. They also can cause your liver and spleen to enlarge. Blood clots in the liver and spleen can cause sudden, intense pain.

Slowed blood flow also prevents enough oxygen-rich blood from reaching your organs. This can lead to angina (chest pain or discomfort) and heart failure. The high levels of red blood cells that PV causes can lead to stomach ulcers, gout, or kidney stones.

Some people who have PV may develop myelofibrosis. This is a condition in which your bone marrow is replaced with scar tissue. Abnormal bone marrow cells may begin to grow out of control.

This abnormal growth can lead to acute myelogenous leukemia (AML), a cancer of the blood and bone marrow. This disease can worsen very quickly.

How Is Polycythemia Vera Diagnosed?

PV may not cause signs or symptoms for years. The disease often is found during routine blood tests done for other reasons. If the results of your blood tests aren't normal, your doctor may want to do more tests.

Your doctor will diagnose PV based on your signs and symptoms, your age and overall health, your medical history, a physical exam, and test results.

During the physical exam, your doctor will look for signs of PV. He or she will check for an enlarged spleen, red skin on your face, and bleeding from your gums.

If your doctor confirms that you have polycythemia, the next step is to find out whether you have primary polycythemia (polycythemia vera) or secondary polycythemia.

Your medical history and physical exam may confirm which type of polycythemia you have. If not, you may have tests that check the level of the hormone erythropoietin (EPO) in your blood.

People who have PV have very low levels of EPO. People who have secondary polycythemia usually have normal or high levels of EPO.

Specialists Involved

If your primary care doctor thinks you have PV, he or she may refer you to a hematologist. A hematologist is a doctor who specializes in diagnosing and treating blood diseases and conditions.

Diagnostic Tests

You may have blood tests to diagnose PV. These tests include a complete blood count (CBC) and other tests, if necessary.

Complete Blood Count

Often, the first test used to diagnose PV is a CBC. The CBC measures many parts of your blood

This test checks your hemoglobin and hematocrit levels. Hemoglobin is an iron-rich protein that helps red blood cells carry oxygen from the lungs to the rest of the body. Hematocrit is a measure of how much space red blood cells take up in your blood. A high level of hemoglobin or hematocrit may be a sign of PV.

The CBC also checks the number of red blood cells, white blood cells, and platelets in your blood. Abnormal results may be a sign of PV, a blood disorder, an infection, or another condition.

In addition to high red blood cell counts, people who have PV also may have high white blood cell and/or platelet counts.

Other Blood Tests

Blood smear. For this test, a small sample of blood is drawn from a vein, usually in your arm. The blood sample is examined under a microscope.

A blood smear can show whether you have a higher than normal number of red blood cells. The test also can show abnormal blood cells that are linked to myelofibrosis and other conditions related to PV.

Erythropoietin level. This blood test measures the level of EPO in your blood. EPO is a hormone that prompts your bone marrow to make new blood cells. People who have PV have very low levels of EPO. People who have secondary polycythemia usually have normal or high levels of EPO.

Bone Marrow Tests

Bone marrow tests can show whether your bone marrow is healthy. These tests also show whether your bone marrow is making normal amounts of blood cells.

The two bone marrow tests are aspiration and biopsy. For aspiration, your doctor removes a small amount of fluid bone marrow through a needle. For a biopsy, your doctor removes a small amount of bone marrow tissue through a larger needle. The samples are then examined under a microscope.

If the tests show that your bone marrow is making too many blood cells, it may be a sign that you have PV.

How Is Polycythemia Vera Treated?

PV doesn't have a cure. However, treatments can help control the disease and its complications. PV is treated with procedures, medicines, and other methods. You may need one or more treatments to manage the disease.

Goals of Treatment

The goals of treating PV are to control symptoms and reduce the risk of complications, especially heart attack and stroke. To do this, PV treatments reduce the number of red blood cells and the level of hemoglobin (an iron-rich protein) in the blood. This brings the thickness of your blood closer to normal.

Blood with normal thickness flows better through the blood vessels. This reduces the chance that blood clots will form and cause a heart attack or stroke.

Blood with normal thickness also ensures that your body gets enough oxygen. This can help reduce some of the signs and symptoms of PV, such as headaches, vision problems, and itching.

Studies show that treating PV greatly improves your chances of living longer.

The goal of treating secondary polycythemia is to control its underlying cause, if possible. For example, if the cause is carbon monoxide exposure, the goal is to find the source of the carbon monoxide and fix or remove it.

Treatments To Lower Red Blood Cell Levels

Phlebotomy

Phlebotomy is a procedure that removes some blood from your body. For this procedure, a needle is inserted into one of your veins. Blood from the vein flows through an airtight tube into a sterile container or bag. The process is similar to the process of donating blood.

Phlebotomy reduces your red blood cell count and starts to bring your blood thickness closer to normal.

Typically, a pint (1 unit) of blood is removed each week until your hematocrit level approaches normal. (Hematocrit is the measure of how much space red blood cells take up in your blood.)

You may need to have phlebotomy done every few months.

Medicines

Your doctor may prescribe medicines to keep your bone marrow from making too many red blood cells. Examples of these medicines include hydroxyurea and interferon-alpha.

Hydroxyurea is a medicine generally used to treat cancer. This medicine can reduce the number of red blood cells and platelets in your blood. As a result, this medicine helps improve your blood flow and bring the thickness of your blood closer to normal.

Interferon-alpha is a substance that your body normally makes. It also can be used to treat PV. Interferon-alpha can prompt your immune system to fight overactive bone marrow cells. This helps lower your red blood cell count and keep your blood flow and blood thickness closer to normal.

Radiation Treatment

Radiation treatment can help suppress overactive bone marrow cells. This helps lower your red blood cell count and keep your blood flow and blood thickness closer to normal.

However, radiation treatment can raise your risk of leukemia (blood cancer) and other blood diseases.

Treatments for Symptoms

Aspirin can relieve bone pain and burning feelings in your hands or feet that you may have as a result of PV. Aspirin also thins your blood, so it reduces the risk of blood clots.

Aspirin can have side effects, including bleeding in the stomach and intestines. For this reason, take aspirin only as your doctor recommends.

If your PV causes itching, your doctor may prescribe medicines to ease the discomfort. Your doctor also may prescribe ultraviolet light treatment to help relieve your itching.

Other ways to reduce itching include:

- **Avoiding hot baths.** Cooler water can limit irritation to your skin.

- **Gently patting yourself dry after bathing.** Vigorous rubbing with a towel can irritate your skin.
- **Taking starch baths.** Add half a box of starch to a tub of luke-warm water. This can help soothe your skin.

How Can Polycythemla Vera Be Prevented?

Primary polycythemia (polycythemia vera) can't be prevented. However, with proper treatment, you can prevent or delay symptoms and complications.

Sometimes you can prevent secondary polycythemia by avoiding things that deprive your body of oxygen for long periods. For example, you can avoid mountain climbing, living at a high altitude, or smoking.

People who have serious heart or lung diseases may develop secondary polycythemia. Treatment for the underlying disease may improve the secondary polycythemia. Following a healthy lifestyle to lower your risk of heart and lung diseases also will help you prevent secondary polycythemia.

Living with Polycythemia Vera

PV develops very slowly. It may not cause signs or symptoms for years. If you have PV, the sooner it's diagnosed, the sooner your doctor can begin treating you. With proper treatment, you can prevent or delay complications.

Preventing Complications

Moderate physical activities, such as walking, can safely increase your heart rate and improve blood flow to your body. Improving blood flow lowers your risk of blood clots. Leg and ankle stretching exercises also can help improve your blood flow.

PV may cause itching all over your body. It's important not to scratch and damage your skin. If bathing or showering causes you to have severe itching, try using cooler water and gentler soap. Carefully and gently dry your skin after baths, and use moisturizing lotion on your skin. Starch baths also may help ease itchy skin.

PV causes poor blood flow in your hands and feet. As a result, you may be more prone to injuries from cold, heat, and pressure. If you have PV, avoid long-term exposure to extremes in temperature or pressure. For example:

- Take extra care of your hands and feet in cold weather. Wear warm gloves, socks, and shoes.

- Avoid extreme heat, and protect yourself from the sun. Drink plenty of liquids. Avoid hot tubs, heated whirlpools, or hot baths of any type. Also, tanning beds, sun lamps, and heat lamps can damage your skin if you have PV.

- Guard against trauma or situations where you may be at high risk of injury, such as during sports or strenuous activities. If you're injured, seek treatment right away. Tell the person treating you that you have PV.

- Check your feet regularly and report any sores to your doctor.

Getting Ongoing Care

If you have PV, you'll need lifelong medical care for the disease. Ask your doctor how often you should schedule followup visits.

Routine care will allow your doctor to detect any changes with your PV and treat them early, if needed. You may need periodic blood tests to show whether the disease is getting worse.

Follow your treatment plan and take all of your medicines exactly as your doctor prescribes.

Section 20.5

Thrombocythemia and Thrombocytosis

This section includes text excerpted from "Thrombocythemia and Thrombocytosis," National Heart, Lung, and Blood Institute (NHLBI), July 31, 2012. Reviewed July 2016.

What Are Thrombocythemia and Thrombocytosis?

Thrombocythemia and thrombocytosis are conditions in which your blood has a higher than normal number of platelets.

Platelets are blood cell fragments. They're made in your bone marrow along with other kinds of blood cells.

Platelets travel through your blood vessels and stick together (clot). Clotting helps stop any bleeding that may occur if a blood vessel is damaged. Platelets also are called thrombocytes because a blood clot also is called a thrombus.

A normal platelet count ranges from 150,000 to 450,000 platelets per microliter of blood.

Other Names for Thrombocythemia and Thrombocytosis

Primary thrombocythemia also is called:

- Essential thrombocythemia. This term is used when a high platelet count occurs alone (that is, without other blood cell disorders)

- Idiopathic thrombocythemia
- Primary or essential thrombocytosis (these are less favored terms)

Thrombocytosis also is known as:

- Secondary or reactive thrombocytosis
- Secondary thrombocythemia (this is a less favored term)

What Causes Thrombocythemia and Thrombocytosis?

Primary Thrombocythemia

In this condition, faulty stem cells in the bone marrow make too many platelets. What causes this to happen usually isn't known. When this process occurs without other blood cell disorders, it's called essential thrombocythemia.

A rare form of thrombocythemia is inherited. ("Inherited" means the condition is passed from parents to children through the genes.) In some cases, a genetic mutation may cause the condition.

In addition to the bone marrow making too many platelets, the platelets also are abnormal in primary thrombocythemia. They may form blood clots or, surprisingly, cause bleeding when they don't work well.

Bleeding also can occur because of a condition that develops called von Willebrand disease. This condition affects the blood clotting process.

After many years, scarring of the bone marrow can occur.

Secondary Thrombocytosis

This condition occurs if another disease, condition, or outside factor causes the platelet count to rise. For example, 35 percent of people who have high platelet counts also have cancer—mostly lung, gastrointestinal, breast, ovarian, and lymphoma. Sometimes a high platelet count is the first sign of cancer.

Other conditions or factors that can cause a high platelet count are:

- iron-deficiency anemia
- hemolytic anemia
- absence of a spleen (after surgery to remove the organ)
- inflammatory or infectious diseases, such as connective tissue disorders, inflammatory bowel disease, and tuberculosis
- reactions to medicine

Some conditions can lead to a high platelet count that lasts for only a short time. Examples of such conditions include:

- recovery from serious blood loss

- recovery from a very low platelet count caused by excessive alcohol use and lack of vitamin B12 or folate

- acute (short-term) infection or inflammation

- response to physical activity

Although the platelet count is high in secondary thrombocytosis, the platelets are normal (unlike in primary thrombocythemia). Thus, people who have secondary thrombocytosis have a lower risk of blood clots and bleeding.

Who Is at Risk for Thrombocythemia or Thrombocytosis?

Primary Thrombocythemia

Thrombocythemia isn't common. The exact number of people who have the condition isn't known. Some estimates suggest that 24 out of every 100,000 people have primary thrombocythemia.

Primary thrombocythemia is more common in people aged 50 to 70, but it can occur at any age. For unknown reasons, more women around the age of 30 have primary thrombocythemia than men of the same age.

Secondary Thrombocytosis

You might be at risk for secondary thrombocytosis if you have a disease, condition, or factor that can cause it.

Secondary thrombocytosis is more common than primary thrombocythemia. Studies have shown that most people who have platelet counts over 500,000 have secondary thrombocytosis.

What Are the Signs and Symptoms of Thrombocythemia and Thrombocytosis?

People who have thrombocythemia or thrombocytosis may not have signs or symptoms. These conditions might be discovered only after routine blood tests.

However, people who have primary thrombocythemia are more likely than those who have secondary thrombocytosis to have serious signs and symptoms.

The signs and symptoms of a high platelet count are linked to blood clots and bleeding. They include weakness, bleeding, headache, dizziness, chest pain, and tingling in the hands and feet.

Blood Clots

In primary thrombocythemia, blood clots most often develop in the brain, hands, and feet. But they can develop anywhere in the body, including in the heart and intestines.

Blood clots in the brain may cause symptoms such as chronic (ongoing) headache and dizziness. In extreme cases, stroke may occur.

Blood clots in the tiny blood vessels of the hands and feet leave them numb and red. This may lead to an intense burning and throbbing pain felt mainly on the palms of the hands and the soles of the feet.

Other signs and symptoms of blood clots may include:

- changes in speech or awareness, ranging from confusion to passing out

- seizures

- upper body discomfort in one or both arms, the back, neck, jaw, or abdomen

- shortness of breath and nausea (feeling sick to your stomach)

In pregnant women, blood clots in the placenta can cause miscarriage or problems with fetal growth and development.

Women who have primary thrombocythemia or secondary thrombocytosis and take birth control pills are at increased risk for blood clots.

Blood clots are related to other conditions and factors as well. Older age, prior blood clots, diabetes, high blood pressure, and smoking also increase your risk for blood clots.

Bleeding

If bleeding occurs, it most often affects people who have platelet counts higher than 1 million platelets per microliter of blood. Signs of bleeding include nosebleeds, bruising, bleeding from the mouth or gums, or blood in the stools.

Although bleeding usually is associated with a low platelet count, it also can occur in people who have high platelet counts. Blood clots that develop in thrombocythemia or thrombocytosis may use up your body's platelets. This means that not enough platelets are left in your bloodstream to seal off cuts or breaks on the blood vessel walls.

Another cause of bleeding in people who have very high platelets counts is a condition called von Willebrand Disease. This condition affects the blood clotting process.

In rare cases of primary thrombocythemia, the faulty bone marrow cells will cause a form of leukemia. Leukemia is a cancer of the blood cells.

How Are Thrombocythemia and Thrombocytosis Diagnosed?

Your doctor will diagnose thrombocythemia or thrombocytosis based on your medical history, a physical exam, and test results. A hematologist also may be involved in your care. This is a doctor who specializes in blood diseases and conditions.

Medical History

Your doctor may ask you about factors that can affect your platelets, such as:

- any medical procedures or blood transfusions you've had

- any recent infections or vaccines you've had

- the medicines you take, including over-the-counter medicines

- your general eating habits, including the amount of alcohol you normally drink

- any family history of high platelet counts

Physical Exam

Your doctor will do a physical exam to look for signs and symptoms of blood clots and bleeding. He or she also will check for signs of conditions that can cause secondary thrombocytosis, such as an infection.

Primary thrombocythemia is diagnosed only after all possible causes of a high platelet count are ruled out. For example, your doctor may recommend tests to check for early, undiagnosed cancer. If another disease, condition, or factor is causing a high platelet count, the diagnosis is secondary thrombocytosis.

Diagnostic Tests

Your doctor may recommend one or more of the following tests to help diagnose a high platelet count.

Complete Blood Count

A complete blood count (CBC) measures the levels of red blood cells, white blood cells, and platelets in your blood. For this test, a small amount of blood is drawn from a blood vessel, usually in your arm.

If you have thrombocythemia or thrombocytosis, the CBC results will show that your platelet count is high.

Blood Smear

A blood smear is used to check the condition of your platelets. For this test, a small amount of blood is drawn from a blood vessel, usually in your arm. Some of your blood is put on a glass slide. A microscope is then used to look at your platelets.

Bone Marrow Tests

Bone marrow tests check whether your bone marrow is healthy. Blood cells, including platelets, are made in the bone marrow. The two bone marrow tests are aspiration and biopsy.

Bone marrow aspiration might be done to find out whether your bone marrow is making too many platelets. For this test, your doctor removes a sample of fluid bone marrow through a needle. He or she examines the sample under a microscope to check for faulty cells.

A bone marrow biopsy often is done right after an aspiration. For this test, your doctor removes a small amount of bone marrow tissue through a needle. He or she examines the tissue to check the number and types of cells in the bone marrow.

With thrombocythemia and thrombocytosis, the bone marrow has a higher than normal number of the very large cells that make platelets.

Other Tests

Your doctor may recommend other blood tests to look for genetic factors that can cause a high platelet count.

How Are Thrombocythemia and Thrombocytosis Treated?

Primary Thrombocythemia

This condition is considered less harmful today than in the past, and its outlook often is good. People who have no signs or symptoms don't need treatment, as long as the condition remains stable.

Taking aspirin may help people who are at risk for blood clots (aspirin thins the blood). However, talk with your doctor about using aspirin because it can cause bleeding.

Doctors prescribe aspirin to most pregnant women who have primary thrombocythemia. This is because it doesn't have a high risk of side effects for the fetus.

Some people who have primary thrombocythemia may need medicines or medical procedures to lower their platelet counts.

Medicines To Lower Platelet Counts

You may need medicines to lower your platelet count if you:

- have a history of blood clots or bleeding

- have risk factors for heart disease, such as high blood cholesterol, high blood pressure, or diabetes

- are older than 60

- have a platelet count over 1 million

You'll need to take these medicines throughout your life.

Hydroxyurea. This platelet-lowering medicine is used to treat cancers and other life-threatening diseases. Hydroxyurea most often is given under the care of doctors who specialize in cancer or blood diseases. Patients on hydroxyurea are closely monitored.

Currently, hydroxyurea plus aspirin is the standard treatment for people who have primary thrombocythemia and are at high risk for blood clots.

Anagrelide. This medicine also has been used to lower platelet counts in people who have thrombocythemia. However, research shows that when compared with hydroxyurea, anagrelide has worse outcomes. Anagrelide also has side effects, such as fluid retention, palpitations, arrhythmias, heart failure, and headaches.

263

Interferon alfa. This medicine lowers platelet counts, but 20 percent of patients can't handle its side effects. Side effects include a flu-like feeling, decreased appetite, nausea (feeling sick to the stomach), diarrhea, seizures, irritability, and sleepiness.

Doctors may prescribe this medicine to pregnant women who have primary thrombocythemia because it's safer for a fetus than hydroxyurea and anagrelide.

Plateletpheresis

Plateletpheresis is a procedure used to rapidly lower your platelet count. This procedure is used only for emergencies. For example, if you're having a stroke due to primary thrombocythemia, you may need plateletpheresis.

An intravenous (IV) needle that's connected to a tube is placed in one of your blood vessels to remove blood. The blood goes through a machine that removes platelets from the blood. The remaining blood is then put back into you through an IV line in one of your blood vessels.

One or two procedures might be enough to reduce your platelet count to a safe level.

Secondary Thrombocytosis

Secondary thrombocytosis is treated by addressing the condition that's causing it.

People who have secondary thrombocytosis usually don't need platelet-lowering medicines or procedures. This is because their platelets usually are normal (unlike in primary thrombocythemia).

Also, secondary thrombocytosis is less likely than primary thrombocythemia to cause serious problems related to blood clots and bleeding.

How Can Thrombocythemia and Thrombocytosis Be Prevented?

You can't prevent primary thrombocythemia. However, you can take steps to reduce your risk for complications. For example, you can control many of the risk factors for blood clots, such as high blood cholesterol, high blood pressure, diabetes, and smoking.

To reduce your risk, quit smoking, adopt healthy lifestyle habits, and work with your doctor to manage your risk factors.

It's not always possible to prevent conditions that lead to secondary thrombocytosis. But, if you have routine medical care, your doctor may detect these conditions before you develop a high platelet count.

Living with Thrombocythemia or Thrombocytosis

If you have thrombocythemia or thrombocytosis:

- See your doctor for ongoing medical care.

- Control risk factors for blood clots—for example, quit smoking and work to manage risk factors such as high blood cholesterol, high blood pressure, and diabetes.

- Watch for signs and symptoms of blood clots and bleeding and report them to your doctor right away.

- Take all medicines as prescribed.

If you're taking medicines to lower your platelet count, tell your doctor or dentist about them before any surgical or dental procedures. These medicines thin your blood and may increase bleeding during these procedures.

Medicines that thin the blood also may cause internal bleeding. Signs of internal bleeding include bruises, bloody or tarry-looking stools, pink or bloody urine, increased menstrual bleeding, bleeding gums, and nosebleeds. Contact your doctor right away if you have any of these signs.

Avoid over-the-counter pain medicines such as ibuprofen (except Tylenol®). These medicines may raise your risk of bleeding in the stomach or intestines and may limit the effect of aspirin. Be aware that cold and pain medicines and other over-the-counter products may contain ibuprofen.

Chapter 21

Plasma Cell Disorders

Chapter Contents

Section 21.1

Amyloidosis

This section includes text excerpted from "Amyloidosis and
Kidney Disease," National Institute of Diabetes and Digestive
and Kidney Diseases (NIDDK), September 2014.

What Is Amyloidosis?

Amyloidosis is a rare disease that occurs when amyloid proteins
are deposited in tissues and organs. Amyloid proteins are abnormal
proteins that the body cannot break down and recycle, as it does with
normal proteins. When amyloid proteins clump together, they form
amyloid deposits. The buildup of these deposits damages a person's
organs and tissues. Amyloidosis can affect different organs and tissues
in different people and can affect more than one organ at the same
time. Amyloidosis most frequently affects the kidneys, heart, nervous
system, liver, and digestive tract. The symptoms and severity of amyloidosis depend on the organs and tissues affected.

What Are the Kidneys and What Do They Do?

The kidneys are two bean-shaped organs, each about the size of a
fist. They are located just below the rib cage, one on each side of the
spine. Every day, the two kidneys filter about 120 to 150 quarts of blood
to produce about 1 to 2 quarts of urine, composed of wastes and extra
fluid. The urine flows from the kidneys to the bladder through tubes
called ureters. The bladder stores urine. When the bladder empties,
urine flows out of the body through a tube called the urethra, located
at the bottom of the bladder. In men, the urethra is long, while in
women it is short.

What Types of Amyloidosis Affect the Kidneys?

Primary amyloidosis and dialysis-related amyloidosis are the types
of amyloidosis that can affect the kidneys.

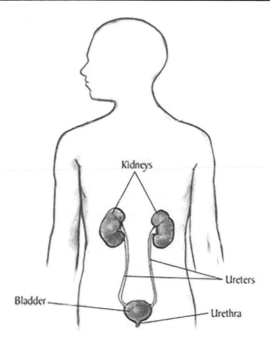

Figure 21.1. *Urinary-Tract*

The kidneys are two bean-shaped organs, each about the size of a fist.

Primary Amyloidosis of the Kidneys

The kidneys are the organs most commonly affected by primary amyloidosis. Amyloid deposits damage the kidneys and make it harder for them to filter wastes and break down proteins. When the kidneys become too damaged, they may no longer be able to function well enough to maintain health, resulting in kidney failure. Kidney failure can lead to problems such as high blood pressure, bone disease, and anemia—a condition in which the body has fewer red blood cells than normal.

Dialysis-Related Amyloidosis

People who suffer from kidney failure and have been on long-term dialysis may develop dialysis-related amyloidosis. This type of amyloidosis occurs when a certain protein, called beta-2 microglobulin, builds up in the blood because dialysis does not remove it completely. The two types of dialysis are

- hemodialysis. Hemodialysis uses a special filter called a dialyzer to remove wastes and extra fluid from the blood.

- peritoneal dialysis. Peritoneal dialysis uses the lining of the abdominal cavity—the space in the body that holds organs such as the stomach, intestines, and liver—to filter the blood.

Dialysis-related amyloidosis is a complication of kidney failure because neither hemodialysis nor peritoneal dialysis effectively filters beta-2 microglobulin from the blood. As a result, elevated amounts of beta-2 microglobulin remain in the blood. Dialysis-related amyloidosis is relatively common in people with kidney failure, especially adults older than 60 years of age, who have been on dialysis for more than 5 years.

What Are the Signs and Symptoms of Primary Amyloidosis of the Kidneys?

The most common sign of primary amyloidosis of the kidneys is nephrotic syndrome—a collection of signs that indicate kidney damage. The signs of nephrotic syndrome include

- albuminuria—an increased amount of albumin, a protein, in the urine. A person with nephrotic syndrome excretes more than half a teaspoon of albumin per day.

- hyperlipidemia—a condition in which a person's blood has more-than-normal amounts of fats and cholesterol.

- edema—swelling, typically in a person's legs, feet, or ankles and less often in the hands or face.

- hypoalbuminemia—a condition in which a person's blood has less-than-normal amounts of albumin.

Other signs and symptoms of primary amyloidosis may include

- fatigue, or feeling tired
- shortness of breath
- low blood pressure
- numbness, tingling, or a burning sensation in the hands or feet
- weight loss

What Are the Symptoms of Dialysis-Related Amyloidosis?

The symptoms of dialysis-related amyloidosis may include

- pain, stiffness, and fluid in the joints.

- abnormal, fluid-containing sacs, called cysts, in some bones.

- carpal tunnel syndrome, caused by unusual buildup of amyloid proteins in the wrists. The symptoms of carpal tunnel syndrome include numbness or tingling, sometimes associated with muscle weakness, in the fingers and hands.

Dialysis-related amyloidosis most often affects bones, joints, and the tissues that connect muscle to bone, called tendons. The disease may also affect the digestive tract and organs such as the heart and lungs. Bone cysts caused by dialysis-related amyloidosis can lead to bone fractures. Dialysis-related amyloidosis can also cause tears in tendons and ligaments. Ligaments are tissues that connect bones to other bones.

How Is Primary Amyloidosis of the Kidneys Diagnosed?

A health care provider diagnoses primary amyloidosis of the kidneys with

- a medical and family history

- a physical exam

- urinalysis

- blood tests

- a kidney biopsy

Medical and Family History

Taking a medical and family history may help a health care provider diagnose amyloidosis of the kidneys. He or she will ask the patient to provide a medical and family history.

Physical Exam

A physical exam may help diagnose primary amyloidosis of the kidneys. During a physical exam, a health care provider usually

- examines a patient's body to check for swelling

- uses a stethoscope to listen to the lungs

- taps on specific areas of the patient's body

Urinalysis

A healthcare provider may use urinalysis—the testing of a urine sample—to check for albumin and amyloid proteins in urine. The patient provides a urine sample in a special container at a health care provider's office or a commercial facility. A nurse or technician can test the sample in the same location or send it to a lab for analysis. More-than-normal amounts of albumin in urine may indicate kidney damage due to primary amyloidosis. Amyloid proteins in urine may indicate amyloidosis.

Blood Tests

The healthcare provider may use blood tests to see how well the kidneys are working and to check for amyloid proteins and hyperlipidemia. A blood test involves drawing a patient's blood at a health care provider's office or a commercial facility and sending the sample to a lab for analysis. Blood tests for kidney function measure the waste products in the blood that healthy kidneys normally filter out. Hyperlipidemia may indicate nephrotic syndrome. Amyloid proteins in blood may indicate amyloidosis.

Kidney Biopsy

Only a biopsy can show the amyloid protein deposits in the kidneys. A health care provider may recommend a kidney biopsy if other tests show kidney damage. A kidney biopsy is a procedure that involves taking a piece of kidney tissue for examination with a microscope. A health care provider performs a kidney biopsy in a hospital with light sedation and local anesthetic. The health care provider uses imaging techniques such as ultrasound or a computerized tomography (CT) scan to guide the biopsy needle into the kidney and take the tissue sample. A pathologist—a doctor who specializes in diagnosing diseases—examines the tissue in a lab for amyloid proteins and kidney damage.

How Is Dialysis-Related Amyloidosis Diagnosed?

A healthcare provider diagnoses dialysis-related amyloidosis with

- urinalysis
- blood tests
- imaging tests

A health care provider can use urinalysis and blood tests to detect the amount of amyloid proteins in urine and blood. Imaging tests, such as X-rays and CT scans, can provide pictures of bone cysts and amyloid deposits in bones, joints, tendons, and ligaments. An X-ray technician performs imaging tests in a health care provider's office, an outpatient center, or a hospital. A radiologist—a doctor who specializes in medical imaging—interprets the images. A patient does not require anesthesia.

How Is Primary Amyloidosis of the Kidneys Treated?

A healthcare provider treats primary amyloidosis of the kidneys with the following:

- medication therapy, including chemotherapy

- a stem cell transplant

- treating other conditions

Medication therapy. The goal of medication therapy, including chemotherapy, is to reduce amyloid protein levels in the blood. Many healthcare providers recommend combination medication therapy such as

- melphalan (Alkeran), a type of chemotherapy

- dexamethasone (Decadron), an anti-inflammatory steroid medication

These medications can stop the growth of the cells that make amyloid proteins. These medications may cause hair loss and serious side effects, such as nausea, vomiting, and fatigue.

Stem cell transplant. A stem cell transplant is a procedure that replaces a patient's damaged stem cells with healthy ones. Stem cells are found in the bone marrow and develop into three types of blood cells the body needs. To prepare for a stem cell transplant, the patient receives high doses of chemotherapy. The actual transplant is like a blood transfusion. The transplanted stem cells travel to the bone marrow to make healthy new blood cells. The chemotherapy a patient receives to prepare for the transplant can have serious side effects, so it is important to talk with the health care provider about the risks of this procedure.

Treating other conditions. Primary amyloidosis has no cure, so treating some of the side effects and other conditions seen with the disease is essential. Other conditions may include

- anemia—treatment may include medications
- depression—treatment may include talking with a mental health counselor and taking medications
- fatigue—treatment may include changes in diet and activity level
- kidney disease—treatment may include medications to help maintain kidney function or slow the progression of kidney disease

A patient and his or her family should talk with the health care provider about resources for support and treatment options.

How Is Dialysis-Related Amyloidosis Treated?

A healthcare provider treats dialysis-related amyloidosis with

- medication therapy
- newer, more effective hemodialysis filters
- surgery
- a kidney transplant

The goal of medication therapy and the use of newer, more effective hemodialysis filters is to reduce amyloid protein levels in the blood. Medication therapy can help reduce symptoms such as pain and inflammation. A health care provider may treat a person with dialysis-related amyloidosis who has bone, joint, and tendon problems, such as bone cysts and carpal tunnel syndrome, using surgery.

Dialysis-related amyloidosis has no cure; however, a successful kidney transplant may stop the disease from progressing.

Eating, Diet, and Nutrition

Researchers have not found that eating, diet, and nutrition play a role in causing or preventing primary amyloidosis of the kidneys or dialysis-related amyloidosis. People with nephrotic syndrome may make dietary changes such as

- limiting dietary sodium, often from salt, to help reduce edema and lower blood pressure
- decreasing liquid intake to help reduce edema and lower blood pressure

- eating a diet low in saturated fat and cholesterol to help control more-than-normal amounts of fats and cholesterol in the blood

Healthcare providers may recommend that people with kidney disease eat moderate or reduced amounts of protein. Proteins break down into waste products that the kidneys filter from the blood. Eating more protein than the body needs may burden the kidneys and cause kidney function to decline faster. However, protein intake that is too low may lead to malnutrition, a condition that occurs when the body does not get enough nutrients.

People with kidney disease on a restricted protein diet should receive blood tests that can show low nutrient levels. People with primary amyloidosis of the kidneys or dialysis-related amyloidosis should talk with a healthcare provider about dietary restrictions to best manage their individual needs.

Section 21.2

Cryoglobulinemia

This section includes text excerpted from "Cryoglobulinemia,"
Genetic and Rare Diseases Information Center (GARD), May 7, 2015.

What Is Cryoglobulinemia?

Cryoglobulinemia is a type of vasculitis that is caused by abnormal proteins (antibodies) in the blood called "cryoglobulins." At cold temperatures, these proteins become solid or gel-like, which can block blood vessels and cause a variety of health problems. Many people affected by this condition will not experience any unusual signs or symptoms. When present, symptoms vary but may include breathing problems; fatigue; glomerulonephritis; joint or muscle pain; purpura; Raynaud phenomenon; skin death; and/or skin ulcers. In some cases, the exact underlying cause is unknown; however, cryoglobulinemia can be associated with a variety of conditions including certain types of infection; chronic inflammatory diseases (such as autoimmune disease); and/or cancers of the blood or immune system. Treatment varies based on the severity of the condition, the symptoms present in each person and the underlying cause.

How Is Cryoglobulinemia Diagnosed?

Cryoglobulinemia can be diagnosed by certain blood tests, examining a sample of skin (skin biopsy), urine tests (urinalysis, particularly to look for blood in the urine), taking images of the arteries (angiogram), a chest X-ray, and/or testing the function of the nerves in the arms or legs.

How Might Cryoglobulinemia Be Treated?

The treatment for cryoglobulinemia depends on the cause and severity of this condition. Avoiding cold temperatures may be enough to treat mild cases. Severe cases may be treated by taking medication to reduce the body's immune response (corticosteroids), by removing some of the blood and replacing it with fluid or donated blood (a process called plasmapheresis), or by specifically treating diseases that may cause cryoglobulinemia (such as hepatitis C).

What Are the Expected Outcomes for Individuals with Cryoglobulinemia?

Cryoglobulinemia is usually not deadly. The outcome usually depends on the disease causing cryoglobulinemia as well as each person's response to treatments. The outcome is not as good when a person's kidneys are affected.

Section 21.3

Gamma Heavy Chain Disease

This section includes text excerpted from "Gamma Heavy Chain Disease," Genetic and Rare Diseases Information Center (GARD), July 25, 2012. Reviewed June 2016.

What Is Gamma Heavy Chain Disease?

Gamma heavy chain disease is characterized by the abnormal production of antibodies. Antibodies are made up of light chains and heavy chains. In this disorder, the heavy chain of the gamma antibody (IgG) is overproduced by the body. Gamma heavy chain disease mainly affects older adults and is similar to aggressive malignant (cancerous) lymphoma. However, some people with this disorder have no symptoms. People with symptoms may respond to chemotherapy drugs, corticosteroids, and radiation therapy. Approximately one-third of individuals with gamma heavy chain disease are also diagnosed with an autoimmune disorder.

What Are the Symptoms of Gamma Heavy Chain Disease?

The severity of symptoms varies widely among people with gamma heavy chain disease. Symptoms include, fever, mild anemia, difficulty swallowing (dysphagia), recurrent upper respiratory infections, and enlarged liver and spleen (hepatosplenomegaly).

What Causes Gamma Heavy Chain Disease?

The causes or risk factors for gamma heavy chain disease are not known.

How Might Gamma Heavy Chain Disease Be Treated?

People with symptoms may respond to chemotherapy drugs, corticosteroids, and radiation therapy. Commonly used chemotherapeutic

277

agents include cyclophosphamide, prednisone, vincristine, chlorambucil and doxorubicin. Patients are most commonly treated and followed by oncologists and/or hematologists.

Section 21.4

Plasma Cell Neoplasms

This section includes text excerpted from "Plasma Cell Neoplasms (Including Multiple Myeloma) Treatment (PDQ®)—Patient Version," National Cancer Institute (NCI), October 1, 2015.

Plasma Cell Neoplasms Are Diseases in Which the Body Makes Too Many Plasma Cells

Plasma cells develop from B lymphocytes (B cells), a type of white blood cell that is made in the bone marrow. Normally, when bacteria or viruses enter the body, some of the B cells will change into plasma cells. The plasma cells make antibodies to fight bacteria and viruses, to stop infection and disease.

Plasma cell neoplasms are diseases in which abnormal plasma cells or myeloma cells form tumors in the bones or soft tissues of the body. The plasma cells also make an antibody protein, called M protein, that is not needed by the body and does not help fight infection. These antibody proteins build up in the bone marrow and can cause the blood to thicken or can damage the kidneys.

Plasma Cell Neoplasms Can Be Benign (Not Cancer) or Malignant (Cancer)

Monoclonal gammopathy of undetermined significance (MGUS) is not cancer but can become cancer. The following types of plasma cell neoplasms are cancer:

- Waldenström's macroglobulinemia

- Plasmacytoma

- Multiple myeloma

There Are Several Types of Plasma Cell Neoplasms

Plasma cell neoplasms include the following:

Monoclonal Gammopathy of Undetermined Significance (MGUS)

In this type of plasma cell neoplasm, less than 10% of the bone marrow is made up of abnormal plasma cells and there is no cancer. The abnormal plasma cells make M protein, which is sometimes found during a routine blood or urine test. In most patients, the amount of M protein stays the same and there are no signs, symptoms, or health problems.

In some patients, MGUS may later become a more serious condition, such as amyloidosis, or cause problems with the kidneys, heart, or nerves. MGUS can also become cancer, such as multiple myeloma, lymphoplasmacytic lymphoma, or chronic lymphocytic leukemia.

Plasmacytoma

In this type of plasma cell neoplasm, the abnormal plasma cells (myeloma cells) are in one place and form one tumor, called a plasmacytoma. Sometimes plasmacytoma can be cured. There are two types of plasmacytoma.

- In isolated plasmacytoma of bone, one plasma cell tumor is found in the bone, less than 10% of the bone marrow is made up of plasma cells, and there are no other signs of cancer. Plasmacytoma of the bone often becomes multiple myeloma.

- In extramedullary plasmacytoma, one plasma cell tumor is found in soft tissue but not in the bone or the bone marrow. Extramedullary plasmacytomas commonly form in tissues of the throat, tonsil, and paranasal sinuses.

Signs and symptoms depend on where the tumor is.

- In bone, the plasmacytoma may cause pain or broken bones.

- In soft tissue, the tumor may press on nearby areas and cause pain or other problems. For example, a plasmacytoma in the throat can make it hard to swallow.

Multiple Myeloma

In multiple myeloma, abnormal plasma cells (myeloma cells) build up in the bone marrow and form tumors in many bones of the body.

These tumors may keep the bone marrow from making enough healthy blood cells. Normally, the bone marrow makes stem cells (immature cells) that become three types of mature blood cells:

- Red blood cells that carry oxygen and other substances to all tissues of the body.

- White blood cells that fight infection and disease.

- Platelets that form blood clots to help prevent bleeding.

As the number of myeloma cells increases, fewer red blood cells, white blood cells, and platelets are made. The myeloma cells also damage and weaken the bone.

Sometimes multiple myeloma does not cause any signs or symptoms. It may be found when a blood or urine test is done for another condition. Signs and symptoms may be caused by multiple myeloma or other conditions. Check with your doctor if you have any of the following:

- bone pain, especially in the back or ribs

- bones that break easily

- fever for no known reason or frequent infections

- easy bruising or bleeding

- trouble breathing

- weakness of the arms or legs

- feeling very tired

A tumor can damage the bone and cause hypercalcemia (too much calcium in the blood). This can affect many organs in the body, including the kidneys, nerves, heart, muscles, and digestive tract, and cause serious health problems.

Hypercalcemia may cause the following signs and symptoms:

- loss of appetite

- nausea or vomiting

- feeling thirsty

- frequent urination

- constipation

- feeling very tired

- muscle weakness

- restlessness

- confusion or trouble thinking

Multiple Myeloma and Other Plasma Cell Neoplasms May Cause a Condition Called Amyloidosis

In rare cases, multiple myeloma can cause peripheral nerves (nerves that are not in the brain or spinal cord) and organs to fail. This may be caused by a condition called amyloidosis. Antibody proteins build up and stick together in peripheral nerves and organs, such as the kidney and heart. This can cause the nerves and organs to become stiff and unable to work the way they should.

Amyloidosis may cause the following signs and symptoms:

- feeling very tired

- purple spots on the skin

- enlarged tongue

- diarrhea

- swelling caused by fluid in your body's tissues

- tingling or numbness in your legs and feet

Age Can Affect the Risk of Plasma Cell Neoplasms

Anything that increases your risk of getting a disease is called a risk factor. Having a risk factor does not mean that you will get cancer; not having risk factors doesn't mean that you will not get cancer. Talk with your doctor if you think you may be at risk.

Plasma cell neoplasms are most common in people who are middle aged or older. For multiple myeloma and plasmacytoma, other risk factors include the following:

- being black

- being male

- having a personal history of MGUS or plasmacytoma

- being exposed to radiation or certain chemicals

Tests That Examine the Blood, Bone Marrow, and Urine Are Used to Detect (Find) and Diagnose Multiple Myeloma and Other Plasma Cell Neoplasms

The following tests and procedures may be used:

- **Physical exam and history**: An exam of the body to check general signs of health, including checking for signs of disease, such as lumps or anything else that seems unusual. A history of the patient's health habits and past illnesses and treatments will also be taken.

- **Blood and urine immunoglobulin studies:** A procedure in which a blood or urine sample is checked to measure the amounts of certain antibodies (immunoglobulins). For multiple myeloma, beta-2-microglobulin, M protein, free light chains, and other proteins made by the myeloma cells are measured. A higher-than-normal amount of these substances can be a sign of disease.

- **Bone marrow aspiration and biopsy:** The removal of bone marrow, blood, and a small piece of bone by inserting a hollow needle into the hipbone or breastbone. A pathologist views the bone marrow, blood, and bone under a microscope to look for abnormal cells.

The following test may be done on the sample of tissue removed during the bone marrow aspiration and biopsy:

- **Cytogenetic analysis:** A test in which cells in a sample of bone marrow are viewed under a microscope to look for certain changes in the chromosomes. Other tests, such as fluorescence in situ hybridization (FISH), may also be done to look for certain changes in the chromosomes.

- **Skeletal bone survey**: In a skeletal bone survey, X-rays of all the bones in the body are taken. The X-rays are used to find areas where the bone is damaged. An X-ray is a type of energy beam that can go through the body and onto film, making a picture of areas inside the body.

- **Complete blood count (CBC) with differential:** A procedure in which a sample of blood is drawn and checked for the following:

  - The number of red blood cells and platelets.

- The number and type of white blood cells.
- The amount of hemoglobin (the protein that carries oxygen) in the red blood cells.
- The portion of the blood sample made up of red blood cells.

- **Blood chemistry studies:** A procedure in which a blood sample is checked to measure the amounts of certain substances, such as calcium or albumin, released into the blood by organs and tissues in the body. An unusual (higher or lower than normal) amount of a substance can be a sign of disease.

- **Twenty-four-hour urine test:** A test in which urine is collected for 24 hours to measure the amounts of certain substances. An unusual (higher or lower than normal) amount of a substance can be a sign of disease in the organ or tissue that makes it. A higher than normal amount of protein may be a sign of multiple myeloma.

- **MRI (magnetic resonance imaging):** A procedure that uses a magnet, radio waves, and a computer to make a series of detailed pictures of areas inside the body. This procedure is also called nuclear magnetic resonance imaging (NMRI). An MRI of the spine may be used to find areas where the bone is damaged.

- **CT scan (CAT scan):** A procedure that makes a series of detailed pictures of areas inside the body, such as the spine, taken from different angles. The pictures are made by a computer linked to an X-ray machine. A dye may be injected into a vein or swallowed to help the organs or tissues show up more clearly. This procedure is also called computed tomography, computerized tomography, or computerized axial tomography.

- **PET-CT scan:** A procedure that combines the pictures from a positron emission tomography (PET) scan and a computed tomography (CT) scan. The PET and CT scans are done at the same time with the same machine. The combined scans give more detailed pictures of areas inside the body, such as the spine, than either scan gives by itself.

Certain Factors Affect Prognosis (Chance of Recovery) and Treatment Options

The prognosis (chance of recovery) depends on the following:

- The type of plasma cell neoplasm.

- The stage of the disease.

- Whether a certain immunoglobulin (antibody) is present.

- Whether there are certain genetic changes.

- Whether the kidney is damaged.

- Whether the cancer responds to initial treatment or recurs (comes back).

Treatment options depend on the following:

- The type of plasma cell neoplasm.

- The age and general health of the patient.

- Whether there are signs, symptoms, or health problems, such as kidney failure or infection, related to the disease.

- Whether the cancer responds to initial treatment or recurs (comes back).

Chapter 22

Rh Incompatibility

What Is Rh Incompatibility?

Rh incompatibility is a condition that occurs during pregnancy if a woman has Rh-negative blood and her baby has Rh-positive blood.

"Rh-negative" and "Rh-positive" refer to whether your blood has Rh factor. Rh factor is a protein on red blood cells. If you have Rh factor, you're Rh-positive. If you don't have it, you're Rh-negative. Rh factor is inherited (passed from parents to children through the genes). Most people are Rh-positive.

Whether you have Rh factor doesn't affect your general health. However, it can cause problems during pregnancy.

Other Names for Rh Incompatibility

- Rh disease

- Rh-induced hemolytic disease of the newborn

What Causes Rh Incompatibility?

A difference in blood type between a pregnant woman and her baby causes Rh incompatibility. The condition occurs if a woman is Rh-negative and her baby is Rh-positive.

This chapter includes text excerpted from "Rh Incompatibility," National Heart, Lung, and Blood Institute (NHLBI), January 1, 2011. Reviewed July 2016.

When you're pregnant, blood from your baby can cross into your bloodstream, especially during delivery. If you're Rh-negative and your baby is Rh-positive, your body will react to the baby's blood as a foreign substance.

Your body will create antibodies (proteins) against the baby's Rh-positive blood. These antibodies can cross the placenta and attack the baby's red blood cells. This can lead to hemolytic anemia in the baby.

Rh incompatibility usually doesn't cause problems during a first pregnancy. The baby often is born before many of the antibodies develop.

However, once you've formed Rh antibodies, they remain in your body. Thus, the condition is more likely to cause problems in second or later pregnancies (if the baby is Rh-positive).

With each pregnancy, your body continues to make Rh antibodies. As a result, each Rh-positive baby you conceive becomes more at risk for serious problems, such as severe hemolytic anemia.

Who Is at Risk for Rh Incompatibility?

An Rh-negative woman who conceives a child with an Rh-positive man is at risk for Rh incompatibility.

Rh factor is inherited (passed from parents to children through the genes). If you're Rh-negative and the father of your baby is Rh-positive, the baby has a 50 percent or more chance of having Rh-positive blood.

Simple blood tests can show whether you and the father of your baby are Rh-positive or Rh-negative.

If you're Rh-negative, your risk of problems from Rh incompatibility is higher if you were exposed to Rh-positive blood before the pregnancy. This may have happened during:

- An earlier pregnancy (usually during delivery). You also may have been exposed to Rh-positive blood if you had bleeding or abdominal trauma (for example, from a car accident) during the pregnancy.

- An ectopic pregnancy, a miscarriage, or an induced abortion. (An ectopic pregnancy is a pregnancy that starts outside of the uterus, or womb.)

- A mismatched blood transfusion or blood and marrow stem cell transplant.

- An injection or puncture with a needle or other object containing Rh-positive blood.

Certain tests also can expose you to Rh-positive blood. Examples include amniocentesis and chorionic villus sampling (CVS).

Amniocentesis is a test that you may have during pregnancy. Your doctor uses a needle to remove a small amount of fluid from the sac around your baby. The fluid is then tested for various reasons.

CVS also may be done during pregnancy. For this test, your doctor threads a thin tube through the vagina and cervix to the placenta. He or she removes a tissue sample from the placenta using gentle suction. The tissue sample is tested for various reasons.

Unless you were treated with the medicine that prevents Rh antibodies (Rh immune globulin) after each of these events, you're at risk for Rh incompatibility during current and future pregnancies.

What Are the Signs and Symptoms of Rh Incompatibility?

Rh incompatibility doesn't cause signs or symptoms in a pregnant woman. In a baby, the condition can lead to hemolytic anemia. Hemolytic anemia is a condition in which red blood cells are destroyed faster than the body can replace them.

Red blood cells contain hemoglobin, an iron-rich protein that carries oxygen to the body. Without enough red blood cells and hemoglobin, the baby won't get enough oxygen.

Hemolytic anemia can cause mild to severe signs and symptoms in a newborn, such as jaundice and a buildup of fluid.

Jaundice is a yellowish color of the skin and whites of the eyes. When red blood cells die, they release hemoglobin into the blood. The hemoglobin is broken down into a compound called bilirubin. This compound gives the skin and eyes a yellowish color. High levels of bilirubin can lead to brain damage in the baby.

The buildup of fluid is a result of heart failure. Without enough hemoglobin-carrying red blood cells, the baby's heart has to work harder to move oxygen-rich blood through the body. This stress can lead to heart failure.

Heart failure can cause fluid to build up in many parts of the body. When this occurs in a fetus or newborn, the condition is called hydrops fetalis.

Severe hemolytic anemia can be fatal to a newborn at the time of birth or shortly after.

How Is Rh Incompatibility Diagnosed?

Rh incompatibility is diagnosed with blood tests. To find out whether a baby is developing hemolytic anemia and how serious it is, doctors may use more advanced tests, such as ultrasound.

Specialists Involved

An obstetrician will screen for Rh incompatibility. This is a doctor who specializes in treating pregnant women. The obstetrician also will monitor the pregnancy and the baby for problems related to hemolytic anemia. He or she also will oversee treatment to prevent problems with future pregnancies.

A pediatrician or hematologist treats newborns who have hemolytic anemia and related problems. A pediatrician is a doctor who specializes in treating children. A hematologist is a doctor who specializes in treating people who have blood diseases and disorders.

Diagnostic Tests

If you're pregnant, your doctor will order a simple blood test at your first prenatal visit to learn whether you're Rh-positive or Rh-negative.

If you're Rh-negative, you also may have another blood test called an antibody screen. This test shows whether you have Rh antibodies in your blood. If you do, it means that you were exposed to Rh-positive blood before and you're at risk for Rh incompatibility.

If you're Rh-negative and you don't have Rh antibodies, your baby's father also will be tested to find out his Rh type. If he's Rh-negative too, the baby has no chance of having Rh-positive blood. Thus, there's no risk of Rh incompatibility.

However, if the baby's father is Rh-positive, the baby has a 50 percent or more chance of having Rh-positive blood. As a result, you're at high risk of developing Rh incompatibility.

If your baby's father is Rh-positive, or if it's not possible to find out his Rh status, your doctor may do a test called amniocentesis.

For this test, your doctor inserts a hollow needle through your abdominal wall into your uterus. He or she removes a small amount of fluid from the sac around the baby. The fluid is tested to learn whether the baby is Rh-positive. (Rarely, an amniocentesis can expose you to Rh-positive blood).

Your doctor also may use this test to measure bilirubin levels in your baby. Bilirubin builds up as a result of red blood cells dying too quickly. The higher the level of bilirubin is, the greater the chance that the baby has hemolytic anemia.

If Rh incompatibility is known or suspected, you'll be tested for Rh antibodies one or more times during your pregnancy. This test often is done at least once at your sixth or seventh month of pregnancy.

The results from this test also can suggest how severe the baby's hemolytic anemia has become. Higher levels of antibodies suggest more severe hemolytic anemia.

To check your baby for hemolytic anemia, your doctor also may use a test called Doppler ultrasound. He or she will use this test to measure how fast blood is flowing through an artery in the baby's head.

Doppler ultrasound uses sound waves to measure how fast blood is moving. The faster the blood flow is, the greater the risk of hemolytic anemia. This is because the anemia will cause the baby's heart to pump more blood.

How Is Rh Incompatibility Treated?

Rh incompatibility is treated with a medicine called Rh immune globulin. Treatment for a baby who has hemolytic anemia will vary based on the severity of the condition.

Goals of Treatment

The goals of treating Rh incompatibility are to ensure that your baby is healthy and to lower your risk for the condition in future pregnancies.

Treatment for Rh Incompatibility

If Rh incompatibility is diagnosed during your pregnancy, you'll receive Rh immune globulin in your seventh month of pregnancy and again within 72 hours of delivery.

You also may receive Rh immune globulin if the risk of blood transfer between you and the baby is high (for example, if you've had a miscarriage, ectopic pregnancy, or bleeding during pregnancy).

Rh immune globulin contains Rh antibodies that attach to the Rh-positive blood cells in your blood. When this happens, your body doesn't react to the baby's Rh-positive cells as a foreign substance. As a result, your body doesn't make Rh antibodies. Rh immune globulin must be given at the correct times to work properly.

Once you have formed Rh antibodies, the medicine will no longer help. That's why a woman who has Rh-negative blood must be treated with the medicine with each pregnancy or any other event that allows her blood to mix with Rh-positive blood.

Rh immune globulin is injected into the muscle of your arm or buttock. Side effects may include soreness at the injection site and a slight fever. The medicine also may be injected into a vein.

Treatment for Hemolytic Anemia

Several options are available for treating hemolytic anemia in a baby. In mild cases, no treatment may be needed. If treatment is needed, the baby may be given a medicine called erythropoietin and iron supplements. These treatments can prompt the body to make red blood cells.

If the hemolytic anemia is severe, the baby may get a blood transfusion through the umbilical cord. If the hemolytic anemia is severe and the baby is almost full-term, your doctor may induce labor early. This allows the baby's doctor to begin treatment right away.

A newborn who has severe anemia may be treated with a blood exchange transfusion. The procedure involves slowly removing the newborn's blood and replacing it with fresh blood or plasma from a donor.

Newborns also may be treated with special lights to reduce the amount of bilirubin in their blood. These babies may have jaundice (a yellowish color of the skin and whites of the eyes). High levels of bilirubin cause jaundice.

Reducing the blood's bilirubin level is important because high levels of this compound can cause brain damage. High levels of bilirubin often are seen in babies who have hemolytic anemia. This is because the compound forms when red blood cells break down.

How Can Rh Incompatibility Be Prevented?

Rh incompatibility can be prevented with Rh immune globulin, as long as the medicine is given at the correct times. Once you have formed Rh antibodies, the medicine will no longer help.

Thus, a woman who has Rh-negative blood must be treated with Rh immune globulin during and after each pregnancy or after any other event that allows her blood to mix with Rh-positive blood.

Early prenatal care also can help prevent some of the problems linked to Rh incompatibility. For example, your doctor can find out early whether you're at risk for the condition.

If you're at risk, your doctor can closely monitor your pregnancy. He or she will watch for signs of hemolytic anemia in your baby and provided treatment as needed.

Living with Rh Incompatibility

If you have Rh-negative blood, injections of Rh immune globulin can reduce your risk of Rh incompatibility in future pregnancies. It's important to get this medicine every time you give birth to an Rh-positive baby or come in contact with Rh-positive blood.

If you're Rh-negative, your risk of problems from Rh incompatibility is higher if you were exposed to Rh-positive blood before your current pregnancy.

You also can be exposed to Rh-positive blood during certain tests, such as amniocentesis and chorionic villus sampling.

Unless you were treated with Rh immune globulin after each of these events, you're at risk for Rh incompatibility during current and future pregnancies.

Let your doctor know about your risk early in your pregnancy. This allows him or her to carefully monitor your pregnancy and promptly treat any problems that arise.

Chapter 23

White Blood Cell Disorders

Chapter Contents

x

Section 23.1

Hypereosinophilic Disorders

This section includes text excerpted from "Eosinophilic Disorders," National Institute of Allergy and Infectious Diseases (NIAID), April 23, 2014.

What Are Eosinophils?

Eosinophils are specialized white blood cells that participate in inflammatory processes such as allergic diseases. They also are involved in tissue repair and remodeling.

Eosinophils belong to a category of white blood cells called granulocytes. Eosinophils contain small particles, called secondary granules, packed with a variety of proteins and chemicals that regulate immune responses. Activation of eosinophils triggers their release of the contents of these granules, a process known as degranulation. In addition to harming intruding pathogens, the substances released during degranulation also can damage the body's cells and tissues.

In healthy people, eosinophils comprise approximately 1 to 6 percent of white blood cells. The body may produce more of these cells in response to parasitic and fungal infections. Certain allergic diseases, skin conditions, autoimmune disorders, cancers, and bone marrow diseases also may result in elevated eosinophil counts. Many people with eosinophilic disorders have high numbers of eosinophils in their blood or tissues over a long period of time. Sometimes, the presence of excess eosinophils in tissue, called "eosinophilic inflammation," can result in tissue damage.

Hypereosinophilic Syndrome

Hypereosinophilic syndrome (HES) describes a group of chronic disorders in which very high numbers of eosinophils are present in the blood and tissues. People diagnosed with HES have elevated blood eosinophil levels on at least two occasions and signs or symptoms of eosinophil infiltration of different tissues. HES can affect any organ in the body and often involves the skin, lungs, gastrointestinal tract, heart, and nervous system.

HES is a rare group of diseases affecting an estimated 0.36 to 6.3 people per 100,000 in the United States. Although HES characteristically develops between the ages of 20 and 50 years, young children and the elderly also can be affected.

Cause

There are many different types of HES. In 10 to 20 percent of cases, HES is caused by a problem in the eosinophil itself. Most of these cases are due to an abnormality in chromosome 4 that leads to the fusion of two genes. This fused gene, called *FIP1L1-PDGFRA*, produces an abnormal protein that may cause changes in bone marrow cells, leading to increased levels of eosinophils. In other cases, HES is caused by abnormalities in a different type of blood cell called a lymphocyte. These abnormal lymphocytes produce substances that lead to increased eosinophil production. A very small number of cases are hereditary. In more than half of cases, the cause of HES is unknown.

Symptoms

HES symptoms are extremely varied and depend on the organs involved and the severity of the disease. People with HES commonly experience fatigue, muscle and joint pains, rashes, itching, abdominal pain, shortness of breath, and cough. Chest pain and symptoms of nervous system involvement, such as weakness or numbness, can be signs of life-threatening complications.

Diagnosis

Currently, there are no specific diagnostic tests for HES. Doctors perform blood tests to measure eosinophil counts. More than 1,500 eosinophils per microliter of blood may indicate HES. Healthy people typically have less than 500 eosinophils per microliter of blood.

To diagnose HES, doctors also conduct tests to measure tissue and organ damage caused by eosinophil invasion and to rule out other known causes of high eosinophil levels, such as parasitic infections and certain bone marrow diseases. These may include more blood tests, ultrasounds, X-rays, or bone marrow biopsies.

Treatment

HES is a life long condition, and there currently is no cure. Treatments for HES aim to prevent or control organ damage by decreasing eosinophil levels.

Corticosteroids

Standard treatment for most variants of HES includes corticosteroids, which often reduce eosinophil counts effectively. However, eosinophil levels may rise and symptoms of organ damage may reappear when the drug is stopped. Long-term use of corticosteroids carries the risk of harmful side effects, including bone loss, fractures, weight gain, depression, and diabetes.

Imatinib Mesylate (Gleevec)

People with HES who have the *FIP1L1-PDGFRA* fusion gene are treated with imatinib mesylate (Gleevec), which blocks the action of the abnormal protein produced from the fusion gene. Studies have indicated that imatinib can reduce eosinophil levels and stop disease progression within one to two weeks of starting treatment. Some people with HES who do not have the fusion gene also respond to imatinib treatment.

Hydroxyurea

Doctors may prescribe hydroxyurea in combination with corticosteroids or other HES therapies. Sometimes, hydroxyurea may be used alone to treat HES patients who do not respond to corticosteroids. Hydroxyurea blocks the growth of cells by interfering with DNA synthesis.

Interferon-Alpha

Interferon-alpha can be an effective and sometimes life-saving treatment for people with certain HES variants who do not respond to corticosteroids or other drugs. Interferon-alpha may sometimes be used in combination with other drugs. However, the drug has several common side effects, including flu-like symptoms, depression, and fatigue.

Section 23.2

Langerhans Cell Histiocytosis

This section includes text excerpted from "Langerhans
Cell Histiocytosis," Genetic and Rare Diseases
Information Center (GARD), October 18, 2014.

What Is Langerhans Cell Histiocytosis?

Langerhans cell histiocytosis (LCH) is a disorder that primarily
affects children, but is also found in adults of all ages. People with
LCH produce too many Langerhans cells or histiocytes, a form of white
blood cell found in healthy people that is supposed to protect the body
from infection. In people with LCH, these cells multiply excessively
and build up in certain areas of the body, causing tumors called gran-
ulomas to form. The symptoms vary among affected individuals, and
the cause of LCH is unknown. In most cases, this condition is not
life-threatening. Some people do experience life-long problems associated with LCH.

What Are the Signs and Symptoms of Langerhans Cell Histiocytosis?

Symptoms of Langerhans cell histiocytosis (LCH) can vary greatly
from person to person depending on how much of the body is involved
and what part(s) are affected. The disease can affect virtually every
organ, including skin, bones, lymph nodes, bone marrow, liver, spleen,
lungs, gastrointestinal tract, thymus, central nervous system, and
hormone glands. The symptoms may range from localized bone lesions
or skin disease to multiple organ involvement and severe dysfunction.

Below are the organs that may be affected as well as the symptoms
that might be observed:

- **Skin** – Red, scaly papules in areas where opposing skin surfaces
  touch or rub (e.g. skin folds) are commonly seen in LCH. Infants
  with the skin presentation on the scalp are often misdiagnosed
  with cradle cap. The skin symptoms usually improve without
  treatment.

- **Bone** – Lesions that cause bone destruction are common, with the skull, lower limbs, ribs, pelvis, and vertebrae usually being affected. Symptoms may include pain, swelling, limited motion, and inability to bear weight.

- **Lymph node** – Lymph node involvement may be limited or associated with a skin or bone lesion or disseminated disease. Although any of the lymph nodes may be affected, the cervical lymph nodes are where the disease commonly occurs. Individuals usually only present with pain of the lymph node affected. If only one lymph node is affected, prognosis is normally good and treatment is unnecessary.

- **Liver** – Liver involvement at the time of diagnosis is generally associated with more severe disease. Symptoms may include ascites, jaundice, low levels of protein, and prolonged clotting time.

- **Central nervous system (CNS) and hormone** – CNS involvement is rare and may be devastating. The most common result of CNS involvement is the altering of hormonal function, with some individuals developing diabetes insipidus.

What Causes Langerhans Cell Histiocytosis?

The cause of Langerhans cell histiocytosis is unknown. It may be triggered by an unusual reaction of the immune system to something commonly found in the environment. It is not considered to be an infection or cancer. It is not known to be hereditary or communicable.

Is Langerhans Cell Histiocytosis Inherited?

Although Langerhans cell histiocytosis is generally considered a sporadic, non-hereditary condition, it has reportedly affected more than one individual in a family in a very limited number of cases (particularly identical twins).

How Is Langerhans Cell Histiocytosis Diagnosed?

Testing for Langerhans cell histiocytosis (LCH) may include bronchoscopy with biopsy, X-ray, skin biopsy, bone marrow biopsy, complete blood count, and pulmonary function tests. Because LCH is sometimes associated with cancer, CT scans and a biopsy may be done to rule out possible cancer.

How Might Langerhans Cell Histiocytosis Be Treated?

Treatment for Langerhans cell histiocytosis (LCH) depends upon the individual patient; it may differ depending on the type and severity of the condition as well as what part(s) of the body are affected. In some cases, the disease will regress without any treatment at all. In other cases, limited surgery and small doses of radiation therapy or chemotherapy will be needed, depending on the extent of the disease. Treatment is planned after complete evaluation of the patient, with the goal of using as little treatment as possible to keep the disease under control.

What Is the Typical Prognosis for People with Langerhans Cell Histiocytosis?

The prognosis (chance of recovery) for people with Langerhans cell histiocytosis can vary greatly from patient to patient, but in the majority of children, the disease resolves itself. Prognosis seems to be dependent mainly on the number of organ systems involved, the severity of organ involvement, and to a lesser rate, the age at which symptoms occur. In general, patients who are young and those with disseminated disease and organ dysfunction tend to have a poorer prognosis. Newborns who present only with skin lesions tend to do well. Therefore, the age at presentation is only important when multiple organs are affected. Additionally, individuals who have liver, spleen, lung, or bone marrow involvement usually have a worse prognosis. In a study looking at patients from several centers, it was shown that the best prognostic indicator was the patient's response to chemotherapy during the first six weeks of therapy. Therefore, it has been recommended by some that individuals who do not respond positively within the first six weeks of treatment should be treated more aggressively.

Other Names for This Disease

- LCH
- Histiocytosis X
- Eosinophilic granuloma (formerly)
- Letterer-Siwe disease (formerly)
- Hand-Schüller-Christian syndrome (formerly)

Section 23.3

Lymphocytopenia

This section includes text excerpted from
"Lymphocytopenia," National Heart, Lung, and Blood
Institute (NHLBI), December 30, 2013.

What Causes Lymphocytopenia?

In general, lymphocytopenia (a low lymphocyte count) occurs
because:

- The body doesn't make enough lymphocytes.

- The body makes enough lymphocytes, but they're destroyed.

- The lymphocytes get stuck in the spleen or lymph nodes.

A combination of these factors also may cause a low lymphocyte
count.

Many diseases, conditions, and factors can lead to a low lymphocyte
count. These conditions can be acquired or inherited. "Acquired" means
you aren't born with the condition, but you develop it. "Inherited"
means your parents passed the gene for the condition on to you.

Exactly how each disease, condition, or factor affects your lymphocyte count isn't known. Some people have low lymphocyte counts with
no underlying cause.

Acquired Causes

Many acquired diseases, conditions, and factors can cause lymphocytopenia. Examples include:

- infectious diseases, such as AIDS, viral hepatitis, tuberculosis,
  and typhoid fever

- autoimmune disorders, such as lupus. (Autoimmune disorders
  occur if the body's immune system mistakenly attacks the body's
  cells and tissues.)

- steroid therapy

- blood cancer and other blood diseases, such as Hodgkin's disease and aplastic anemia

- radiation and chemotherapy (treatments for cancer)

Inherited Causes

Certain inherited diseases and conditions can lead to lymphocytopenia. Examples include DiGeorge anomaly, Wiskott-Aldrich syndrome, severe combined immunodeficiency syndrome, and ataxia-telangiectasia. These inherited conditions are rare.

Who Is at Risk for Lymphocytopenia?

People at highest risk for lymphocytopenia have one of the diseases, conditions, or factors that can cause a low lymphocyte count. This includes people who have:

- AIDS or other infectious diseases

- Autoimmune disorders

- Blood cancers or other blood diseases

- Certain inherited diseases or conditions

People who have had steroid therapy or radiation or chemotherapy (treatments for cancer) also are at increased risk.

What Are the Signs and Symptoms of Lymphocytopenia?

A low lymphocyte count alone may not cause any signs or symptoms. The condition usually is found when a person is tested for other diseases or conditions, such as AIDS.

If you have unusual infections, repeat infections, and/or infections that won't go away, your doctor may suspect that you have lymphocytopenia. Fever is the most common symptom of infection.

How Is Lymphocytopenia Diagnosed?

Your doctor will diagnose lymphocytopenia based on your medical history, a physical exam, and test results.

A low lymphocyte count alone may not cause any signs or symptoms. Thus, the condition often is diagnosed during testing for other diseases or conditions.

Specialists Involved

Your primary care doctor may notice that you have unusual infections, repeat infections, and/or infections that won't go away. These infections may be signs of lymphocytopenia. Your primary care doctor may refer you to an infectious disease specialist to find out what's causing the infections.

You also may see a hematologist (blood disease specialist) or an immunologist (immune disorders specialist). Blood diseases and immune disorders can cause lymphocytopenia.

Medical History

To assess your risk for a low lymphocyte count, your doctor may ask:

- About your risk for AIDS, including questions about blood transfusions, sexual partners, intravenous (IV) drug use, and exposure to infectious blood or bodily fluids at work.

- Whether you've ever had radiation or chemotherapy (treatments for cancer).

- Whether you've ever been diagnosed with a blood disease or immune disorder, or whether you have a family history of such illnesses.

Physical Exam

Your doctor will do a physical exam to look for signs of infection, such as fever. He or she may check your abdomen for signs of an enlarged spleen and your neck for signs of enlarged lymph nodes.

Your doctor also will look for signs and symptoms of diseases and conditions that can affect your lymphocyte count, such as AIDS and blood cancers.

Diagnostic Tests

Your doctor may recommend one or more of the following tests to help diagnose a low lymphocyte count.

Complete Blood Count with Differential

A complete blood count (CBC) measures many parts of your blood. The test checks the number of red blood cells, white blood cells, and platelets in your blood. The CBC will show whether you have a low number of white blood cells.

Lymphocytes account for 20 to 40 percent of all white blood cells. Although a CBC will show an overall low white blood cell count, it won't show whether the number of lymphocytes is low.

You may need a more detailed test, called a CBC with differential, to find out whether you have a low lymphocyte count. This test shows whether you have low levels of certain types of white blood cells, such as lymphocytes. The test results can help your doctor diagnose lymphocytopenia.

Flow Cytometry

Flow cytometry looks at many types of blood cells. It's even more detailed than a CBC with differential. Flow cytometry can measure the levels of the different types of lymphocytes—T cells, B cells, and natural killer cells.

The test can help diagnose the underlying cause of lymphocytopenia. Some underlying conditions cause low levels of T cells. Others may cause low levels of B cells or natural killer cells.

Tests for Underlying Conditions

Many diseases and conditions can cause lymphocytopenia. Your doctor will want to find the cause of the disorder. You may be tested for HIV/AIDS, tuberculosis, blood diseases, and immune disorders.

Tests for these underlying conditions might include blood tests, bone marrow tests, and lymph node tests.

Lymph nodes are part of the immune system. They're found in many places in your body. During a physical exam, your doctor may find that certain lymph nodes are swollen. In lymphocytopenia, the lymph nodes may hold onto too many lymphocytes instead of releasing them into the bloodstream.

To test a lymph node, you may need to have it removed. Removing a lymph node involves minor surgery.

How Is Lymphocytopenia Treated?

If you have mild lymphocytopenia with no underlying cause, you may not need treatment. The disorder may improve on its own.

If you have unusual infections, repeat infections, and/or infections that won't go away due to lymphocytopenia, you'll need treatment for the infections.

If you have a disease or condition that's causing lymphocytopenia, your doctor will prescribe treatment for that illness. Treating the underlying problem will help treat the lymphocytopenia.

Treatment for Infections

A low lymphocyte count makes it hard for your body to fight infections. You may get infections caused by viruses, fungi, parasites, or bacteria.

Treatment for an infection will depend on its cause. You also may need treatment after an infection is gone to help prevent repeat infections.

Children who have serious, ongoing bacterial infections may get a medicine called immune globulin. This medicine helps boost the immune system and fight infections.

Treatment for Underlying Diseases or Conditions

Many diseases and conditions can cause lymphocytopenia. Examples include infectious diseases, such as AIDS; blood diseases, such as aplastic anemia; and inherited diseases, such as Wiskott-Aldrich syndrome.

Your treatment will depend on your underlying disease or condition.

Emerging Treatments

Researchers are looking at ways to increase lymphocyte production in people who have lymphocytopenia with serious underlying conditions.

For example, some studies are looking into blood and marrow stem cell transplants. This procedure may help treat or cure some of the conditions that can cause a low lymphocyte count.

Other studies are looking at medicines and other substances that can help the body make more lymphocytes.

How Can Lymphocytopenia Be Prevented?

You can't prevent lymphocytopenia that's caused by an inherited condition. However, you can take steps to control lymphocytopenia. Follow your treatment plan and take all medicines as your doctor advises.

Early diagnosis also can help control lymphocytopenia. In the United States, newborns are routinely screened for an immune condition that can lead to lymphocytopenia. This allows doctors to diagnose the disorder before serious problems develop.

Living with Lymphocytopenia

Treating and Preventing Infections

The main risk of lymphocytopenia is getting unusual infections, repeat infections, and/or infections that won't go away. If you have the disorder, you may get treatments to prevent infections or to treat infections you already have.

You also can take other steps to prevent infections. For example:

- Stay away from people who are sick, and avoid large crowds of people.

- Avoid foods that can expose you to bacteria, such as uncooked foods.

- Wash your hands often.

- Brush and floss your teeth and get regular dental care to reduce the risk of infection in your mouth and throat.

- Ask your doctor whether you should get a yearly flu shot and the pneumonia vaccine.

Know the signs of an infection, such as a fever. Call your doctor right away if you think you have an infection.

Treating an Underlying Disease or Condition

If you have a disease or condition that's causing lymphocytopenia, you'll need treatment for that condition.

You'll likely have regular tests to show how the treatment is working. For example, you may have blood tests to check the number of lymphocytes in your blood.

If the treatments for the underlying condition are working, the number of lymphocytes in your blood may go up.

Physical Activity

Talk with your doctor about what types and amounts of physical activity are safe for you. You may want to avoid activities that could result in injuries or increase your risk of infections.

Section 23.4

Neutropenia

This section is excerpted from "Neutropenia and
Risk for Infection," Centers for Disease Control and
Prevention (CDC), October 20, 2011. Reviewed July 2016.

What Is Neutropenia?

Neutropenia, is a decrease in the number of white blood cells. These
cells are the body's main defense against infection. Neutropenia is common after receiving chemotherapy and increases your risk for infections.

Why Does Chemotherapy Cause Neutropenia?

These cancer-fighting drugs work by killing fast-growing cells in
the body—both good and bad. These drugs kill cancer cells as well as
healthy white blood cells.

How Do I Know If I Have Neutropenia?

Your doctor or nurse will tell you. Because neutropenia is common
after receiving chemotherapy, your doctor may draw some blood to
look for neutropenia.

When Will I Be Most Likely to Have Neutropenia?

Neutropenia often occurs between 7 and 12 days after you receive
chemotherapy. This period can be different depending upon the chemotherapy you get. Your doctor or nurse will let you know exactly when
your white blood cell count is likely to be at its lowest. You should
carefully watch for signs and symptoms of infection during this time.

How Can I Prevent Neutropenia?

There is not much you can do to prevent neutropenia from occurring, but you can decrease your risk for getting an infection while your
white blood cell count is low.

How Can I Prevent an Infection?

In addition to receiving treatment from your doctor, the following suggestions can help prevent infections:

- Clean your hands frequently.
- Try to avoid crowded places and contact with people who are sick.
- Do not share food, drink cups, utensils or other personal items, such as toothbrushes.
- Shower or bathe daily and use an unscented lotion to prevent your skin from becoming dry and cracked.
- Cook meat and eggs all the way through to kill any germs.
- Carefully wash raw fruits and vegetables.
- Protect your skin from direct contact with pet bodily waste (urine or feces) by wearing vinyl or household cleaning gloves when cleaning up after your pet. Wash your hands immediately afterwards.
- Use gloves for gardening.
- Clean your teeth and gums with a soft toothbrush, and if your doctor or nurse recommends one, use a mouthwash to prevent mouth sores.
- Try and keep all your household surfaces clean.
- Get the seasonal flu shot as soon as it is available.

What If I Have to Go to the Emergency Room?

Cancer patients receiving chemotherapy should not sit in a waiting room for a long time. While you are receiving chemotherapy, fever may be a sign of infection. Infections can become serious very quickly. When you check in, tell them right away that you are getting chemotherapy and have a fever. This may be an indication of an infection.

What Are the Signs and Symptoms of an Infection?

For patients with neutropenia, even a minor infection can quickly become serious. Call your doctor right away if you have:

- fever that is 100.4°F (38°C) or higher for more than one hour, or a one-time temperature of 101° F or higher

- chills and sweats
- change in cough or new cough
- sore throat or new mouth sore
- shortness of breath
- nasal congestion
- stiff neck
- burning or pain with urination
- unusual vaginal discharge or irritation
- increased urination
- redness, soreness, or swelling in any area, including surgical wounds and ports
- diarrhea
- vomiting
- pain in the abdomen or rectum
- new onset of pain
- changes in skin, urination, or mental status

Part Four

Bleeding and Clotting Disorders

Chapter 24

What Are Hereditary Bleeding and Clotting Disorders?

Bleeding Disorders

The blood clotting process, known as coagulation, occurs when an injury causes a wound to bleed. When a healthy person is injured and begins to bleed, blood platelets immediately begin bonding together to form a blood clot, stopping further blood loss. Bleeding disorders interfere with the body's ability to form blood clots. This can result in excessive or abnormal bleeding internally or externally, depending upon the nature of the wound.

In most cases, bleeding disorders are inherited. Certain chronic health conditions can also result in a person developing an acquired bleeding disorder. Bleeding disorders can result from anemia, HIV, low red blood cell count, liver disease, leukemia, vitamin K deficiency, and use of certain medications known as anti-coagulants.

Types of Bleeding Disorders

Bleeding disorders are primarily caused by insufficient levels or absence of blood proteins known as clotting factors. There are 13 blood clotting factors that help blood clots to form. Bleeding disorders are diagnosed and categorized according to the specific clotting factor that is deficient in a person's blood.

Hemophilia A (factor VIII deficiency) and Hemophilia B (factor IX deficiency) are bleeding disorders that result in excessive bleeding after injury to deep tissue (for example, in joints and muscles).

Von Willebrand disease is an inherited bleeding disorder affecting the body's ability to form blood clots due to lack of the von Willebrand factor. People who live with von Willebrand disease experience excessive bleeding after injuries to skin or mucous membranes (for example, inside the nose, mouth, and intestines).

Bleeding disorders due to deficiencies in the remaining clotting factors occur more rarely than hemophilia and von Willebrand's disease.

Symptoms and Risks

Bleeding disorder symptoms tend to be different for each condition. Most bleeding disorders share primary symptoms such as frequent unexplained bruising, frequent nosebleeds, excessive bleeding after minor cuts, scrapes, or dental surgery, bleeding into joints or pooling blood in joints, and excessive or prolonged menstrual bleeding.

Bleeding disorders can expose a person to serious health risks if left undiagnosed and/or untreated. Some bleeding disorders result in unseen complications such as internal bleeding in the intestines, the brain, or joints. Women with untreated bleeding disorders can be at greater risk for developing anemia, a condition in which the body lacks sufficient levels of red blood cells. Anemia can result in dizziness, shortness of breath, and persistent general fatigue.

Diagnosis

Most bleeding disorders are diagnosed through blood tests. These tests measure the levels of certain blood components such as red and white blood cells, platelet function, and bleeding time. Health professionals typically analyze blood test results while also considering a person's medical history. A medical history interview may be conducted, with a focus on the frequency of episodes of excessive bleeding, how long it usually takes to stop bleeding after a wound, and whether any family members have been diagnosed with bleeding disorders.

Clotting Disorders

Clotting disorders are similar to bleeding disorders in that both types of conditions affect the body's ability to form blood clots properly.

However, where bleeding disorders indicate a lack of proper blood clot formation, clotting disorders result in unnecessary or excessive blood clot formation.

Clotting disorders can be inherited or acquired. Acquired clotting disorders can result from traumatic injury, surgery, certain chronic health conditions, and the use of certain medications.

Types of Clotting Disorders

Clotting disorders are typically caused by abnormal levels of the blood proteins that prevent blood clotting. Like bleeding disorders, clotting disorders are also categorized and diagnosed according to the specific blood protein that is affected. The most common form of inherited clotting disorder is Factor V Leiden, a condition that results in excessive blood clots. Other inherited clotting disorders are indicated by abnormal levels of antithrombin, protein C, protein S, homocysteine, fibrinogen, or factors VIII, IX, and XI. A genetic disorder known as Prothrombin gene mutation also produces excessive blood clotting.

Many health conditions and treatments can result in acquired clotting disorder. These include cancer and cancer treatments, central venous catheter placements, deep vein thrombosis, heart attack, heart failure, HIV/AIDS, hormone replacement therapy, inflammatory bowel syndrome (IBS), liver disease, nephrotic syndrome, obesity, oral contraceptives (birth control pills), pregnancy, prolonged immobility due to bed rest or other reason, traumatic injury, stroke, and surgery. Clotting disorders can also arise from frequent, lengthy airplane travel.

Symptoms and Risks

Clotting disorders, also known as hypercoagulable state or thrombophilia, can be dangerous if left undiagnosed and/or untreated. Clotting disorders can cause blood clots to form within blood vessels as blood travels through the body. This type of blood clot is known as a thrombus or embolus and can result in a clotting disorder known as disseminated intravascular coagulation. Blood clots that form in blood vessels can move throughout the body's bloodstream, resulting in serious complications if the clot lodges in the lungs, liver, intestines, kidneys, or veins in the legs and arms. Blood clots that move through or become lodged in arteries can cause stroke, heart attack, or loss of a limb due to restricted blood supply.

Clotting disorder symptoms vary according to each specific condition. Some common symptoms include pain or swelling of arms or legs, changes in skin color or temperature (redness, warmth), chest pain, shortness of breath, rapid heartbeat, heart attack or stroke at a young age, and multiple pregnancies that end in miscarriage or stillbirth.

Diagnosis

Clotting disorders are most often diagnosed through a medical history interview, various blood tests, diagnostic imaging such as magnetic resonance imaging (MRI), ultrasound, or computed tomography (CT scan). Some important medical history considerations in the diagnosis of clotting disorders are unexplained or recurring blood clots, history of frequent miscarriages, stroke or heart attack at a young age, and family members who have been diagnosed with a clotting disorder.

References

1. Kahn, April. "What is a Bleeding Disorder?" Health Line. December 3, 2015.

2. "Bleeding Disorders," National Hemophilia Foundation.

3. "Blood Clotting Disorders (Hypercoagulable States)," Cleveland Clinic. December 2015.

4. "Coagulation Disorders," Riley Children's Health.

Chapter 25

Hemophilia

What Is Hemophilia?

Hemophilia is an inherited bleeding disorder in which the blood does not clot properly. This can lead to spontaneous bleeding as well as bleeding following injuries or surgery.

Blood contains many proteins called clotting factors that can help to stop bleeding. People with hemophilia have low levels of either factor VIII (8) or factor IX (9). The severity of hemophilia that a person has is determined by the amount of factor in the blood. The lower the amount of the factor, the more likely it is that bleeding will occur which can lead to serious health problems.

Causes

Hemophilia is caused by a mutation or change, in one of the genes, that provides instructions for making the clotting factor proteins needed to form a blood clot. This change or mutation can prevent the clotting protein from working properly or to be missing altogether. These genes are located on the X chromosome. Males have one X and one Y chromosome (XY) and females have two X chromosomes (XX). Males inherit the X chromosome from their mothers and the Y chromosome from their fathers. Females inherit one X chromosome from each parent.

This chapter includes text excerpted from "Hemophilia," Centers for Disease Control and Prevention (CDC), August 26, 2014.

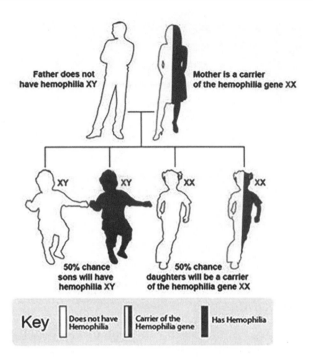

Figure 24.1. *Hemophilia Mutation*

The X chromosome contains many genes that are not present on the Y chromosome. This means that males only have one copy of most of the genes on the X chromosome, whereas females have 2 copies. Thus, males can have a disease like hemophilia if they inherit an affected X chromosome that has a mutation in either the factor VIII or factor IX gene. Females can also have hemophilia, but this is much rarer. In such cases both X chromosomes are affected or one is affected and the other is missing or inactive. In these females, bleeding symptoms may be similar to males with hemophilia.

A female with one affected X chromosome is a "carrier" of hemophilia. Sometimes a female who is a carrier can have symptoms of hemophilia. In addition, she can pass the affected X chromosome with the clotting factor gene mutation on to her children.

Even though hemophilia runs in families, some families have no prior history of family members with hemophilia. Sometimes, there are carrier females in the family, but no affected boys, just by chance. However, about one-third of the time, the baby with hemophilia is the first one in the family to be affected with a mutation in the gene for the clotting factor.

Hemophilia can result in:

- Bleeding within joints that can lead to chronic joint disease and pain
- Bleeding in the head and sometimes in the brain which can cause long term problems, such as seizures and paralysis
- Death can occur if the bleeding cannot be stopped or if it occurs in a vital organ such as the brain.

Types

There are several different types of hemophilia. The following two are the most common:

1. Hemophilia A (Classic Hemophilia: This type is caused by a lack or decrease of clotting factor VIII).

2. Hemophilia B (Christmas Disease: This type is caused by a lack or decrease of clotting factor IX).

Signs and Symptoms

Common signs of hemophilia include:

- Bleeding into the joints. This can cause swelling and pain or tightness in the joints; it often affects the knees, elbows, and ankles.
- Bleeding into the skin (which is bruising) or muscle and soft tissue causing a build-up of blood in the area (called a hematoma).
- Bleeding of the mouth and gums, and bleeding that is hard to stop after losing a tooth.
- Bleeding after circumcision (surgery performed on male babies to remove the hood of skin, called the foreskin, covering the head of the penis).
- Bleeding after having shots, such as vaccinations.
- Bleeding in the head of an infant after a difficult delivery.
- Blood in the urine or stool.
- Frequent and hard-to-stop nosebleeds.

Who Is Affected?

Hemophilia occurs in about 1 of every 5,000 male births. Currently, about 20,000 males in the United States are living with the disorder.

Hemophilia A is about four times as common as hemophilia B, and about half of those affected have the severe form. Hemophilia affects people from all racial and ethnic groups.

Diagnosis

Many people who have or have had family members with hemophilia will ask that their baby boys get tested soon after birth.

About one-third of babies who are diagnosed with hemophilia have a new mutation not present in other family members. In these cases, a doctor might check for hemophilia if a newborn is showing certain signs of hemophilia.

To make a diagnosis, doctors would perform certain blood tests to show if the blood is clotting properly. If it does not, then they would do clotting factor tests, also called factor assays, to diagnose the cause of the bleeding disorder. These blood tests would show the type of hemophilia and the severity.

Treatment

The best way to treat hemophilia is to replace the missing blood clotting factor so that the blood can clot properly. This is done by infusing (administering through a vein) commercially prepared factor concentrates. People with hemophilia can learn how to perform these infusions themselves so that they can stop bleeding episodes and, by performing the infusions on a regular basis, can even prevent most bleeding episodes.

Good quality medical care from doctors and nurses who know a lot about the disorder can help prevent some serious problems. Often the best choice for care is to visit a comprehensive Hemophilia Treatment Center (HTC). A HTC not only provides care to address all issues related to the disorder, but also provides health education that helps people with hemophilia stay healthy.

Inhibitors

About 15–20 percent of people with hemophilia develop an antibody (called an inhibitor) that stops the clotting factors from being able to clot the blood and stop bleeding. Treatment of bleeding episodes becomes extremely difficult, and the cost of care for a person with an inhibitor can skyrocket because more clotting factor or a different type of clotting factor is needed. People with inhibitors often experience more joint disease and other problems from bleeding that result in a reduced quality of life.

Chapter 26

Von Willebrand Disease (VWD)

Facts about von Willebrand Disease

Von Willebrand disease (VWD) is a blood disorder in which the blood does not clot properly. Blood contains many proteins that help the body stop bleeding. One of these proteins is called von Willebrand factor (VWF). People with VWD either have a low level of VWF in their blood or the VWF protein doesn't work the way it should.

Normally, when a person is injured and starts to bleed, the VWF in the blood attaches to small blood cells called platelets. This helps the platelets stick together, like glue, to form a clot at the site of injury and stop the bleeding. When a person has VWD, because the VWF doesn't work the way it should, the clot might take longer to form or not form the way it should, and bleeding might take longer to stop. This can lead to heavy, hard-to-stop bleeding. Although rare, the bleeding can be severe enough to damage joints or internal organs, or even be life-threatening.

Types of VWD

Type 1

This is the most common and mildest form of VWD, in which a person has lower than normal levels of VWF. A person with Type 1 VWD

This chapter includes text excerpted from "Von Willebrand Disease (VWD)," Centers for Disease Control and Prevention (CDC), March 2, 2016.

also might have low levels of factor VIII, another type of blood-clotting protein. This should not be confused with hemophilia, in which there are low levels or a complete lack of factor VIII but normal levels of VWF.

Type 2

With this type of VWD, although the body makes normal amounts of the VWF, the factor does not work the way it should. Type 2 is further broken down into four subtypes–2A, 2B, 2M, and 2N–depending on the specific problem with the person's VWF. Because the treatment is different for each type, it is important that a person know which subtype he or she has.

Type 3

This is the most severe form of VWD, in which a person has very little or no VWF and low levels of factor VIII.

Causes

Most people who have VWD are born with it. It almost always is inherited, or passed down, from a parent to a child. VWD can be passed down from either the mother or the father, or both, to the child.

While rare, it is possible for a person to get VWD without a family history of the disease. This happens when a "spontaneous mutation" occurs. That means there has been a change in the person's gene. Whether the child received the affected gene from a parent or as a result of a mutation, once the child has it, the child can later pass it along to his or her children. Rarely, a person who is not born with VWD can acquire it or have it first occur later in life. This can happen when a person's own immune system destroys his or her VWF, often as a result of use of a medication or as a result of another disease. If VWD is acquired, meaning it was not inherited from a parent, it cannot be passed along to any children.

Signs and Symptoms

The major signs of VWD are:

Frequent or Hard-to-Stop Nosebleeds

People with VWD might have nosebleeds that:

- start without injury (spontaneous)

- occur often, usually five times or more in a year
- last more than 10 minutes
- need packing or cautery to stop the bleeding

Easy Bruising

People with VWD might experience easy bruising that:

- Occurs with very little or no trauma or injury.
- Occurs often (one to four times per month).
- Is larger than the size of a quarter.
- Is not flat and has a raised lump.

Heavy Menstrual Bleeding

Women with VWD might have heavy menstrual periods during which:

- Clots larger than the size of a quarter are passed.
- More than one pad is soaked through every 2 hours.
- A diagnosis of anemia (not having enough red blood cells) is made as a result of bleeding from heavy periods.

Longer than Normal Bleeding after Injury, Surgery, Childbirth, or Dental Work

People with VWD might have longer than normal bleeding after injury, surgery, or childbirth, for example:

- After a cut to the skin, the bleeding lasts more than 5 minutes.
- Heavy or longer bleeding occurs after surgery. Bleeding sometimes stops, but starts up again hours or days later.
- Heavy bleeding occurs during or after childbirth.

People with VWD might have longer than normal bleeding during or after dental work, for example:

- Heavy bleeding occurs during or after dental surgery.
- The surgery site oozes blood longer than 3 hours after the surgery.
- The surgery site needs packing or cautery to stop the bleeding.

The amount of bleeding depends on the type and severity of VWD. Other common bleeding events include:

- Blood in the stool (feces) from bleeding into the stomach or intestines.
- Blood in the urine from bleeding into the kidneys or bladder.
- Bleeding into joints or internal organs in severe cases (Type 3).

Diagnosis

To find out if a person has VWD, the doctor will ask questions about personal and family histories of bleeding. The doctor also will check for unusual bruising or other signs of recent bleeding and order some blood tests that will measure how the blood clots. The tests will provide information about the amount of clotting proteins present in the blood and if the clotting proteins are working properly. Because certain medications can cause bleeding, even among people without a bleeding disorder, the doctor will ask about recent or routine medications taken that could cause bleeding or make bleeding symptoms worse.

Treatments

The type of treatment prescribed for VWD depends on the type and severity of the disease. For minor bleeds, treatment might not be needed.

The most commonly used types of treatment are:

Desmopressin Acetate Injection

This medicine (DDAVP®) is injected into a vein to treat people with milder forms of VWD (mainly type 1). It works by making the body release more VWF into the blood. It helps increase the level of factor VIII in the blood as well.

Desmopressin Acetate Nasal Spray

This high-strength nasal spray (Stimate®) is used to treat people with milder forms of VWD. It works by boosting the levels of VWF and factor VIII in the blood.

Factor Replacement Therapy

The medicines used in this treatment are rich in VWF and factor VIII (for example, Humate P®, Alphanate®, or Koate DVI®) and are used to treat people with more severe forms of VWD or people with milder forms of VWD who do not respond well to the nasal spray. These medicines are injected into a vein in the arm to replace the missing factor in the blood.

Antifibrinolytic Drugs

These drugs (for example, Amicar®, Lysteda®) are either injected or taken orally to help slow or prevent the breakdown of blood clots.

Birth Control Pills

Birth control pills can increase the levels of VWF and factor VIII in the blood and reduce menstrual blood loss. A doctor can prescribe these pills for women who have heavy menstrual bleeding.

Who Is Affected?

VWD is the most common bleeding disorder, found in up to 1% of the U.S. population. This means that 3.2 million (or about 1 in every 100) people in the United States have the disease. Although VWD occurs among men and women equally, women are more likely to notice the symptoms because of heavy or abnormal bleeding during their menstrual periods and after childbirth.

Chapter 27

Factor V Leiden (Thrombophilia)

What Is Factor V Leiden?

Factor V Leiden thrombophilia is an inherited disorder that results in an increased risk of developing abnormal blood clots. Factor V Leiden is the name of a specific gene mutation in the *F5* gene. This gene plays a critical role in the normal formation of blood clots in response to an injury. People can inherit one or two copies of the factor V Leiden gene mutation. Those who inherit one copy are called heterozygotes. People who inherit two copies of the mutation, one from each parent, are called homozygotes. Having the factor V Leiden mutation increases your risk for developing a clot in your legs called a deep venous thrombosis (DVT). It also increases your risk of developing a clot that travels through the bloodstream and lodges in the lungs, called a pulmonary embolism (PE).

What Are the Signs and Symptoms of Factor V Leiden Thrombophilia?

Individuals affected by factor V Leiden thrombophilia have an increased risk of developing blood clots. The severity of factor V Leiden

This chapter includes text excerpted from "Factor V Leiden Thrombophilia," Genetic and Rare Diseases Information Center (GARD), June 29, 2012. Reviewed July 2016.

thrombophilia is extremely variable. Many individuals with the factor V Leiden allele never develop a blood clot. Although most individuals with factor V thrombophilia do not experience their first thrombotic event until adulthood, some have recurrent thromboembolism before age 30 years. The chance a person will develop a blood clot is affected by the number of factor V Leiden mutations, the presence of coexisting genetic abnormalities, and non-genetic risk factors. Non-genetic risk factors include surgery, long periods of not moving (like sitting on a long airplane ride), birth control pills and other female hormones, childbirth within the last 6 months, and traumas or fractures.

Individuals who inherit one copy of the factor V Leiden mutation have a fourfold to eightfold increase in the chance of developing a clot. Homozygotes (people who inherit two factor V Leiden mutations) may have up to 80 times the usual risk of developing a blood clot. Considering that the risk of developing an abnormal blood clot averages about 1 in 1,000 per year in the general population, the presence of one copy of the factor V Leiden mutation increases that risk to 4 to 8 in 1,000, and having two copies of the mutation may raise the risk as high as 80 in 1,000. People with factor V Leiden have an increased chance of having a blood clot that forms in large veins in the legs (deep venous thrombosis, or DVT) or a clot that travels through the bloodstream and lodges in the lungs (pulmonary embolism, or PE). Symptoms of deep vein thrombosis usually include leg pain, tenderness, swelling, increased warmth or redness in one leg. The symptoms of pulmonary embolism usually include cough, chest pain, shortness of breath or rapid heartbeat or breathing.

What Causes Factor V Leiden Thrombophilia?

Factor V Leiden thrombophilia is caused by a specific mutation in the Factor V gene. Factor V plays a critical role in the formation of blood clots in response to injury. Genes are our body's instructions for making proteins. The factor V gene instructs the body how to make a protein called coagulation factor V. Coagulation factor V is involved in a series of chemical reactions that hold blood clots together. A molecule called activated protein C (APC) prevents blood clots from growing too large by inactivating factor V.

How Is Factor V Leiden Inherited?

Factor V Leiden is a genetic condition and can be inherited from a parent. It is important to understand that each person inherits two copies of every gene, one from their mother and the other copy from their father. Individuals who inherit one copy of the factor V Leiden mutation from a parent are called heterozygotes. Heterozygotes have a 50% chance with each pregnancy of passing the mutated gene to their offspring (and therefore they also have a 50% chance of having a child who does not inherit the gene mutation). People who inherit two copies of the mutation, one from each parent, are called homozygotes. Homozygotes will always pass one copy of the mutated gene to their offspring.

If both parents are heterozygotes (carry one factor V Leiden mutation) than they would have a 25% chance of having a child with two factor V Leiden mutations, a 25% chance of having a child with no mutations, and a 50% chance of having a child with one mutation.

How Is Factor V Leiden Thrombophilia Diagnosed?

No clinical features (signs and/or symptoms) are specific for factor V Leiden thrombophilia. The diagnosis of factor V Leiden thrombophilia requires a coagulation screening test or DNA analysis of *F5*, the gene for factor V, to identify the specific mutation that causes this condition. The APC (activated protein C) resistance assay, a coagulation screening test, measures the anticoagulant response to APC. This screening test has a sensitivity and specificity for factor V Leiden approaching 100%. The sensitivity of a test is a measure of the test's ability to detect a positive result when someone has the condition, while the specificity is a measure of the test's ability to identify negative results. Targeted mutation analysis (a type of DNA test) of the *F5* gene for the Leiden mutation is considered definitive and has a mutation detection frequency of approximately 100%. This means that approximately all individuals who have the factor V Leiden mutation will be detected by this genetic test. It is generally recommended that individuals who test positive by another means should then have the DNA test both for confirmation and to distinguish heterozygotes (individuals with a mutation in one copy of the gene) from homozygotes (individuals with mutations in both copies of the gene).

How Might Factor V Leiden Be Treated?

The management of individuals with factor V Leiden depends on the clinical circumstances. People with factor V Leiden who have had a deep venous thrombosis (DVT) or pulmonary embolism (PE) are usually treated with blood thinners, or anticoagulants. Anticoagulants such as heparin and warfarin are given for varying amounts of time depending on the person's situation. It is not usually recommended that people with factor V Leiden be treated lifelong with anticoagulants if they have had only one DVT or PE, unless there are additional risk factors present. Having had a DVT or PE in the past increases a person's risk for developing another one in the future, but having factor V Leiden does not seem to add to the risk of having a second clot. In general, individuals who have factor V Leiden but have never had a blood clot are not routinely treated with an anticoagulant. Rather, these individuals are counseled about reducing or eliminating other factors that may add to one's risk of developing a clot in the future. In addition, these individuals may require temporary treatment with an anticoagulant during periods of particularly high risk, such as major surgery. Factor V Leiden increases the risk of developing a DVT during pregnancy by about seven-fold. Women with factor V Leiden who are planning pregnancy should discuss this with their obstetrician and/ or hematologist. Most women with factor V Leiden have normal pregnancies and only require close follow-up during pregnancy. For those with a history of DVT or PE, treatment with an anticoagulant during a subsequent pregnancy can prevent recurrent problems.

How Common Is Factor V Leiden Thrombophilia?

The factor V Leiden mutation is the most common inherited predisposition to abnormal blood clotting in the United States. It has a prevalence of about 5% in the Caucasian population. A person with a factor V Leiden mutation may be heterozygous or, more rarely, homozygous. Those who are heterozygous have a 3 to 8 fold greater risk of developing a venous thromboembolism than those who don't carry the mutation; while those who are homozygous have a 50 to 80 fold increased risk of thrombosis.

Chapter 28

Factor Deficiencies

Chapter Contents

Section 28.1

Factor V Deficiency

This section includes text excerpted from "Factor
V Deficiency," Genetic and Rare Diseases Information
Center (GARD), July 22, 2013.

What Is Factor V Deficiency?

Factor V deficiency is an inherited blood disorder that involves abnormal blood clotting (coagulation). This disorder is caused by the deficiency of a blood protein called factor V. The reduced amount of factor V leads to episodes of abnormal bleeding that range from mild to severe. Factor V deficiency is inherited in an autosomal recessive manner, which means that both copies of the *F5* gene in each cell have mutations.

What Are the Signs and Symptoms of Factor V Deficiency?

The symptoms of factor V deficiency may include:

- bleeding into the skin
- excessive bruising
- nose bleeds
- bleeding of the gums
- excessive menstrual bleeding
- prolonged or excessive loss of blood with surgery or trauma
- umbilical stump bleeding

What Causes Factor V Deficiency?

Factor V deficiency is caused by mutations in the *F5* gene that prevent the production of a functional factor V protein or decrease the amount of the protein in the bloodstream. Mutations are present in both copies of the *F5* gene in each cell, which prevents blood from clotting normally.

How Is Factor V Deficiency Treated?

Resources state that fresh plasma or fresh frozen plasma infusions will correct the deficiency temporarily and may be administered daily during a bleeding episode or after surgery. Individuals with factor V deficiency should discuss treatment options with their primary health-care provider and a hematologist.

Section 28.2

Hemophilia A (Factor VIII Deficiency)

This section includes text excerpted from "Hemophilia A," Genetic and Rare Diseases Information Center (GARD), March 18, 2015.

What Is Factor VIII (Hemophilia A)?

Hemophilia A is a bleeding disorder in which the blood does not clot normally. People with this disorder have prolonged bleeding or oozing after an injury, surgery, or tooth extraction. In severe cases, heavy bleeding occurs after minor injury or even when there is no injury (spontaneous bleeding). Serious complications can result from bleeding into the joints, muscles, brain, or other internal organs. In milder forms there is no spontaneous bleeding, and the disorder may not become apparent until after a surgery or serious injury. Hemophilia A is inherited in an X-linked recessive manner and is caused by changes (mutations) in the *F8* gene. The main treatment is called replacement therapy, during which clotting factor VIII is dripped or injected into a vein.

What Are the Signs and Symptoms of Hemophilia A?

The Human Phenotype Ontology (HPO) provides the following list of signs and symptoms for Hemophilia A.

- bruising susceptibility

- degenerative joint disease

- joint hemorrhage

- persistent bleeding after trauma

- prolonged partial thromboplastin time

- reduced factor VIII activity

- X-linked recessive inheritance

How Does Hemophilia a Run in Families?

Hemophilia A is inherited in an X-linked recessive pattern. This means that hemophilia A nearly always affects males. Females who have the hemophilia A gene mutation are called carriers. Most carriers have no signs or symptoms, however about 10% of female carriers experience some abnormal bleeding, particularly after an injury, surgery, or tooth extraction.

Family history is an important tool for assessing family members risks for hemophilia A and carrier status. For example, when a woman has one affected child and another affected male relative (e.g., a sibling), it is assumed that she is a carrier. In this scenario, each of the woman's children would have a 1 in 2 or 50% chance of inheriting the gene mutation. Sons who inherit the gene mutation are affected, daughter's who inherit the mutation are carriers.

When a male child is the first and only person in a family with hemophilia A, further testing may be needed to determine if the child inherited the condition from his mother, or if the mutation occurred by chance for the first time in the child. In this scenario, the mother has an estimated 80% chance (or higher) to be a carrier for hemophilia A. Once the mother's carrier status is known, risks to siblings can be determined.

When a father has hemophilia A, none of his sons will inherit the condition, but all of his daughters will be carriers.

To find a genetics professional, we recommend that you contact your primary healthcare provider for a referral. The following online resources can also help you find a genetics professional in your community:

- GeneTests offers a searchable directory of U.S. and international genetics and prenatal diagnosis clinics.

- The National Society of Genetic Counselors provides a searchable directory of U.S. and international genetic counseling services.

- The American College of Medical Genetics has a searchable database of U.S. genetics clinics.

- The American Society of Human Genetics maintains a database of its members, which includes individuals who live outside of the United States.

How Might Hemophilia a Be Treated?

People with inherited hemophilia A require life-long care, preferably through a specialized hemophilia treatment center. Although there is no cure for hemophilia A, current treatments usually work well. Treatment primarily consists of replacing the missing clotting factor VIII (replacement therapy) and preventing complications that are associated with the disorder. The type and frequency of treatment often depends on the severity of the disorder in each person.

People with mild or moderate hemophilia A may be treated with replacement therapy as needed (for example, when a specific bleeding episode occurs). This is called episodic therapy. Some people with mild hemophilia A may be treated with desmopressin (DDAVP). Desmopressin raises the levels of factor VIII in the blood and may be taken intravenously or through a nasal spray. Drugs known as antifibrinolytics, which slow the breakdown of clotting factors in the blood, can also be used to treat those with a mild form of the disorder.

Some people with severe hemophilia A may receive periodic factor VIII infusions to prevent bleeding episodes and associated complications such as joint damage. This is referred to as prophylactic therapy.

People can be trained to give infusions at home. This is especially important for people with severe disease because the infusion works the best within one hour of a bleeding episode. In general, rapid treatment is important because it reduces pain and damage to the joints, muscles or other affected tissues or organs.

What Is the Long-Term Outlook for People with Hemophilia A?

Hemophilia can be mild, moderate, or severe, depending on how much clotting factor is in an affected person's blood. However, about 70% of patients have the severe form of the disorder.

With appropriate education and treatment, people with hemophilia can live full and productive lives. Prophylaxis (preventive measures) and early treatment have dramatically improved the long-term outlook (prognosis) for people with severe hemophilia. Replacement therapy has significantly improved life expectancy, and the availability of therapy at home has improved quality of life. About 25% of people with severe disease between 6–18 years of age do have below-normal motor skills and academic performance, and have more emotional and behavioral problems than others.

The most important life-threatening complications of hemophilia are intracranial hemorrhage (bleeding within the skull) and hemorrhages into the soft tissue around vital areas (such as the airway or internal organs). The lifetime risk of intracranial bleeding in affected people is 2–8% and accounts for one third of deaths due to hemorrhage. About 10% of those with severe hemophilia have intracranial bleeding, with a mortality rate of 30%. Chronic, debilitating joint disease can also develop.

Overall, the mortality rate for affected people is about twice that of the healthy male population. For severe hemophilia, the rate is about 4–6 times higher. In some cases the mortality rate depends on whether any other underlying diseases or conditions are present.

Section 28.3

Hemophilia B (Factor IX Deficiency)

This section includes text excerpted from "Hemophilia B," Genetic and Rare Diseases Information Center (GARD), February 8, 2016.

What Is Factor IX (Hemophilia B)?

Hemophilia B is a bleeding disorder that slows the blood clotting process. People with this disorder experience prolonged bleeding or oozing following an injury or surgery. In severe cases of hemophilia, heavy bleeding occurs after minor injury or even in the absence of injury. Serious complications can result from bleeding into the joints, muscles, brain, or other internal organs. Milder forms may not become apparent until abnormal bleeding occurs following surgery or a serious injury. People with an unusual form of hemophilia B, known as hemophilia B Leyden, experience episodes of excessive bleeding in childhood but have few bleeding problems after puberty. Hemophilia

B is inherited in an X-linked recessive pattern and is caused by mutations in the *F9* gene.

What Are the Signs and Symptoms of Hemophilia B?

The Human Phenotype Ontology provides the following list of signs and symptoms for Hemophilia B.

- abnormal bleeding
- degenerative joint disease
- gastrointestinal hemorrhage
- joint hemorrhage
- persistent bleeding after trauma
- prolonged partial thromboplastin time
- prolonged whole-blood clotting time
- reduced factor IX activity
- X-linked recessive inheritance

Section 28.4

Factor X Deficiency

This section includes text excerpted from "Factor X Deficiency," Genetic and Rare Diseases Information Center (GARD), November 12, 2015.

What Is Factor X Deficiency?

Factor X deficiency is a rare condition that affects the blood's ability to clot. The severity of the condition and the associated signs and symptoms can vary significantly from person to person. Common features of factor X deficiency may include easy bruising, frequent nosebleeds, bleeding gums, blood in the urine, and prolonged bleeding after minor injuries. Affected women may also experience heavy menstrual bleeding and may have an increased risk for first trimester miscarriages. Acquired (non-inherited) factor X deficiency, which is the most common form of the condition, generally occurs sporadically in people with no family history of the condition. Acquired factor X deficiency has a variety of causes including liver disease, vitamin K deficiency, exposure to certain medications that affect clotting, and cancers. The inherited form of factor X deficiency (also called congenital factor X deficiency) is caused by changes (mutations) in the *F10* gene and is inherited in an autosomal recessive manner. Treatment aims to control bleeding through intravenous (IV) infusions of plasma or concentrates of clotting factors.

What Are the Signs and Symptoms of Factor X Deficiency?

The Human Phenotype Ontology provides the following list of signs and symptoms for Factor X deficiency.

- autosomal recessive inheritance
- epistaxis
- gingival bleeding
- intracranial hemorrhage
- intramuscular hematoma
- joint hemorrhage
- menorrhagia
- prolonged partial thromboplastin time
- prolonged prothrombin time
- variable expressivity

Section 28.5

Factor XI Deficiency

This section includes text excerpted from "Factor XI Deficiency," Genetic and Rare Diseases Information Center (GARD), February 5, 2016.

What Is Factor XI Deficiency?

Factor XI deficiency is a bleeding disorder that interferes with the body's clotting process. As a result, people affected by this condition may have difficulty stopping the flow of blood following dental extractions, trauma or surgery. Women with factor XI deficiency may also experience heavy menstrual periods or heavy postpartum bleeding. Within affected people and their families, highly variable bleeding patterns occur, and bleeding risk can not be predicted by the level of factor XI (a clotting factor) in the blood. Although the condition can affect people of all heritages, it is most common in people of Ashkenazi Jewish descent. Most cases of factor XI deficiency are inherited and caused by changes (mutations) in the *F11* gene. The condition is generally inherited in an autosomal recessive manner; however, it may follow an autosomal dominant pattern in some families. Treatment is often only recommended during periods of high bleeding risk (i.e. surgery) and may include fresh frozen plasma and/ or antifibrinolytics (medications that improve blood clotting). Factor XI concentrates may be available for factor replacement in some countries.

What Are the Signs and Symptoms of Factor XI Deficiency?

The Human Phenotype Ontology provides the following list of signs and symptoms for Factor XI deficiency.

- abnormal bleeding
- autosomal dominant inheritance
- autosomal recessive inheritance
- prolonged partial thromboplastin time
- reduced factor XI activity

337

Chapter 29

Hereditary Hemorrhagic Telangiectasia

Facts about Hereditary Hemorrhagic Telangiectasia (HHT)

HHT is a disorder in which some blood vessels do not develop properly. A person with HHT may form blood vessels without the capillaries (tiny blood vessels that pass blood from arteries to veins) that are usually present between arteries and veins. The space between an artery and a vein is often fragile and can burst and bleed much more easily than other blood vessels. Men, women, and children from all racial and ethnic groups can be affected by HHT and experience the problems associated with this disorder, some of which are serious and potentially life-threatening. Fortunately, if HHT is discovered early, effective treatments are available. However, there is no cure for HHT.

This chapter contains text excerpted from the following sources: Text beginning with the heading "Facts about Hereditary Hemorrhagic Telangiectasia (HHT)" is excerpted from "Blood Disorders," Centers for Disease Control and Prevention (CDC), February 23, 2016; Text under the heading "How Might Hereditary Hemorrhagic Telangiectasia (HHT) Be Treated?" is excerpted from "Hereditary Hemorrhagic Telangiectasia," Centers for Disease Control and Prevention (CDC), April 20, 2016.

Signs

Nosebleeds are the most common sign of HHT, resulting from small abnormal blood vessels within the inside layer of the nose. Abnormal blood vessels in the skin can appear on the hands, fingertips, face, lips, lining of the mouth, and nose as delicate red or purplish spots that lighten briefly when touched. Bleeding within the stomach or intestines is another possible indicator of HHT that occurs because of abnormal blood vessels lining the digestive tract. Additional signs of HHT include abnormal artery-vein connections within the brain, lungs, and liver, which often do not display any warning signs before rupturing.

Causes of HHT

HHT is a genetic disorder. Each person with HHT has one gene that is altered (mutated), which causes HHT, as well as one normal gene. It takes only one mutant gene to cause HHT. When someone with HHT has children, each child has a 50% chance to receive the mutant gene from his/her parent, and therefore to have HHT, as well. Each child also has a 50% chance to receive the normal gene and not be affected with HHT. At least five different genes can cause HHT, three of which are known.

Diagnosis

HHT can be diagnosed by performing genetic testing. Genetic testing can detect a gene mutation in about three-fourth of families with signs of HHT, which if found can establish the diagnosis of HHT in individuals and families who are unsure about whether they have HHT. HHT can also be diagnosed by using clinical criteria (presence of signs and a history of signs in a parent, sibling, or child).

Complications and Treatments

The complications of HHT can vary widely, even among people affected by HHT in the same family. Complications and treatment of HHT depend on the parts of the body that are affected by this disorder. Treatment may include controlling bleeding and anemia and preventing complications from abnormal artery-vein connections in the lungs and brain.

How Might Hereditary Hemorrhagic Telangiectasia (HHT) Be Treated?

Although there is not yet a way to prevent the telangiectases or AVMs associated with HHT, most can be treated once they occur. Management includes surveillance for undiagnosed AVMs and treatment for identified complications such as nosebleeds, gastrointestinal bleeding, anemia, pulmonary AVMs, cerebral AVMs, and hepatic AVMs.

Treatment of nosebleeds with humidification and nasal lubricants, laser ablation, septal dermoplasty, or estrogen-progesterone therapy can prevent anemia and allow individuals with HHT to pursue normal activities. In more severe cases, coagulation therapy may be needed.

Individuals with GI bleeding are treated with iron therapy to maintain hemoglobin concentration; endoscopic application of a heater probe, bicap, or laser; surgical removal of bleeding sites; and estrogen-progesterone therapy. Iron replacement and red blood cell transfusions are used to treat anemia.

Treatment of pulmonary AVMs is indicated for dyspnea, exercise intolerance, hypoxemia, and prevention of lung hemorrhage and the neurologic complications of brain abscess and stroke. Pulmonary AVMs with feeding vessels that exceed 1.0 mm in diameter require consideration of occlusion. Preventive measures should be undertaken by those who have pulmonary AVMs, including antibiotics prior to dental or surgical procedures, the implementation of IV filters, avoidance of blood thinners and non-steroidal anti-inflammatory medications, and regular monitoring by a qualified medical professional.

Cerebral AVMs greater than 1.0 cm in diameter are usually treated by surgery, embolotherapy, and/or stereotactic radiosurgery. Liver AVMs are currently treated only if a patient shows signs of heart failure or other significant health problems. Treatments might include liver transplantation or medications like bevacizumab.

Surveillance includes annual evaluations for anemia and neurologic conditions and re-evaluation for pulmonary AVMs every one to two years during childhood and every five years thereafter. Women with HHT considering pregnancy are screened and treated for pulmonary AVMs; if pulmonary AVMs are discovered during pregnancy, they are treated during the second trimester.

Chapter 30

Bruises

What Is a Bruise?

A bruise, also called a **contusion** or an **ecchymosis**, happens when a part of the body is struck and the muscle fibers and connective tissue underneath are crushed but the skin doesn't break. When this occurs, blood from the ruptured **capillaries** (small blood vessels) near the skin's surface escapes by leaking out under the skin. With no place to go, the blood gets trapped, forming a red or purplish mark that's tender when you touch it—a bruise.

Bruises can happen for many reasons, but most are the result of bumping and banging into things—or having things bump and bang into you. Fortunately, as anyone who's ever sported a shiner knows, the mark isn't permanent.

How Long Do Bruises Last?

You know how a bruise changes color over time? That's your body fixing the bruise by breaking down and reabsorbing the blood, which causes the bruise to go through many colors of the rainbow before it eventually disappears. You can pretty much guess the age of a bruise just by looking at its color:

- When you first get a bruise, it's kind of reddish as the blood appears under the skin.

- Within 1 or 2 days, the hemoglobin (an iron-containing substance that carries oxygen) in the blood changes and your bruise turns bluish-purple or even blackish.

- After 5 to 10 days, the bruise turns greenish or yellowish.

- Then, after 10 or 14 days, it turns yellowish-brown or light brown.

Finally, after about 2 weeks, your bruise fades away.

Who Gets Bruises?

Anyone can get a bruise. Some people bruise easily, whereas others don't. Why? Bruising depends on several things, such as:

- how tough the skin tissue is

- whether someone has certain diseases or conditions

- whether a person's taking certain medications

Also, blood vessels tend to become fragile as people get older, which is why elderly people tend to bruise more easily.

How Can I Help Myself Feel Better?

It's hard to prevent bruises, but you can help speed the healing process. When you get a bruise, you can use stuff you find right in your freezer to help the bruise go away faster. Applying cold when you first get a bruise helps reduce its size by slowing down the blood that's flowing to the area, which decreases the amount of blood that ends up leaking into the tissues. It also keeps the inflammation and swelling down. All you have to do is apply cold to the bruise for 15 to 20 minutes at a time for a day or two after the bruise appears.

You don't need to buy a special cold pack, although they're great to keep on hand in the freezer. Just get some ice, put it in a plastic bag, and wrap the bag in a cloth or a towel and place it on the bruise (it isn't a good idea to apply the ice directly to the skin).

Another trick is to use a bag of frozen vegetables. It doesn't matter what kind—carrots, peas, lima beans, whatever—as long as they're frozen. A bag of frozen vegetables is easy to apply to the bruise because it can form to the shape of the injured area. Also, like a cold pack, it can be used and refrozen again and again (just pick your least-favorite vegetables and label the bag—you don't want to keep thawing and freezing veggies that you plan to eat!).

To reduce swelling and bruising, elevate the bruised area above the level of your heart. In other words, if the bruise is on your shin, lie down on a couch or bed and prop up your leg. This will help prevent blood from pooling in the area because more of the blood will flow back toward your heart. If you keep standing, more blood will flow to your bruised shin and the bruise will be larger.

Take acetaminophen for pain, if needed.

When to See a Doctor

Minor bruises are easily treated, but it's probably best to talk to a doctor if:

- A bruise isn't improving after 2 weeks.
- You bruise often and bruises seem to develop for no known reasons.
- Your bruise is swelling and very painful.
- You can't move a joint or you think you may have a broken bone.
- The bruise is near your eye and you have difficulty moving your eyes or seeing.

Can Bruises Be Prevented?

Bruises are kind of hard to avoid completely, but if you're playing sports, riding your bike, inline skating, or doing anything where you might bump, bang, crash, or smash into something—or something might bump, bang, crash, or smash into you—it's smart to wear protective gear like pads, shin guards, and helmets. Taking just a few extra seconds to put on that gear might save you from a couple of weeks of aches and pains (not to mention save your life if the accident's really serious)!

Chapter 31

Antiphospholipid Antibody Syndrome

What Is Antiphospholipid Antibody Syndrome?

Antiphospholipid antibody syndrome (APS) is an autoimmune disorder. Autoimmune disorders occur if the body's immune system makes antibodies that attack and damage tissues or cells.

Antibodies are a type of protein. They usually help defend the body against infections. In APS, however, the body makes antibodies that mistakenly attack phospholipids—a type of fat.

Phospholipids are found in all living cells and cell membranes, including blood cells and the lining of blood vessels.

When antibodies attack phospholipids, cells are damaged. This damage causes blood clots to form in the body's arteries and veins. (These are the vessels that carry blood to your heart and body.)

Usually, blood clotting is a normal bodily process. Blood clots help seal small cuts or breaks on blood vessel walls. This prevents you from losing too much blood. In APS, however, too much blood clotting can block blood flow and damage the body's organs.

This section includes text excerpted from "Antiphospholipid Antibody Syndrome," National Heart, Lung, and Blood Institute (NHLBI), May 17, 2012. Reviewed July 2016

Other Names for Antiphospholipid Antibody Syndrome

- Anticardiolipin antibody syndrome, or aCL syndrome
- Antiphospholipid syndrome
- aPL syndrome
- Hughes syndrome
- Lupus anticoagulant syndrome

What Causes Antiphospholipid Antibody Syndrome?

Antiphospholipid antibody syndrome (APS) occurs if the body's immune system makes antibodies (proteins) that attack phospholipids.

Phospholipids are a type of fat found in all living cells and cell membranes, including blood cells and the lining of blood vessels. What causes the immune system to make antibodies against phospholipids isn't known.

APS causes unwanted blood clots to form in the body's arteries and veins. Usually, blood clotting is a normal bodily process. It helps seal small cuts or breaks on blood vessel walls. This prevents you from losing too much blood. In APS, however, too much blood clotting can block blood flow and damage the body's organs.

Researchers don't know why APS antibodies cause blood clots to form. Some believe that the antibodies damage or affect the inner lining of the blood vessels, which causes blood clots to form. Others believe that the immune system makes antibodies in response to blood clots damaging the blood vessels.

Who Is at Risk for Antiphospholipid Antibody Syndrome?

Antiphospholipid antibody syndrome (APS) can affect people of any age. The disorder is more common in women than men, but it affects both sexes.

APS also is more common in people who have other autoimmune or rheumatic disorders, such as lupus. ("Rheumatic" refers to disorders that affect the joints, bones, or muscles.)

About 10 percent of all people who have lupus also have APS. About half of all people who have APS also have another autoimmune or rheumatic disorder.

Some people have APS antibodies, but don't ever have signs or symptoms of the disorder. The mere presence of APS antibodies doesn't mean that you have APS. To be diagnosed with APS, you must have APS antibodies and a history of health problems related to the disorder.

However, people who have APS antibodies but no signs or symptoms are at risk of developing APS. Health problems, other than auto-immune disorders, that can trigger blood clots include:

- smoking
- prolonged bed rest
- pregnancy and the postpartum period
- birth control pills and hormone therapy
- cancer and kidney disease

What Are the Signs and Symptoms of Antiphospholipid Antibody Syndrome?

The signs and symptoms of antiphospholipid antibody syndrome (APS) are related to abnormal blood clotting. The outcome of a blood clot depends on its size and location.

Blood clots can form in, or travel to, the arteries or veins in the brain, heart, kidneys, lungs, and limbs. Clots can reduce or block blood flow. This can damage the body's organs and may cause death.

Major Signs and Symptoms

Major signs and symptoms of blood clots include:

- chest pain and shortness of breath
- pain, redness, warmth, and swelling in the limbs
- ongoing headaches
- speech changes
- upper body discomfort in the arms, back, neck, and jaw
- nausea (feeling sick to your stomach)

Blood clots can lead to stroke, heart attack, kidney damage, deep vein thrombosis, and pulmonary embolism.

Pregnant women who have APS can have successful pregnancies. However, they're at higher risk for miscarriages, stillbirths, and other pregnancy-related problems, such as preeclampsia.

Preeclampsia is high blood pressure that occurs during pregnancy. This condition may progress to eclampsia. Eclampsia is a serious condition that causes seizures in pregnant women.

Some people who have APS may develop thrombocytopenia. This is a condition in which your blood has a lower than normal number of blood cell fragments called platelets.

Mild to serious bleeding causes the main signs and symptoms of thrombocytopenia. Bleeding can occur inside the body (internal bleeding) or underneath or from the skin (external bleeding).

Other Signs and Symptoms

Other signs and symptoms of APS include chronic (ongoing) headaches, memory loss, and heart valve problems. Some people who have APS also get a lacy-looking red rash on their wrists and knees.

How Is Antiphospholipid Antibody Syndrome Diagnosed?

Specialists Involved

A hematologist often is involved in the care of people who have APS. This is a doctor who specializes in diagnosing and treating blood diseases and disorders.

You may have APS and another autoimmune disorder, such as lupus. If so, a doctor who specializes in that disorder also may provide treatment.

Many autoimmune disorders that occur with APS also affect the joints, bones, or muscles. Rheumatologists specialize in treating these types of disorders.

Medical History

Some people have APS antibodies but no signs or symptoms of the disorder. Having APS antibodies doesn't mean that you have APS. To be diagnosed with APS, you must have APS antibodies and a history of health problems related to the disorder.

APS can lead to many health problems, including stroke, heart attack, kidney damage, deep vein thrombosis, and pulmonary embolism.

APS also can cause pregnancy-related problems, such as multiple miscarriages, a miscarriage late in pregnancy, or a premature birth due to eclampsia. (Eclampsia, which follows preeclampsia, is a serious condition that causes seizures in pregnant women.)

Blood Tests

Your doctor can use blood tests to confirm a diagnosis of APS. These tests check your blood for any of the three APS antibodies: anticardiolipin, beta-2 glycoprotein I (□2GPI), and lupus anticoagulant.

The term "anticoagulant" refers to a substance that prevents blood clotting. It may seem odd that one of the APS antibodies is called lupus anticoagulant. The reason for this is because the antibody slows clotting in lab tests. However, in the human body, it increases the risk of blood clotting.

To test for APS antibodies, a small blood sample is taken. It's often drawn from a vein in your arm using a needle. The procedure usually is quick and easy, but it may cause some short-term discomfort and a slight bruise.

You may need a second blood test to confirm positive results. This is because a single positive test can result from a short-term infection. The second blood test often is done 12 weeks or more after the first one.

How Is Antiphospholipid Antibody Syndrome Treated?

Antiphospholipid antibody syndrome (APS) has no cure. However, medicines can help prevent complications. The goals of treatment are to prevent blood clots from forming and keep existing clots from getting larger.

You may have APS and another autoimmune disorder, such as lupus. If so, it's important to control that condition as well. When the other condition is controlled, APS may cause fewer problems.

Research is ongoing for new ways to treat APS.

Medicines

Anticoagulants, or "blood thinners," are used to stop blood clots from forming. They also may keep existing blood clots from getting larger. These medicines are taken as either a pill, an injection under the skin, or through a needle or tube inserted into a vein (called intravenous, or IV, injection).

Warfarin and heparin are two blood thinners used to treat APS. Warfarin is given in pill form. (Coumadin® is a common brand name for warfarin.) Heparin is given as an injection or through an IV tube. There are different types of heparin. Your doctor will discuss the options with you.

Your doctor may treat you with both heparin and warfarin at the same time. Heparin acts quickly. Warfarin takes 2 to 3 days before it starts to work. Once the warfarin starts to work, the heparin is stopped.

Aspirin also thins the blood and helps prevent blood clots. Sometimes aspirin is used with warfarin. Other times, aspirin might be used alone.

Blood thinners don't prevent APS. They simply reduce the risk of further blood clotting. Treatment with these medicines is long term. Discuss all treatment options with your doctor.

Side Effects

The most common side effect of blood thinners is bleeding. This happens if the medicine thins your blood too much. This side effect can be life threatening.

Sometimes the bleeding is internal (inside your body). People treated with blood thinners usually need regular blood tests, called PT and PTT tests, to check how well their blood is clotting.

These tests also show whether you're taking the right amount of medicine. Your doctor will check to make sure that you're taking enough medicine to prevent clots, but not so much that it causes bleeding.

Talk with your doctor about the warning signs of internal bleeding and when to seek emergency care.

Treatment during Pregnancy

Pregnant women who have APS can have successful pregnancies. With proper treatment, these women are more likely to carry their babies to term.

Pregnant women who have APS usually are treated with heparin or heparin and low-dose aspirin. Warfarin is not used as a treatment during pregnancy because it can harm the fetus.

Babies whose mothers have APS are at higher risk for slowed growth while in the womb. If you're pregnant and have APS, you may need to have extra ultrasound tests (sonograms) to check your baby's growth. An ultrasound test uses sound waves to look at the growing fetus.

Treatment for Other Medical Conditions

People who have APS are at increased risk for thrombocytopenia. This is a condition in which your blood has a lower than normal number of blood cell fragments called platelets. Platelets help the blood clot.

If you have APS, you'll need regular complete blood counts (a type of blood test) to count the number of platelets in your blood.

Thrombocytopenia is treated with medicines and medical procedures.

If you have other health problems, such as heart disease or diabetes, work with your doctor to manage them.

Living with Antiphospholipid Antibody Syndrome

Antiphospholipid antibody syndrome (APS) has no cure. However, you can take steps to control the disorder and prevent complications.

Take all medicines as your doctor prescribes and get ongoing medical care. Talk with your doctor about healthy lifestyle changes and any concerns you have.

Medicines

You may need to take anticoagulants, or "blood thinners," to prevent blood clots or to keep them from getting larger. You should take these medicines exactly as your doctor prescribes.

Tell your doctor about all other medicines you're taking, including over-the-counter or herbal medicines. Some medicines, including over-the-counter ibuprofen or aspirin, can thin your blood. Your doctor may not want you to take two medicines that thin your blood because of the risk of bleeding.

Women who have APS shouldn't use birth control or hormone therapy that contains estrogen. Estrogen increases the risk of blood clots. Talk with your doctor about other options.

Ongoing Medical Care

If you have APS, getting regular medical checkups is important. Have blood tests done as your doctor directs. These tests help track how well your blood is clotting.

The medicines used to treat APS increase the risk of bleeding. Bleeding might occur inside your body (internal bleeding) or underneath the skin or from the surface of the skin (external bleeding). Know the warning signs of bleeding, so you can get help right away. They include:

- unexplained bleeding from the gums and nose
- increased menstrual flow
- bright red vomit or vomit that looks like coffee grounds
- bright red blood in your stools or black, tarry stools

- pain in your abdomen or severe pain in your head

- sudden changes in vision

- sudden loss of movement in your limbs

- memory loss or confusion

A lot of bleeding after a fall or injury or easy bruising or bleeding also might mean that your blood is too thin. Ask your doctor about these warning signs and when to seek emergency care.

Lifestyle Changes

Talk with your doctor about lifestyle changes that can help you stay healthy. Ask him or her whether your diet may affect your medicines. Some foods or drinks may increase or decrease the effects of warfarin.

Ask your doctor what amount of alcohol is safe for you to drink if you're taking medicine. If you smoke, talk with your doctor about programs and products that can help you quit. Smoking can damage your blood vessels and raise your risk for many health problems.

APS medicines might increase your risk of bleeding. Thus, your doctor may advise you to avoid activities that have a high risk of injury, such as some contact sports.

Other Concerns

Pregnancy

APS can raise the risk of pregnancy-related problems. Talk with your doctor about how to manage your APS if you're pregnant or planning a pregnancy.

With proper treatment, women who have APS are more likely to carry babies to term than women whose APS isn't treated.

Surgery

If you need surgery, your doctor may adjust your medicines before, during, and after the surgery to prevent dangerous bleeding.

Chapter 32

Disseminated Intravascular Coagulation

What Is Disseminated Intravascular Coagulation?

Disseminated intravascular coagulation, or DIC, is a condition in which blood clots form throughout the body's small blood vessels. These blood clots can reduce or block blood flow through the blood vessels, which can damage the body's organs.

In DIC, the increased clotting uses up platelets and clotting factors in the blood. Platelets are blood cell fragments that stick together to seal small cuts and breaks on blood vessel walls and stop bleeding. Clotting factors are proteins needed for normal blood clotting.

With fewer platelets and clotting factors in the blood, serious bleeding can occur. DIC can cause internal and external bleeding.

Internal bleeding occurs inside the body. External bleeding occurs underneath or from the skin or mucosa. (The mucosa is the tissue that lines some organs and body cavities, such as your nose and mouth.)

DIC can cause life-threatening bleeding.

This chapter includes text excerpted from "Disseminated Intravascular Coagulation," National Heart, Lung, and Blood Institute (NHLBI), November 2, 2011. Reviewed July 2016.

Other Names for Disseminated Intravascular Coagulation

- Consumption coagulopathy
- Defibrination syndrome

What Causes Disseminated Intravascular Coagulation?

Some diseases and conditions can disrupt the body's normal blood clotting process and lead to disseminated intravascular coagulation (DIC). These diseases and conditions include:

- sepsis (an infection in the bloodstream)
- surgery and trauma
- cancer
- serious complications of pregnancy and childbirth

Examples of less common causes of DIC are bites from poisonous snakes (such as rattlesnakes and other vipers), frostbite, and burns.

The two types of DIC are acute and chronic. Acute DIC begins with clotting in the small blood vessels and quickly leads to serious bleeding. Chronic DIC causes blood clotting, but it usually doesn't lead to bleeding. Cancer is the most common cause of chronic DIC.

Similar Clotting Conditions

Two other conditions cause blood clotting in the small blood vessels. However, their causes and treatments differ from those of DIC.

These conditions are thrombotic thrombocytopenic purpura, or TTP, and hemolytic-uremic syndrome (HUS). HUS is more common in children than adults. It's also more likely to cause kidney damage than TTP.

What Are the Signs and Symptoms of Disseminated Intravascular Coagulation?

Signs and symptoms of disseminated intravascular coagulation (DIC) depend on its cause and whether the condition is acute or chronic.

Acute DIC develops quickly (over hours or days) and is very serious. Chronic DIC develops more slowly (over weeks or months). It lasts longer and usually isn't recognized as quickly as acute DIC.

With acute DIC, blood clotting in the blood vessels usually occurs first, followed by bleeding. However, bleeding may be the first obvious sign. Serious bleeding can occur very quickly after developing acute DIC. Thus, emergency treatment in a hospital is needed.

Blood clotting also occurs with chronic DIC, but it usually doesn't lead to bleeding. Sometimes chronic DIC has no signs or symptoms.

Signs and Symptoms of Excessive Blood Clotting

In DIC, blood clots form throughout the body's small blood vessels. These blood clots can reduce or block blood flow through the blood vessels. This can cause the following signs and symptoms:

- Chest pain and shortness of breath if blood clots form in the blood vessels in your lungs and heart.

- Pain, redness, warmth, and swelling in the lower leg if blood clots form in the deep veins of your leg.

- Headaches, speech changes, paralysis (an inability to move), dizziness, and trouble speaking and understanding if blood clots form in the blood vessels in your brain. These signs and symptoms may indicate a stroke.

- Heart attack and lung and kidney problems if blood clots lodge in your heart, lungs, or kidneys. These organs may even begin to fail.

Signs and Symptoms of Bleeding

In DIC, the increased clotting activity uses up the platelets and clotting factors in the blood. As a result, serious bleeding can occur. DIC can cause internal and external bleeding.

Internal Bleeding

Internal bleeding can occur in your body's organs, such as the kidneys, intestines, and brain. This bleeding can be life threatening. Signs and symptoms of internal bleeding include:

- Blood in your urine from bleeding in your kidneys or bladder.

- Blood in your stools from bleeding in your intestines or stomach. Blood in your stools can appear red or as a dark, tarry color. (Taking iron supplements also can cause dark, tarry stools.)

- Headaches, double vision, seizures, and other symptoms from bleeding in your brain.

External Bleeding

External bleeding can occur underneath or from the skin, such as at the site of cuts or an intravenous (IV) needle. External bleeding also can occur from the mucosa. (The mucosa is the tissue that lines some organs and body cavities, such as your nose and mouth.)

External bleeding may cause purpura or petechiae. Purpura are purple, brown, and red bruises. This bruising may happen easily and often. Petechiae are small red or purple dots on your skin.

Other signs of external bleeding include:

- Prolonged bleeding, even from minor cuts.

- Bleeding or oozing from your gums or nose, especially nosebleeds or bleeding from brushing your teeth.

- Heavy or extended menstrual bleeding in women.

How Is Disseminated Intravascular Coagulation Diagnosed?

Your doctor will diagnose disseminated intravascular coagulation (DIC) based on your medical history, a physical exam, and test results. Your doctor also will look for the cause of DIC.

Acute DIC requires emergency treatment. The condition can be life threatening if it's not treated right away. If you have signs or symptoms of severe bleeding or blood clots, call 9–1–1 right away.

Medical History and Physical Exam

Your doctor will ask whether you have or have had any diseases or conditions that can trigger DIC.

Your doctor will ask about signs and symptoms of blood clots and bleeding. He or she also will do a physical exam to look for signs and symptoms of blood clots and internal and external bleeding. For example, your doctor may look for bleeding from your gums.

Diagnostic Tests

To diagnose DIC, your doctor may recommend blood tests to look at your blood cells and the clotting process. For these tests, a small amount of blood is drawn from a blood vessel, usually in your arm.

Complete Blood Count and Blood Smear

A complete blood count (CBC) measures the number of red blood cells, white blood cells, and platelets in your blood.

Platelets are blood cell fragments that help with blood clotting. Abnormal platelet numbers may be a sign of a bleeding disorder (not enough clotting) or a thrombotic disorder (too much clotting).

A blood smear is a test that may reveal whether your red blood cells are damaged.

Tests for Clotting Factors and Clotting Time

The following tests examine the proteins active in the blood clotting process and how long it takes them to form a blood clot.

- **PT and PTT tests.** These tests measure how long it takes blood clots to form.

- **Serum fibrinogen.** Fibrinogen is a protein that helps the blood clot. This test measures how much fibrinogen is in your blood.

- **Fibrin degradation.** After blood clots dissolve, substances called fibrin degradation products are left behind in the blood. This test measures the amount of these substances in the blood.

How Is Disseminated Intravascular Coagulation Treated?

Treatment for disseminated intravascular coagulation (DIC) depends on its severity and cause. The main goals of treating DIC are to control bleeding and clotting problems and treat the underlying cause.

Acute Disseminated Intravascular Coagulation

People who have acute DIC may have severe bleeding that requires emergency treatment in a hospital. Treatment may include blood transfusions, medicines, and oxygen therapy. (Oxygen is given through nasal prongs, a mask, or a breathing tube.)

A blood transfusion is a safe, common procedure. You receive blood through an intravenous (IV) line in one of your blood vessels. Blood transfusions are done to replace blood loss due to an injury, surgery, or illness.

Blood is made up of various parts, including red blood cells, white blood cells, platelets, and plasma. Some blood transfusions involve whole blood (blood with all of its parts). More often though, only some parts of blood are transfused.

If you have DIC, you may be given platelets and clotting factors, red blood cells, and plasma (the liquid part of blood).

Chronic Disseminated Intravascular Coagulation

People who have chronic DIC are more likely to have blood clotting problems than bleeding. If you have chronic DIC, your doctor may treat you with medicines called anticoagulants, or blood thinners.

Blood thinners help prevent blood clots from forming. They also keep existing blood clots from getting larger.

Living with Disseminated Intravascular Coagulation

If you have disseminated intravascular coagulation (DIC), ask your doctor how often you should schedule followup care and blood tests. Blood tests help track how well your blood is clotting.

You may need to take blood-thinning medicines (blood thinners) to help prevent blood clots or to keep existing clots from getting larger. If you take blood thinners, let everyone on your healthcare team know.

Blood thinners may thin your blood too much and cause bleeding. A lot of bleeding after a fall or injury or easy bruising or bleeding may mean that your blood is too thin.

Call your doctor right away if you have any signs of bleeding. If you have severe bleeding, call 9–1–1 right away.

Also, you should talk with your doctor before using any over-the-counter medicines or products, such as vitamins, supplements, or herbal remedies. Some of these products also can affect blood clotting and bleeding. For example, aspirin and ibuprofen may thin your blood too much. This can increase your risk of bleeding.

If you need surgery, your doctor may adjust the amount of medicine you take before, during, and after the surgery to prevent bleeding. This also may happen for dental work, but it's less common.

Chapter 33

Hypercoagulation

Chapter Contents

Section 33.1

Excessive Blood Clotting

Excessive blood clotting is a medical disorder known as hypercoagulation. In healthy people, a wound that causes bleeding triggers an immediate response in the body. Blood platelets begin to stick together in masses called blood clots. This process is known as coagulation and is the body's primary means of stopping blood loss. Hypercoagulation means that the body has an abnormal blood clotting response. Hypercoagulation can manifest as an overactive blood clot response, in which blood clots form too easily or too often. It can also refer to persistent blood clots that are not dissolved by the body, or blood clots that form inside blood vessels or arteries.

Causes

Excessive blood clotting disorders can be inherited or acquired. Acquired clotting disorders can result from traumatic injury, surgery, long-term bed rest, pregnancy, obesity, smoking, severe dehydration, certain chronic health conditions, and the use of certain medications. Excessive blood clotting can also be caused by sitting for long periods of time during car or airplane trips. Certain medical history factors can also indicate a person's likelihood of having an excessive blood clotting disorder. These include family members who have been diagnosed with an excessive blood clotting disorder, a history of excessive blood clots before age 40, and a history of pregnancies that ended in miscarriage.

Symptoms and Risks

Symptoms of excessive blood clotting disorders vary depending on where excessive blood clots form in the body.

Chest pain, shortness of breath, and pain in the upper arms, back, neck, or jaw can be symptoms of a blood clot in the heart or lungs. This type of blood clot can result in a heart attack, which restricts or blocks blood flow to part of the heart. An undiagnosed or untreated heart attack can result in serious long-term complications, including death.

Persistent headaches, changes in ability to speak, difficulty understanding others talking, dizziness, or paralysis can indicate a blood clot in the brain. This type of blood clot can result in a stroke. A stroke causes restricted blood flow to the brain, which can result in serious complications including death if left undiagnosed or untreated.

Swelling, pain, redness, or warm skin on the arms or legs can indicate a type of blood clot known as a deep vein thrombosis. These types of blood clots can travel through the blood stream and cause serious complications if they reach the brain, heart, or lungs.

Excessive blood clots during pregnancy can cause complications such as high blood pressure (hypertension), miscarriage, or stillbirth.

Diagnosis

Excessive blood clotting disorders are diagnosed through physical exam, medical history interview, and diagnostic blood tests. Blood tests for excessive clotting measure the levels of various blood components such as red and white blood cells, platelets, and blood clotting protein factors. Blood tests also analyze the clotting behavior of the blood samples to identify normal or abnormal clotting function. Medical history factors are evaluated to assess a person's risk for excessive blood clotting disorder. Some factors that indicate a possible blood clotting disorder diagnosis include family members who have been diagnosed with a blood clotting disorder, a history of blood clots before age 40, frequent unexplained bruising, or multiple pregnancies that ended in miscarriage.

References

1. "What Is Excessive Blood Clotting (Hypercoagulation)?" American Heart Association. November 30, 2015.

2. "Hypercoagulation," FamilyDoctor.org. March 2014.

Section 33.2

Deep Vein Thrombosis and Pulmonary Embolism (DVT/PE)

This section includes text excerpted from "Venous Thromboembolism (Blood Clots)," Centers for Disease Control and Prevention (CDC), February 24, 2016.

What Is Deep Vein Thrombosis and Pulmonary Embolism?

Deep vein thrombosis and pulmonary embolism (DVT/PE) are often underdiagnosed and serious, but preventable medical conditions.

Deep vein thrombosis (DVT) is a medical condition that occurs when a blood clot forms in a deep vein. These clots usually develop in the lower leg, thigh, or pelvis, but they can also occur in the arm.

It is important to know about DVT because it can happen to anybody and can cause serious illness, disability, and in some cases, death. The good news is that DVT is preventable and treatable if discovered early.

Complications of DVT

The most serious complication of DVT happens when a part of the clot breaks off and travels through the bloodstream to the lungs, causing a blockage called pulmonary embolism (PE). If the clot is small, and with appropriate treatment, people can recover from PE. However, there could be some damage to the lungs. If the clot is large, it can stop blood from reaching the lungs and is fatal.

In addition, nearly one-third of people who have a DVT will have long-term complications caused by the damage the clot does to the valves in the vein called post-thrombotic syndrome (PTS). People with PTS have symptoms such as swelling, pain, discoloration, and in severe cases, scaling or ulcers in the affected part of the body. In some cases, the symptoms can be so severe that a person becomes disabled.

For some people, DVT and PE can become a chronic illness; about 30% of people who have had a DVT or PE are at risk for another episode.

Risk Factors for DVT

Almost anyone can have a DVT. However, certain factors can increase the chance of having this condition. The chance increases even more for someone who has more than one of these factors at the same time.

Following is a list of factors that increase the risk of developing DVT:

- Injury to a vein, often caused by:

- fractures

- severe muscle injury, or

- major surgery (particularly involving the abdomen, pelvis, hip, or legs)

- Slow blood flow, often caused by:

- confinement to bed (e.g., due to a medical condition or after surgery)

- limited movement (e.g., a cast on a leg to help heal an injured bone)

- sitting for a long time, especially with crossed legs, or

- paralysis

- Increased estrogen, often caused by:

- birth control pills

- hormone replacement therapy, sometimes used after menopause

- pregnancy, for up to 6 weeks after giving birth

- Certain chronic medical illnesses, such as:

- heart disease

- lung disease

- cancer and its treatment

- inflammatory bowel disease (Crohn disease or ulcerative colitis)

- Other factors that increase the risk of DVT include:

- previous DVT or PE

- family history of DVT or PE

- age (risk increases as age increases)
- obesity
- a catheter located in a central vein
- inherited clotting disorders

Preventing DVT

The following tips can help prevent DVT:

- Move around as soon as possible after having been confined to bed, such as after surgery, illness, or injury.
- If you're at risk for DVT, talk to your doctor about:
- graduated compression stockings (sometimes called "medical compression stockings")
- medication (anticoagulants) to prevent DVT.
- When sitting for long periods of time, such as when traveling for more than four hours:
- Get up and walk around every 2 to 3 hours.
- Exercise your legs while you're sitting by:
- Raising and lowering your heels while keeping your toes on the floor
- Raising and lowering your toes while keeping your heels on the floor
- Tightening and releasing your leg muscles
- Wear loose-fitting clothes.
- You can reduce your risk by maintaining a healthy weight, avoiding a sedentary lifestyle, and following your doctor's recommendations based on your individual risk factors.

Symptoms

Know the Signs. Know your Risk. Seek Care.

Everybody should know the signs and symptoms of DVT/PE, their risk for DVT/PE, to talk to their health care provider about their risk, and to seek care immediately if they have any sign or symptom of DVT/PE.

Deep Vein Thrombosis

About half of people with DVT have no symptoms at all. The following are the most common symptoms of DVT that occur in the affected part of the body:

- swelling
- pain
- tenderness
- redness of the skin

If you have any of these symptoms, you should see your doctor as soon as possible.

Pulmonary Embolism

You can have a PE without any symptoms of a DVT.
Signs and symptoms of PE can include:

- difficulty breathing
- faster than normal or irregular heartbeat
- chest pain or discomfort, which usually worsens with a deep breath or coughing
- coughing up blood
- very low blood pressure, lightheadedness, or fainting

If you have any of these symptoms, you should seek medical help immediately.

Diagnosis

There are other conditions with signs and symptoms similar to those of DVT and PE. For example, muscle injury, cellulitis (a bacterial skin infection), and inflammation (swelling) of veins that are just under the skin can mimic the signs and symptoms of DVT. It is important to know that heart attack and pneumonia can have signs and symptoms similar to those of PE. Therefore, special tests that can look for clots in the veins or in the lungs (imaging tests) are needed to diagnose DVT or PE.

DVT

- **Duplex ultrasonography** is an imaging test that uses sound waves to look at the flow of blood in the veins. It can detect blockages or blood clots in the deep veins. It is the standard imaging test to diagnose DVT.

- A **D-dimer blood test** measures a substance in the blood that is released when a clot breaks up. If the D-dimer test is negative, it means that the patient probably does not have a blood clot.

- **Contrast venography** is a special type of X-ray where contrast material (dye) is injected into a large vein in the foot or ankle so that the doctor can see the deep veins in the leg and hip. It is the most accurate test for diagnosing blood clots but it is an invasive procedure, which means it is a medical test that requires doctors to use instruments to enter the body. Therefore this test has been largely replaced by duplex ultrasonography, and it is used only in certain patients.

- **Magnetic resonance imaging (MRI)**—a test that uses radio waves and a magnetic field to provide images of the body—and computed tomography (CT) scan—a special X-ray test—are imaging tests that help doctors diagnose and treat a variety of medical conditions. These tests can provide images of veins and clots, but they are not generally used to diagnose DVT.

PE

- **Computed tomographic pulmonary angiography (CTPA)** is a special type of X-ray test that includes injection of contrast material (dye) into a vein. This test can provide images of the blood vessels in the lungs. It is the standard imaging test to diagnose PE.

- **Ventilation-perfusion (V/Q) scan** is a specialized test that uses a radioactive substance to show the parts of the lungs that are getting oxygen (ventilation scan) and getting blood flow (perfusion scan) to see if there are portions of the lungs with differences between ventilation and perfusion. For example, if there are clots in some of the blood vessels in the lungs, the V/Q scan might show normal amounts of oxygen, but low blood flow to the portions of the lungs served by the clotted blood vessels. This test is used when CTPA is not available or when the CPTA test should not be done because it might be harmful to the particular patient.

- **Pulmonary angiography** is a special type of X-ray test that requires insertion of a large catheter (a long, thin hollow tube) into a large vein (usually in the groin) and into the arteries within the lung, followed by injection of contrast material (dye) through the catheter. It provides images of the blood vessels in the lung and it is the most accurate test to diagnose PE. However, it is an invasive test so it is used only in certain patients.

- **Magnetic resonance imaging (MRI)** uses radio waves and a magnetic field to provide images of the lung, but this test is usually reserved for certain patients, such as for pregnant women or in patients where the use of contrast material could be harmful.

Treatment

Anticoagulants

- Anticoagulants (commonly referred to as "blood thinners") are the medications most commonly used to treat DVT or PE. Although called blood thinners, these medications do not actually thin the blood. They reduce the ability of the blood to clot, preventing the clot from becoming larger while the body slowly reabsorbs it, and reducing the risk of further clots developing.

- The most frequently used injectable anticoagulants are

- unfractionated heparin (injected into a vein)

- low molecular weight heparin (LMWH) (injected under the skin), and

- fondaparinux (injected under the skin)

- Anticoagulants that are taken orally (swallowed) include

- warfarin

- dabigatran

- rivaroxaban

- apixaban, and

- edoxaban

- All of the anticoagulants can cause bleeding, so people taking them have to be monitored to prevent unusual bleeding.

Thrombolytics

- Thrombolytics (commonly referred to as "clot busters") work by dissolving the clot. They have a higher risk of causing bleeding compared to the anticoagulants, so they are reserved for severe cases.

Inferior Vena Cava Filter

- When anticoagulants cannot be used or don't work well enough, a filter can be inserted inside the inferior vena cava (a large vein that brings blood back to the heart) to capture or trap an embolus (a clot that is moving through the vein) before it reaches the lungs.

Thrombectomy / Embolectomy

In rare cases, a surgical procedure to remove the clot may be necessary. Thrombectomy involves removal of the clot in a patient with DVT. Embolectomy involves removal of the blockage in the lungs caused by the clot in a patient with PE.

Did You Know?

DVT does not cause heart attack or stroke.

There are two main types of blood clots. How a clot affects the body depends on the type and location of the clot:

- A blood clot in a deep vein of the leg, pelvis, and sometimes arm, is called deep vein thrombosis (DVT). This type of blood clot does not cause heart attack or stroke.

- A blood clot in an artery, usually in the heart or brain, is called arterial thrombosis. This type of blood clot can cause heart attack or stroke.

Both types of clots can cause serious health problems, but the causes and steps you can take to protect yourself are different.

Healthcare-Associated Venous Thromboembolism (HA-VTE)

People who are currently or recently hospitalized, recovering from surgery, or being treated for cancer are at increased risk of developing serious and potentially deadly blood clots in the form of venous thromboembolism (VTE). A blood clot that occurs as a result of hospitalization, surgery, or other healthcare treatment or procedure is called healthcare-associated venous thromboembolism (HA-VTE).

Why is HA-VTE a Public Health Problem?

Each year VTE affects as many as 900,000 Americans, resulting in about 100,000 premature deaths. The associated health care costs $10 billion or more each year in the United States. More and more people living in the United States have factors that increase their risk for a VTE. Without improvements and consistent use of strategies to prevent VTE, we expect the number of people affected by VTE to increase. Although anyone can develop a blood clot, over half of blood clots are related to a recent hospitalization or surgery and most of these do not occur until after discharge.

Fortunately, many cases of HA-VTE can be prevented. However, proven strategies to prevent HA-VTE are not being consistently or regularly applied across and within healthcare settings. Reports suggest that as many as 70% of cases of HA-VTE in patients could be prevented. Despite this finding, fewer than half of hospitalized patients receive appropriate prevention measures.

What Is Being Done to Reduce HA-VTE?

Preventing HA-VTE in patients can result in a major decrease in overall VTE occurrence, illness, financial costs, and death. Reducing HA-VTE has been the subject of a number of patient safety and public health programs developed and promoted by federal agencies including Healthy People 2020.

Currently, CDC is focusing on three main areas to promote, translate and implement strategies to prevent HA-VTE:

1. **Strengthen Healthcare Monitoring of HA-VTE:** Advance and promote methods and tools to improve and support monitoring of HA-VTE occurrence and prevention.

2. **Identify and Promote Best Practices for HA-VTE Prevention:** Identify and share proven prevention tools and resources for partners and stakeholders.

3. **Increase Education and Awareness of HA-VTE:** Share evidence-based education tools and strategies to increase awareness of risks for and prevention of HA-VTE.

Data and Statistics on HA-VTE

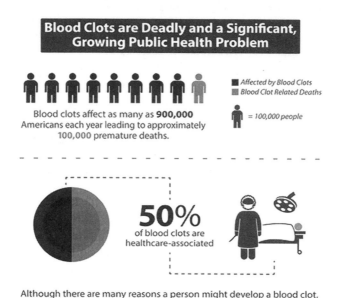

Figure 33.1. *Blood Clot Statistics*

- VTE is a leading cause of preventable hospital death in the United States.

- More than half of blood clots occurring in the outpatient setting (after discharge) are directly linked to a recent hospitalization or surgery.

- VTE is the fifth most frequent reason for unplanned hospital readmissions after surgery, overall, and the third most frequent among patients undergoing total hip or knee joint replacement.

- As many as 70% of cases of HA-VTE are preventable through prevention measures, such as use of blood thinning medications called anticoagulants, which help prevent blood from clotting, or use of compression stockings. Yet fewer than half of hospital patients receive these measures.

- A recent study of U.S. hospitalizations found that hospitalized adults with certain pre-existing health conditions (such as AIDS, anemia, arthritis, or congestive heart failure) are almost 3 times more likely to be diagnosed with VTE than hospitalized adults without any of these conditions.

- A recent study of almost 500,000 surgeries performed at Department of Veterans Affairs (VA) hospitals found that about 4 in 10 patients that developed VTE after surgery had it occur while they were still in the hospital, but approximately 6 in 10 patients with VTE after surgery developed the VTE up to 90 days after having left the hospital. This finding shows that looking at hospital discharge data alone to track how often VTE occurs after surgery would lead to a serious understatement of the true size and scope of the problem.

Section 33.3

Preventing and Treating Blood Clots

This section includes text excerpted from "Your Guide to Preventing and Treating Blood Clots," Agency for Healthcare Research and Quality (AHRQ), September 2012. Reviewed July 2016.

Blood clots (also called deep vein thrombosis) most often occur in people who can't move around well or who have had recent surgery or an injury. Blood clots are serious. It is important to know the signs and get treated right away. This section tells about ways to prevent and treat blood clots.

Preventing Blood Clots

You can help prevent blood clots if you:

- Wear loose-fitting clothes, socks, or stockings.

- Raise your legs 6 inches above your heart from time to time.

- Wear special stockings (called compression stockings) if your doctor prescribes them.

- Do exercises your doctor gives you.

- Change your position often, especially during a long trip.

- Do not stand or sit for more than 1 hour at a time.

- Eat less salt.

- Try not to bump or hurt your legs and try not to cross them.

- Do not use pillows under your knees.

- Raise the bottom of your bed 4 to 6 inches.

- Take all medicines the doctor prescribes you.

Treatment for Blood Clots

If you have been told you have a blood clot, your doctor may give you medicine to treat it. This type of medicine is called a blood thinner (also called an anticoagulant). In most cases, your doctor will tell you to follow this treatment plan:

- For the first week you will receive medicine called heparin that works quickly.

- This medicine is injected under the skin. You will learn how to give yourself these shots, or a family member or friend may do it for you.

- You will also start taking Coumadin®—generic name: warfarin—pills by mouth. After about a week of taking both the shots and the pills, you will stop taking the shots. You will continue to take the Coumadin®/warfarin pills for about 3 to 6 months or longer.

Side Effects of Blood Thinners

Blood thinners can cause side effects. Bleeding is the most common problem. Your doctor will watch you closely. If you notice something wrong that you think may be caused by your medication, call your doctor.

Section 33.4

Prothrombin Thrombophilia

This section includes text excerpted from "Prothrombin Thrombophilia," Genetics Home Reference (GHR), July 19, 2016.

What Is Prothrombin thrombophilia?

Prothrombin thrombophilia is an inherited disorder of blood clotting. Thrombophilia is an increased tendency to form abnormal blood clots in blood vessels. People who have prothrombin thrombophilia are at somewhat higher than average risk for a type of clot called a deep venous thrombosis, which typically occurs in the deep veins of the legs. Affected people also have an increased risk of developing a pulmonary embolism, which is a clot that travels through the bloodstream and lodges in the lungs. Most people with prothrombin thrombophilia never develop abnormal blood clots, however.

Some research suggests that prothrombin thrombophilia is associated with a somewhat increased risk of pregnancy loss (miscarriage) and may also increase the risk of other complications during pregnancy. These complications may include pregnancy-induced high blood pressure (preeclampsia), slow fetal growth, and early separation of the placenta from the uterine wall (placental abruption). It is important to note, however, that most women with prothrombin thrombophilia have normal pregnancies.

Frequency

Prothrombin thrombophilia is the second most common inherited form of thrombophilia after factor V Leiden thrombophilia. Approximately 1 in 50 people in the white population in the United States and Europe has prothrombin thrombophilia. This condition is less common in other ethnic groups, occurring in less than one percent of African American, Native American, or Asian populations.

Genetic Changes

Prothrombin thrombophilia is caused by a particular mutation in the *F2* gene. The *F2* gene plays a critical role in the formation of blood clots in response to injury. The protein produced from the *F2* gene, prothrombin (also called coagulation factor II), is the precursor to a protein called thrombin that initiates a series of chemical reactions in order to form a blood clot. The particular mutation that causes pro-thrombin thrombophilia results in an overactive *F2* gene that causes too much prothrombin to be produced. An abundance of prothrombin leads to more thrombin, which promotes the formation of blood clots.

Other factors also increase the risk of blood clots in people with prothrombin thrombophilia. These factors include increasing age, obe-sity, trauma, surgery, smoking, the use of oral contraceptives (birth control pills) or hormone replacement therapy, and pregnancy. The combination of prothrombin thrombophilia and mutations in other genes involved in blood clotting can also influence risk.

Inheritance Pattern

The risk of developing an abnormal clot in a blood vessel depends on whether a person inherits one or two copies of the *F2* gene mutation that causes prothrombin thrombophilia. In the general population, the risk of developing an abnormal blood clot is about 1 in 1,000 people per year. Inheriting one copy of the *F2* gene mutation increases that risk to 2 to 3 in 1,000. People who inherit two copies of the mutation, one from each parent, may have a risk as high as 20 in 1,000.

Chapter 34

Thrombocytopenia

What Is Thrombocytopenia?

Thrombocytopenia is a condition in which your blood has a lower than normal number of blood cell fragments called platelets.

Platelets are made in your bone marrow along with other kinds of blood cells. They travel through your blood vessels and stick together (clot) to stop any bleeding that may happen if a blood vessel is damaged. Platelets also are called thrombocytes because a clot also is called a thrombus.

What Causes Thrombocytopenia?

Many factors can cause thrombocytopenia (a low platelet count). The condition can be inherited or acquired. "Inherited" means your parents pass the gene for the condition to you. "Acquired" means you aren't born with the condition, but you develop it. Sometimes the cause of thrombocytopenia isn't known.

In general, a low platelet count occurs because:

- The body's bone marrow doesn't make enough platelets.

- The bone marrow makes enough platelets, but the body destroys them or uses them up.

- The spleen holds on to too many platelets.

This chapter includes text excerpted from "Thrombocytopenia," National Heart, Lung, and Blood Institute (NHLBI), September 25, 2012. Reviewed July 2016.

A combination of the above factors also may cause a low platelet count.

The Bone Marrow Doesn't Make Enough Platelets

Bone marrow is the sponge-like tissue inside the bones. It contains stem cells that develop into red blood cells, white blood cells, and platelets. When stem cells are damaged, they don't grow into healthy blood cells. Many conditions and factors can damage stem cells.

Cancer

Cancer, such as leukemia or lymphoma, can damage the bone marrow and destroy blood stem cells. Cancer treatments, such as radiation and chemotherapy, also destroy the stem cells.

Aplastic Anemia

Aplastic anemia is a rare, serious blood disorder in which the bone marrow stops making enough new blood cells. This lowers the number of platelets in your blood.

Toxic Chemicals

Exposure to toxic chemicals—such as pesticides, arsenic, and benzene—can slow the production of platelets.

Medicines

Some medicines, such as diuretics and chloramphenicol, can slow the production of platelets. Chloramphenicol (an antibiotic) rarely is used in the United States.

Common over-the-counter medicines, such as aspirin or ibuprofen, also can affect platelets.

Alcohol

Alcohol also slows the production of platelets. A temporary drop in the platelet count is common among heavy drinkers, especially if they're eating foods that are low in iron, vitamin B12, or folate.

Viruses

Chickenpox, mumps, rubella, Epstein-Barr virus, or parvovirus can decrease your platelet count for a while. People who have AIDS often develop thrombocytopenia.

Genetic Conditions

Some genetic conditions can cause low numbers of platelets in the blood. Examples include Wiskott-Aldrich and May-Hegglin syndromes.

The Body Destroys Its Own Platelets

A low platelet count can occur even if the bone marrow makes enough platelets. The body may destroy its own platelets due to auto-immune diseases, certain medicines, infections, surgery, pregnancy, and some conditions that cause too much blood clotting.

Autoimmune Diseases

Autoimmune diseases occur if the body's immune system mistakenly attacks healthy cells in the body. If an autoimmune disease destroys the body's platelets, thrombocytopenia can occur.

One example of this type of autoimmune disease is immune thrombocytopenia (ITP). ITP is a bleeding disorder in which the blood doesn't clot as it should. An autoimmune response is thought to cause most cases of ITP.

Normally, your immune system helps your body fight off infections and diseases. But if you have ITP, your immune system attacks and destroys its own platelets. Why this happens isn't known. (ITP also may occur if the immune system attacks your bone marrow, which makes platelets.)

Other autoimmune diseases that destroy platelets include lupus and rheumatoid arthritis.

Medicines

A reaction to medicine can confuse your body and cause it to destroy its platelets. Examples of medicines that may cause this to happen include quinine; antibiotics that contain sulfa; and some medicines for seizures, such as Dilantin®, vancomycin, and rifampin. (Quinine is a substance often found in tonic water and nutritional health products.)

Heparin is a medicine commonly used to prevent blood clots. But an immune reaction may trigger the medicine to cause blood clots and thrombocytopenia. This condition is called heparin-induced thrombocytopenia (HIT). HIT rarely occurs outside of a hospital.

In HIT, the body's immune system attacks a substance formed by heparin and a protein on the surface of the platelets. This attack activates the platelets and they start to form blood clots.

Blood clots can form deep in the legs (deep vein thrombosis), or they can break loose and travel to the lungs (pulmonary embolism).

Infection

A low platelet count can occur after blood poisoning from a widespread bacterial infection. A virus, such as mononucleosis or cytomegalovirus, also can cause a low platelet count.

Surgery

Platelets can be destroyed when they pass through man-made heart valves, blood vessel grafts, or machines and tubing used for blood transfusions or bypass surgery.

Pregnancy

About 5 percent of pregnant women develop mild thrombocytopenia when they're close to delivery. The exact cause isn't known for sure.

Rare and Serious Conditions That Cause Blood Clots

Some rare and serious conditions can cause a low platelet count. Two examples are thrombotic thrombocytopenic purpura (TTP) and disseminated intravascular coagulation (DIC).

TTP is a rare blood condition. It causes blood clots to form in the body's small blood vessels, including vessels in the brains, kidneys, and heart.

DIC is a rare complication of pregnancy, severe infections, or severe trauma. Tiny blood clots form suddenly throughout the body.

In both conditions, the blood clots use up many of the blood's platelets.

The Spleen Holds On to Too Many Platelets

Usually, one-third of the body's platelets are held in the spleen. If the spleen is enlarged, it will hold onto too many platelets. This means that not enough platelets will circulate in the blood.

An enlarged spleen often is due to cancer or severe liver disease, such as cirrhosis. Cirrhosis is a disease in which the liver is scarred. This prevents it from working well.

An enlarged spleen also might be due to a bone marrow condition, such as myelofibrosis. With this condition, the bone marrow is scarred and isn't able to make blood cells.

Who Is at Risk for Thrombocytopenia?

People who are at highest risk for thrombocytopenia are those affected by one of the conditions or factors discussed in "What Causes Thrombocytopenia?" This includes people who:

- have certain types of cancer, aplastic anemia, or autoimmune diseases

- are exposed to certain toxic chemicals

- have a reaction to certain medicines

- have certain viruses

- have certain genetic conditions

People at highest risk also include heavy alcohol drinkers and pregnant women.

What Are the Signs and Symptoms of Thrombocytopenia?

Mild to serious bleeding causes the main signs and symptoms of thrombocytopenia. Bleeding can occur inside your body (internal bleeding) or underneath your skin or from the surface of your skin (external bleeding).

Signs and symptoms can appear suddenly or over time. Mild thrombocytopenia often has no signs or symptoms. Many times, it's found during a routine blood test.

Check with your doctor if you have any signs of bleeding. Severe thrombocytopenia can cause bleeding in almost any part of the body. Bleeding can lead to a medical emergency and should be treated right away.

External bleeding usually is the first sign of a low platelet count. External bleeding may cause purpura or petechiae. Purpura are purple, brown, and red bruises. This bruising may happen easily and often. Petechiae are small red or purple dots on your skin.

Other signs of external bleeding include:

- prolonged bleeding, even from minor cuts

- bleeding or oozing from the mouth or nose, especially nosebleeds or bleeding from brushing your teeth

- Abnormal vaginal bleeding (especially heavy menstrual flow)

A lot of bleeding after surgery or dental work also might suggest a bleeding problem.

Heavy bleeding into the intestines or the brain (internal bleeding) is serious and can be fatal. Signs and symptoms include:

- Blood in the urine or stool or bleeding from the rectum. Blood in the stool can appear as red blood or as a dark, tarry color. (Taking iron supplements also can cause dark, tarry stools.)

- Headaches and other neurological symptoms. These problems are very rare, but you should discuss them with your doctor.

How Is Thrombocytopenia Diagnosed?

Your doctor will diagnose thrombocytopenia based on your medical history, a physical exam, and test results. A hematologist also may be involved in your care. This is a doctor who specializes in diagnosing and treating blood diseases and conditions.

Once thrombocytopenia is diagnosed, your doctor will begin looking for its cause.

Medical History

Your doctor may ask about factors that can affect your platelets, such as:

- The medicines you take, including over-the-counter medicines and herbal remedies, and whether you drink beverages that contain quinine.

- Your general eating habits, including the amount of alcohol you normally drink.

- Your risk for AIDS, including questions about blood transfusions, sexual partners, intravenous (IV) drugs, and exposure to infectious blood or bodily fluids at work.

- Any family history of low platelet counts.

Physical Exam

Your doctor will do a physical exam to look for signs and symptoms of bleeding, such as bruises or spots on the skin. He or she will check your abdomen for signs of an enlarged spleen or liver. You also will be checked for signs of infection, such as a fever.

Diagnostic Tests

Your doctor may recommend one or more of the following tests to help diagnose a low platelet count.

Complete Blood Count

A complete blood count (CBC) measures the levels of red blood cells, white blood cells, and platelets in your blood. For this test, a small amount of blood is drawn from a blood vessel, usually in your arm.

If you have thrombocytopenia, the results of this test will show that your platelet count is low.

Blood Smear

A blood smear is used to check the appearance of your platelets under a microscope. For this test, a small amount of blood is drawn from a blood vessel, usually in your arm.

Bone Marrow Tests

Bone marrow tests check whether your bone marrow is healthy. Blood cells, including platelets, are made in your bone marrow. The two bone marrow tests are aspiration and biopsy.

Bone marrow aspiration might be done to find out why your bone marrow isn't making enough blood cells. For this test, your doctor removes a sample of fluid bone marrow through a needle. He or she examines the sample under a microscope to check for faulty cells.

A bone marrow biopsy often is done right after an aspiration. For this test, your doctor removes a sample of bone marrow tissue through a needle. He or she examines the tissue to check the number and types of cells in the bone marrow.

Other Tests

If a bleeding problem is suspected, you may need other blood tests as well. For example, your doctor may recommend PT and PTT tests to see whether your blood is clotting properly.

Your doctor also may suggest an ultrasound to check your spleen. An ultrasound uses sound waves to create pictures of your spleen. This will allow your doctor to see whether your spleen is enlarged.

How Is Thrombocytopenia Treated?

Treatment for thrombocytopenia depends on its cause and severity. The main goal of treatment is to prevent death and disability caused by bleeding.

If your condition is mild, you may not need treatment. A fully normal platelet count isn't necessary to prevent bleeding, even with severe cuts or accidents.

Thrombocytopenia often improves when its underlying cause is treated. People who inherit the condition usually don't need treatment.

If a reaction to a medicine is causing a low platelet count, your doctor may prescribe another medicine. Most people recover after the initial medicine has been stopped. For heparin-induced thrombocytopenia (HIT), stopping the heparin isn't enough. Often, you'll need another medicine to prevent blood clotting.

If your immune system is causing a low platelet count, your doctor may prescribe medicines to suppress the immune system.

Severe Thrombocytopenia

If your thrombocytopenia is severe, your doctor may prescribe treatments such as medicines, blood or platelet transfusions, or splenectomy.

Medicines

Your doctor may prescribe corticosteroids, also called steroids for short. Steroids may slow platelet destruction. These medicines can be given through a vein or by mouth. One example of this type of medicine is prednisone.

The steroids used to treat thrombocytopenia are different from illegal steroids taken by some athletes to enhance performance.

Your doctor may prescribe immunoglobulins or medicines like rituximab to block your immune system. These medicines are given through a vein. He or she also may prescribe other medicines, such as eltrombopag or romiplostim, to help your body make more platelets. The former comes as a tablet to take by mouth and the latter is given as an injection under the skin.

Blood or Platelet Transfusions

Blood or platelet transfusions are used to treat people who have active bleeding or are at a high risk of bleeding. During this procedure, a needle is used to insert an intravenous (IV) line into one of your blood vessels. Through this line, you receive healthy blood or platelets.

Splenectomy

A splenectomy is surgery to remove the spleen. This surgery may be used if treatment with medicines doesn't work. This surgery mostly is used for adults who have immune thrombocytopenia (ITP). However, medicines often are the first course of treatment.

How Can Thrombocytopenia Be Prevented?

Whether you can prevent thrombocytopenia depends on its specific cause. Usually the condition can't be prevented. However, you can take steps to prevent health problems associated with thrombocytopenia. For example:

- Avoid heavy drinking. Alcohol slows the production of platelets.

- Try to avoid contact with toxic chemicals. Chemicals such as pesticides, arsenic, and benzene can slow the production of platelets.

- Avoid medicines that you know have decreased your platelet count in the past.

- Be aware of medicines that may affect your platelets and raise your risk of bleeding. Two examples of such medicines are aspirin and ibuprofen. These medicines may thin your blood too much.

- Talk with your doctor about getting vaccinated for viruses that can affect your platelets. You may need vaccines for mumps, measles, rubella, and chickenpox. You may want to have your child vaccinated for these viruses as well. Talk with your child's doctor about these vaccines.

Living with Thrombocytopenia

If you have thrombocytopenia, watch for any signs and symptoms of bleeding. Report these signs and symptoms to your doctor right away.

Symptoms can appear suddenly or over time. Severe thrombocytopenia can cause bleeding in almost any part of the body. Bleeding can lead to a medical emergency and should be treated right away.

You can take steps to avoid health problems associated with thrombocytopenia. Be aware of the medicines you're taking, avoid injuries, and contact your doctor if you have a fever or other signs or symptoms of an infection.

Medicines

Avoid medicines that may affect your platelets and raise your risk of bleeding. Two examples of such medicines are aspirin and ibuprofen. These medicines may thin your blood too much. Be careful when using over-the-counter medicines—many contain aspirin or ibuprofen.

Tell your doctor about all of the medicines you take, including over-the-counter medicines, vitamins, supplements, and herbal remedies.

Injuries

Avoid injuries that can cause bruising and bleeding. Don't take part in contact sports such as boxing, football, or karate. These sports are likely to lead to injuries that can cause bleeding.

Other sports, such as skiing or horseback riding, also put you at risk for injuries that can cause bleeding. Ask your doctor about physical activities that are safe for you.

Take safety precautions, such as using a seatbelt while riding in a car and wearing gloves when working with knives and other tools.

If your child has thrombocytopenia, try to protect him or her from injuries, especially head injuries that can cause bleeding in the brain. Ask your child's doctor whether you need to restrict your child's activities.

Infection

If you've had your spleen removed, you may be more likely to become ill from certain types of infection. Watch for fever or other signs of infection and report them to your doctor promptly. People who have had their spleens removed may need vaccines to prevent certain infections.

Chapter 35

Immune (Idiopathic) Thrombocytopenic Purpura

What Is Immune Thrombocytopenia?

Immune thrombocytopenia, or ITP, is a bleeding disorder. In ITP, the blood doesn't clot as it should. This is due to a low number of blood cell fragments called platelets or thrombocytes.

Platelets are made in your bone marrow along with other kinds of blood cells. They stick together (clot) to seal small cuts or breaks on blood vessel walls and stop bleeding.

Other Names for Immune Thrombocytopenia

- Idiopathic thrombocytopenic purpura
- Immune thrombocytopenic purpura
- Autoimmune thrombocytopenic purpura

What Causes Immune Thrombocytopenia?

In most cases, an autoimmune response is thought to cause immune thrombocytopenia (ITP).

This chapter includes text excerpted from "Immune Thrombocytopenia," National Heart, Lung, and Blood Institute (NHLBI), March 14, 2012. Reviewed July 2016.

Normally, your immune system helps your body fight off infections and diseases. In ITP, however, your immune system attacks and destroys your body's platelets by mistake. Why this happens isn't known.

In some people, ITP may be linked to viral or bacterial infections, such as HIV, hepatitis C, or *H. pylori*.

Children who have acute (short-term) ITP often have had recent viral infections. These infections may "trigger" or set off the immune reaction that leads to ITP.

Who Is at Risk for Immune Thrombocytopenia?

Immune thrombocytopenia (ITP) is a fairly common blood disorder. Both children and adults can develop ITP.

Children usually have the acute (short-term) type of ITP. Acute ITP often develops after a viral infection.

Adults tend to have the chronic (long-lasting) type of ITP. Women are two to three times more likely than men to develop chronic ITP.

The number of cases of ITP is rising because routine blood tests that can detect a low platelet count are being done more often.

ITP can't be passed from one person to another.

What Are the Signs and Symptoms of Immune Thrombocytopenia?

Immune thrombocytopenia (ITP) may not cause any signs or symptoms. However, ITP can cause bleeding inside the body (internal bleeding) or underneath or from the skin (external bleeding). Signs of bleeding may include:

- Bruising or purplish areas on the skin or mucous membranes (such as in the mouth). These bruises are called purpura. They're caused by bleeding under the skin, and they may occur for no known reason.

- Pinpoint red spots on the skin called petechiae. These spots often are found in groups and may look like a rash. Bleeding under the skin causes petechiae.

- A collection of clotted or partially clotted blood under the skin that looks or feels like a lump. This is called a hematoma.

- Nosebleeds or bleeding from the gums (for example, during dental work).

- Blood in the urine or stool (bowel movement).

Any kind of bleeding that's hard to stop could be a sign of ITP. This includes menstrual bleeding that's heavier than normal. Bleeding in the brain is rare, and its symptoms may vary.

A low platelet count doesn't directly cause pain, problems concentrating, or other symptoms. However, a low platelet count might be associated with fatigue (tiredness).

How Is Immune Thrombocytopenia Diagnosed?

Your doctor will diagnose immune thrombocytopenia (ITP) based on your medical history, a physical exam, and test results.

Your doctor will want to make sure that your low platelet count isn't due to another condition (such as an infection) or medicines you're taking (such as chemotherapy medicines or aspirin).

Medical History

Your doctor may ask about:

- Your signs and symptoms of bleeding and any other signs or symptoms you're having

- Whether you have illnesses that could lower your platelet count or cause bleeding

- Medicines or any over-the-counter supplements or remedies you take that could cause bleeding or lower your platelet count

Physical Exam

During a physical exam, your doctor will look for signs of bleeding and infection. For example, your doctor may look for purplish areas on the skin or mucous membranes and pinpoint red spots on the skin. These are signs of bleeding under the skin.

Diagnostic Tests

You'll likely have blood tests to check your platelet count. These tests usually include:

- **A complete blood count.** This test checks the number of red blood cells, white blood cells, and platelets in your blood. In ITP, the red and white blood cell counts are normal, but the platelet count is low.

389

- **A blood smear.** For this test, some of your blood is put on a slide. A microscope is used to look at your platelets and other blood cells.

You also may have a blood test to check for the antibodies (proteins) that attack platelets.

If blood tests show that your platelet count is low, your doctor may recommend more tests to confirm a diagnosis of ITP. For example, bone marrow tests can show whether your bone marrow is making enough platelets.

If you're at risk for HIV, hepatitis C, or *H. pylori*, your doctor may screen you for these infections, which might be linked to ITP.

Some people who have mild ITP have few or no signs of bleeding. They may be diagnosed only if a blood test done for another reason shows that they have low platelet counts.

How Is Immune Thrombocytopenia Treated?

Treatment for immune thrombocytopenia (ITP) is based on how much and how often you're bleeding and your platelet count.

Adults who have mild ITP may not need any treatment, other than watching their symptoms and platelet counts. Adults who have ITP with very low platelet counts or bleeding problems often are treated.

The acute (short-term) type of ITP that occurs in children often goes away within a few weeks or months. Children who have bleeding symptoms, other than merely bruising (purpura), usually are treated.

Children who have mild ITP may not need treatment other than monitoring and follow-up to make sure their platelet counts return to normal.

Medicines

Medicines often are used as the first course of treatment for both children and adults.

Corticosteroids, such as prednisone, are commonly used to treat ITP. These medicines, called steroids for short, help increase your platelet count. However, steroids have many side effects. Some people relapse (get worse) when treatment ends.

The steroids used to treat ITP are different from the illegal steroids that some athletes take to enhance performance. Corticosteroids aren't habit-forming, even if you take them for many years.

Other medicines also are used to raise the platelet count. Some are given through a needle inserted into a vein. These medicines include rituximab, immune globulin, and anti-Rh (D) immunoglobulin.

Medicines also may be used with a procedure to remove the spleen called splenectomy.

If medicines or splenectomy don't help, two newer medicines— eltrombopag and romiplostim—can be used to treat ITP.

Removal of the Spleen (Splenectomy)

If needed, doctors can surgically remove the spleen. This organ is located in the upper left abdomen. The spleen is about the size of a golf ball in children and a baseball in adults.

The spleen makes antibodies (proteins) that help fight infections. In ITP, these antibodies destroy platelets by mistake.

If ITP hasn't responded to medicines, removing the spleen will reduce the destruction of platelets. However, it also may raise your risk for infections. Before you have the surgery, your doctor may give you vaccines to help prevent infections.

If your spleen is removed, your doctor will explain what steps you can take to help avoid infections and what symptoms to watch for.

Other Treatments

Platelet Transfusions

Some people who have ITP with severe bleeding may need to have platelet transfusions and be hospitalized. Some people will need platelet transfusions before having surgery.

For a platelet transfusion, donor platelets from a blood bank are injected into the recipient's bloodstream. This increases the platelet count for a short time.

Treating Infections

Some infections can briefly lower your platelet count. Treating the infection may help increase your platelet count and reduce bleeding problems.

Stopping Medicines

Some medicines can lower your platelet count or cause bleeding. Stopping the medicine can sometimes help raise your platelet count or prevent bleeding.

For example, aspirin and ibuprofen are common medicines that increase the risk of bleeding. If you have ITP, your doctor may suggest that you avoid these medicines.

How Can Immune Thrombocytopenia Be Prevented?

You can't prevent immune thrombocytopenia (ITP), but you can prevent its complications.

- Talk with your doctor about which medicines are safe for you. Your doctor may advise you to avoid medicines that can affect your platelets and increase your risk of bleeding. Examples of such medicines include aspirin and ibuprofen.

- Protect yourself from injuries that can cause bruising or bleeding.

- Seek treatment right away if you develop any infections. Report any symptoms of infection, such as a fever, to your doctor. This is very important for people who have ITP and have had their spleens removed.

Living with Immune Thrombocytopenia

If you have immune thrombocytopenia (ITP), you can take steps to prevent complications. Lifestyle changes and ongoing care can help you manage the condition.

Lifestyle Changes

Try to avoid injuries, especially head injuries, that can cause bleeding in the brain. For example, don't take part in contact sports, such as boxing, football, or karate. Other sports, such as skiing or horseback riding, also put you at risk for injuries that can cause bleeding.

Some safe activities are swimming, biking (with a helmet), and walking. Ask your doctor about physical activities that are safe for you.

Take precautions such as regular use of seatbelts and wearing gloves while working with knives and other tools.

If your child has ITP, ask his or her doctor whether you need to restrict your child's activities.

Ongoing Care

You may want to find a doctor who is familiar with treating people who have ITP. For example, hematologists are doctors who specialize in diagnosing and treating blood disorders. Discuss with your doctor how to manage ITP and when to seek medical care.

Talk with your doctor before taking prescription medicines or over-the-counter medicines, supplements, vitamins, or herbal remedies. Some medicines and supplements can affect platelets and increase your chance of bleeding. Common examples are aspirin or ibuprofen. Your doctor may advise you to avoid these medicines.

Watch for symptoms of infection, such as a fever, and report them to your doctor promptly. If you've had your spleen removed, you may be more likely to become ill from certain infections.

Immune Thrombocytopenia in Pregnancy

In women who are pregnant and have ITP, the ITP usually doesn't affect the baby. However, some babies may be born with or develop low platelet counts soon after birth.

The babies' platelet counts almost always return to normal without any treatment. Treatment can speed up recovery in the babies whose platelet counts are very low.

Treatment for ITP during pregnancy depends on a woman's platelet count. If treatment is needed, the doctor will take a close look at the possible effects of the treatment on the unborn baby.

Women who have mild cases of ITP usually can go through pregnancy without treatment. Pregnant women who have very low platelet counts or a lot of bleeding are more likely to have heavy bleeding during delivery or afterward. To prevent heavy bleeding, these women usually are treated.

Chapter 36

Thrombotic Thrombocytopenic Purpura

What Is Thrombotic Thrombocytopenic Purpura?

Thrombotic thrombocytopenic purpura (TTP) is a rare blood disorder. In TTP, blood clots form in small blood vessels throughout the body.

The clots can limit or block the flow of oxygen-rich blood to the body's organs, such as the brain, kidneys, and heart. As a result, serious health problems can develop.

The increased clotting that occurs in TTP also uses up platelets in the blood. Platelets are blood cell fragments that help form blood clots. These cell fragments stick together to seal small cuts and breaks on blood vessel walls and stop bleeding.

With fewer platelets available in the blood, bleeding problems can occur. People who have TTP may bleed inside their bodies, underneath the skin, or from the surface of the skin. When cut or injured, they also may bleed longer than normal.

"Thrombotic" refers to the blood clots that form. "Thrombocytopenic" means the blood has a lower than normal number of platelets. "Purpura" refers to purple bruises caused by bleeding under the skin.

This chapter includes text excerpted from "Thrombotic Thrombocytopenic Purpura," National Heart, Lung, and Blood Institute (NHLBI), March 21, 2014.

Bleeding under the skin also can cause tiny red or purple dots on the skin. These pinpoint-sized dots are called petechiae. Petechiae may look like a rash.

TTP also can cause red blood cells to break apart faster than the body can replace them. This leads to hemolytic anemia—a rare form of anemia. Anemia is a condition in which the body has a lower than normal number of red blood cells.

A lack of activity in the *ADAMTS13* enzyme (a type of protein in the blood) causes TTP. The *ADAMTS13* gene controls the enzyme, which is involved in blood clotting. The enzyme breaks up a large protein called von Willebrand factor that clumps together with platelets to form blood clots.

Other Names for Thrombotic Thrombocytopenic Purpura

Inherited Thrombotic Thrombocytopenic Purpura

- Familial thrombotic thrombocytopenic purpura

- Upshaw-Schulman syndrome (USS)

Acquired Thrombotic Thrombocytopenic Purpura

- Moschcowitz disease

- Microangiopathic hemolytic anemia

If you have TTP, you may sometimes hear it referred to as TTP–HUS. HUS, or hemolytic-uremic syndrome, is a disorder that resembles TTP, but is more common in children. Kidney problems also tend to be worse in HUS. Although some researchers think TTP and HUS are two forms of a single syndrome, recent evidence suggests that each has different causes.

What Causes Thrombotic Thrombocytopenic Purpura?

A lack of activity in the *ADAMTS13* enzyme (a type of protein in the blood) causes thrombotic thrombocytopenic purpura (TTP). The ADAMTS13 gene controls the enzyme, which is involved in blood clotting.

Not having enough enzyme activity causes overactive blood clotting. In TTP, blood clots form in small blood vessels throughout the body. These clots can limit or block the flow of oxygen-rich blood to the body's organs, such as the brain, kidneys, and heart. As a result, serious health problems can develop.

The increased clotting that occurs in TTP also uses up many of the blood's platelets. With fewer platelets available in the blood, bleeding problems can occur.

People who have TTP may bleed inside their bodies, underneath the skin, or from the surface of the skin. When cut or injured, they also may bleed longer than normal.

TTP also can cause red blood cells to break apart faster than the body can replace them. This leads to hemolytic anemia.

Inherited Thrombotic Thrombocytopenic Purpura

In inherited TTP, the *ADAMTS13* gene is faulty. It doesn't prompt the body to make a normal *ADAMTS13* enzyme. As a result, enzyme activity is lacking or changed.

"Inherited" means that the condition is passed from parents to children through genes. A person who inherits TTP is born with two copies of the faulty gene—one from each parent.

Most often, the parents each have one copy of the faulty gene, but have no signs or symptoms TTP.

Acquired Thrombotic Thrombocytopenic Purpura

In acquired TTP, the *ADAMTS13* gene isn't faulty. Instead, the body makes antibodies (proteins) that block the activity of the ADAMTS13 enzyme.

"Acquired" means you aren't born with the condition, but you develop it sometime after birth.

Who Is at Risk for Thrombotic Thrombocytopenic Purpura?

Thrombotic thrombocytopenic purpura (TTP) is a rare disorder. Most cases of TTP are acquired. Acquired TTP mostly occurs in adults, but it can affect children. The condition occurs more often in women and in Black people than in other groups.

Inherited TTP mainly affects newborns and children. Most people who have inherited TTP begin to have symptoms soon after birth. Some, however, don't have symptoms until they're adults.

It isn't clear what triggers inherited and acquired TTP, but some factors may play a role. These factors may include:

- Some diseases and conditions, such as pregnancy, cancer, HIV, lupus, and infections

- Some medical procedures, such as surgery and blood and marrow stem cell transplant

- Some medicines, such as chemotherapy, ticlopidine, clopidogrel, cyclosporine A, and hormone therapy and estrogens

- Quinine, which is a substance often found in tonic water and nutritional health products

What Are the Signs and Symptoms of Thrombotic Thrombocytopenic Purpura?

Blood clots, a low platelet count, and damaged red blood cells cause the signs and symptoms of thrombotic thrombocytopenic purpura (TTP). The signs and symptoms include:

- Purplish bruises on the skin or mucous membranes (such as in the mouth). These bruises, called purpura, are caused by bleeding under the skin.

- Pinpoint-sized red or purple dots on the skin. These dots, called petechiae, often are found in groups and may look like a rash. Bleeding under the skin causes petechiae.

- Paleness or jaundice (a yellowish color of the skin or whites of the eyes).

- Fatigue (feeling very tired and weak).

- Fever.

- A fast heart rate or shortness of breath.

- Headache, speech changes, confusion, coma, stroke, or seizure.

- A low amount of urine, or protein or blood in the urine.

If you've had TTP and have any of these signs or symptoms, you may be having a relapse (flareup). Ask your doctor when to call him or her or seek emergency care.

How Is Thrombotic Thrombocytopenic Purpura Diagnosed?

Your doctor will diagnose thrombotic thrombocytopenic purpura (TTP) based on your medical history, a physical exam, and test results.

If TTP is suspected or diagnosed, a hematologist will be involved in your care. A hematologist is a doctor who specializes in diagnosing and treating blood disorders.

Medical History

Your doctor will ask about factors that may affect TTP. For example, he or she may ask whether you:

- Have certain diseases or conditions, such as cancer, HIV, lupus, or infections (or whether you're pregnant).
- Have had previous medical procedures, such as a blood and marrow stem cell transplant.
- Take certain medicines, such as ticlopidine, clopidogrel, cyclosporine A, or hormone therapy and estrogens, or whether you've had chemotherapy.
- Have used any products that contain quinine.

Physical Exam

As part of the medical history and physical exam, your doctor will ask about any signs or symptoms you've had. He or she will look for signs such as:

- bruising and bleeding under your skin
- fever
- paleness or jaundice (a yellowish color of the skin or whites of the eyes)
- a fast heart rate
- speech changes or changes in awareness that can range from confusion to passing out
- changes in urine

Diagnostic Tests

Your doctor also may recommend tests to help find out whether you have TTP.

Complete Blood Count

This test measures the number of red blood cells, white blood cells, and platelets in your blood. For this test, a sample of blood is drawn from a vein, usually in your arm.

If you have TTP, you'll have a lower than normal number of platelets and red blood cells (anemia).

Blood Smear

For this test, a sample of blood is drawn from a vein, usually in your arm. Some of your blood is put on a glass slide. A microscope is then used to look at your red blood cells. In TTP, the red blood cells are torn and broken.

Platelet Count

This test counts the number of platelets in a blood smear. People who have TTP have a lower than normal number of platelets in their blood. This test is used with the blood smear to help diagnose TTP.

Bilirubin Test

When red blood cells die, they release a protein called hemoglobin into the bloodstream. The body breaks down hemoglobin into a compound called bilirubin. High levels of bilirubin in the bloodstream cause jaundice.

For this blood test, a sample of blood is drawn from a vein, usually in your arm. The level of bilirubin in the sample is checked. If you have TTP, your bilirubin level may be high because your body is breaking down red blood cells faster than normal.

Kidney Function Tests and Urine Tests

These tests show whether your kidneys are working well. If you have TTP, your urine may contain protein or blood cells. Also, your blood creatinine level may be high. Creatinine is a blood product that's normally removed by the kidneys.

Coombs Test

This blood test is used to find out whether TTP is the cause of hemolytic anemia. For this test, a sample of blood is drawn from a vein, usually in your arm.

In TTP, hemolytic anemia occurs because red blood cells are broken into pieces as they try to squeeze around blood clots.

When TTP is the cause of hemolytic anemia, the Coombs test is negative. The test is positive if antibodies (proteins) are destroying your red blood cells.

Lactate Dehydrogenase Test

This blood test measures a protein called lactate dehydrogenase (LDH). For this test, a sample of blood is drawn from a vein, usually in your arm.

Hemolytic anemia causes red blood cells to break down and release LDH into the blood. LDH also is released from tissues that are injured by blood clots as a result of TTP.

ADAMTS13 Assay

A lack of activity in the *ADAMTS13* enzyme causes TTP. For this test, a sample of blood is drawn from a vein, usually in your arm. The blood is sent to a special lab to test for the enzyme's activity.

How Is Thrombotic Thrombocytopenic Purpura Treated?

Thrombotic thrombocytopenic purpura (TTP) can be fatal or cause lasting damage, such as brain damage or a stroke, if it's not treated right away.

In most cases, TTP occurs suddenly and lasts for days or weeks, but it can go on for months. Relapses (flareups) can occur in up to 60 percent of people who have acquired TTP. flareups also occur in most people who have inherited TTP.

Plasma treatments are the most common way to treat TTP. Other treatments include medicines and surgery. Treatments are done in a hospital.

Plasma Therapy

Plasma is the liquid part of your blood. It carries blood cells, hormones, enzymes, and nutrients to your body.

TTP is treated with plasma therapy. This includes:

- Fresh frozen plasma for people who have inherited TTP

- Plasma exchange for people who have acquired TTP

Plasma therapy is started in the hospital as soon as TTP is diagnosed or suspected.

For inherited TTP, fresh frozen plasma is given through an intravenous (IV) line inserted into a vein. This is done to replace the missing or changed *ADAMTS13* enzyme.

401

Plasma exchange (also called plasmapheresis) is used to treat acquired TTP. This is a lifesaving procedure. It removes antibodies (proteins) from the blood that damage your *ADAMTS13* enzyme. Plasma exchange also replaces the *ADAMTS13* enzyme.

If plasma exchange isn't available, you may be given fresh frozen plasma until it is available.

During plasma exchange, an IV needle or tube is placed in a vein in your arm to remove blood. The blood goes through a cell separator, which removes plasma from the blood. The nonplasma part of the blood is saved, and donated plasma is added to it.

Then, the blood is put back into you through an IV line inserted into one of your blood vessels. The time required to complete the procedure varies, but it often takes about 2 hours.

Treatments of fresh frozen plasma or plasma exchange usually continue until your blood tests results and signs and symptoms improve. This can take days or weeks, depending on your condition. You'll stay in the hospital while you recover.

Some people who recover from TTP have flareups. This can happen in the hospital or after you go home. If you have a flareup, your doctor will restart plasma therapy.

Other Treatments

Other treatments are used if plasma therapy doesn't work well or if flareups occur often.

For acquired TTP, medicines can slow or stop antibodies to the *ADAMTS13* enzyme from forming. Medicines used to treat TTP include glucocorticoids, vincristine, rituximab, and cyclosporine A.

Sometimes surgery to remove the spleen (an organ in the abdomen) is needed. This is because cells in the spleen make the antibodies that block *ADAMTS13* enzyme activity.

How Can Thrombotic Thrombocytopenic Purpura Be Prevented?

Both inherited and acquired thrombotic thrombocytopenic purpura (TTP) occur suddenly with no clear cause. You can't prevent either type.

If you've had TTP, watch for signs and symptoms of a relapse (flareup).

Ask your doctor about factors that may trigger TTP or a flareup.

Living with Thrombotic Thrombocytopenic Purpura

Some people fully recover from thrombotic thrombocytopenic purpura (TTP). However, relapses (flareups) can occur in many people who have acquired and inherited TTP.

If you've had TTP, call your doctor right away if you have signs or symptoms of a relapse.

If you've been treated for TTP, ask your doctor about medicines that may raise your risk of bleeding during a relapse, such as aspirin and ibuprofen.

Also, tell your doctor about all over-the-counter medicines you take, including vitamins, supplements, and herbal remedies.

Your doctor may ask whether you're using any products that contain quinine.

If your child has inherited TTP, ask the doctor whether you need to restrict your child's activities.

Report any symptoms of infection, such as a fever, to your doctor. This is very important for people who have had their spleens removed.

Talk with your doctor about changing medicines that may raise your risk of TTP, such as ticlopidine and clopidogrel.

Chapter 37

Vitamin K Deficiency Bleeding

Vitamins

- **Vitamins** are substances our bodies need, which we get from either the foods we eat or from a multivitamin.

- Vitamins are normally stored in the body. A person without enough of a vitamin stored in the body is **"vitamin deficient"** or has a **"vitamin deficiency."**

What Is Vitamin K and Why Is It Important?

Vitamin K is a substance that our body needs to form clots and to stop bleeding. We get vitamin K from the food we eat. Some vitamin K is also made by the good bacteria that live in our intestines. Babies are born with very small amounts of vitamin K stored in their bodies, which can lead to serious bleeding problems if not supplemented.

What is Vitamin K Deficiency Bleeding or VKDB?

Vitamin K deficiency bleeding or VKDB, occurs when babies cannot stop bleeding because their blood does not have enough Vitamin K to form a clot. The bleeding can occur anywhere on the inside or outside

This chapter includes text excerpted from "Vitamin K Deficiency Bleeding," Centers for Disease Control and Prevention (CDC), January 4, 2016.

of the body. When the bleeding occurs inside the body, it can be difficult to notice. Commonly, a baby with VKDB will bleed into his or her intestines, or into the brain, which can lead to brain damage and even death. Infants who do not receive the vitamin K shot at birth can develop VKDB at any time up to 6 months of age. There are three types of VKDB, based on the age of the baby when the bleeding problems start: early, classical and late.

Why Are Babies More Likely to Have Vitamin K Deficiency and to Get VKDB?

All infants, regardless of sex, race, or ethnic background, are at higher risk for VKDB until they start eating regular foods, usually at age 4-6 months, and until the normal intestinal bacteria start making vitamin K. This is because:

- At birth, babies have very little vitamin K stored in their bodies because only small amounts pass to them through the placenta from their mothers.

- The good bacteria that produce vitamin K are not yet present in the newborn's intestines.

- Breast milk contains low amounts of vitamin K, so exclusively breastfed babies don't get enough vitamin K from the breast milk, alone.

What Can I Do to Prevent My Baby from Getting Vitamin K Deficiency and VKDB?

The good news is that VKDB is easily prevented by giving babies a vitamin K shot into a muscle in the thigh. One shot given just after birth will protect your baby from VKDB. In order to provide for immediate bonding and contact between the newborn and mother, giving the vitamin K shot can be delayed up to 6 hours after birth.

Is the Vitamin K Shot Safe?

Yes. Many studies have shown that vitamin K is safe when given to newborns.

What Might Cause Babies to Be Deficient in Vitamin K and Have Bleeding Problems?

Some things can put infants at a higher risk for developing VKDB.

Babies at greater risk include:

- Babies who do not receive a vitamin K shot at birth. The risk is even higher if they are exclusively breastfed.

- Babies whose mothers used certain medications, like isoniazid or medicines to treat seizures. These drugs interfere with how the body uses vitamin K.

- Babies who have liver disease; often they cannot use the vitamin K their body stores.

- Babies who have diarrhea, celiac disease, or cystic fibrosis often have trouble absorbing vitamins, including vitamin K, from the foods they eat.

How Often Are Babies Affected with Vitamin K Deficiency Bleeding?

Since babies can be affected until they are 6 months old, healthcare providers divide VKDB into three types; early, classical and late. Table 36.1 helps explain these three different types.

1. Early and classical VKDB are more common, occurring in 1 in 60 to 1 in 250 newborns, although the risk is much higher for early VKDB among those infants whose mothers used certain medications during the pregnancy.

2. Late VKDB is rarer, occurring in 1 in 14,000 to 1 in 25,000 infants.

3. Infants who do not receive a vitamin K shot at birth are 81 times more likely to develop late VKDB than infants who do receive a vitamin K shot at birth.

Table 37.1. Types of Vitamin K Deficiency Bleeding (VKDB)

Type of VKDB	When it Occurs	Characteristics
Early	0–24 hours after birth	• Severe
		• Mainly found in infants whose mothers used certain medications (like medicines to treat seizures or isoniazid) that interfere with how the body uses vitamin K

Table 37.1. Continued

Type of VKDB	When it Occurs	Characteristics
Classical	1–7 days after birth	• Bruising
		• Bleeding from the umbilical cord
Late	2–12 weeks after birth is typical, but can occur up to 6 months of age in previously healthy infants	• 30–60% of infants have bleeding within the brain
		• Tends to occur in breastfed only babies who have not received the vitamin K shot
		• Warning bleeds are rare

What Things Should I Look for in My Baby If I Think He or She Might Have VKDB?

Unfortunately, in the majority of cases of VKDB, there are NO WARNING SIGNS before a life-threatening event starts. Babies with VKDB might develop any of the following signs:

- bruises, especially around the baby's head and face.

- bleeding from the nose or umbilical cord.

- skin color that is paler than before. For darker skinned babies, the gums may appear pale.

- after the first 3 weeks of life, the white parts of your baby's eyes may turn yellow.

- stool that has blood in it, is black or dark and sticky (also called 'tarry'), or vomiting blood.

- irritability, seizures, excessive sleepiness, or a lot of vomiting may all be signs of bleeding in the brain.

Remember, VKDB is easily preventable with just a single vitamin K shot at birth.

Part Five

Circulatory Disorders

Chapter 38

Aneurysm

What Is an Aneurysm?

An aneurysm is a balloon-like bulge in an artery. Arteries are blood vessels that carry oxygen-rich blood to your body.

Arteries have thick walls to withstand normal blood pressure. However, certain medical problems, genetic conditions, and trauma can damage or injure artery walls. The force of blood pushing against the weakened or injured walls can cause an aneurysm.

An aneurysm can grow large and rupture (burst) or dissect. A rupture causes dangerous bleeding inside the body. A dissection is a split in one or more layers of the artery wall. The split causes bleeding into and along the layers of the artery wall.

Both rupture and dissection often are fatal.

Types of Aneurysms

Aortic Aneurysms

The two types of aortic aneurysm are abdominal aortic aneurysm and thoracic aortic aneurysm. Some people have both types.

This chapter includes text excerpted from "Aneurysm," National Heart, Lung, and Blood Institute (NHLBI), April 1, 2011. Reviewed July 2016.

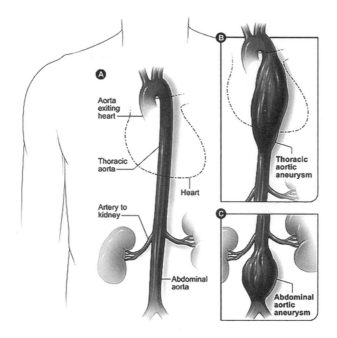

Figure 38.1. *Aortic Aneurysms*

Figure A shows a normal aorta. Figure B shows a thoracic aortic aneurysm, which is located behind the heart. Figure C shows an abdominal aortic aneurysm, which is located below the arteries that supply blood to the kidneys.

Abdominal Aortic Aneurysms

An aneurysm that occurs in the abdominal portion of the aorta is called an abdominal aortic aneurysm (AAA). Most aortic aneurysms are AAAs.

These aneurysms are found more often now than in the past because of computed tomography scans, or CT scans, done for other medical problems.

Small AAAs rarely rupture. However, AAAs can grow very large without causing symptoms. Routine checkups and treatment for an AAA can help prevent growth and rupture.

Thoracic Aortic Aneurysms

An aneurysm that occurs in the chest portion of the aorta (above the diaphragm, a muscle that helps you breathe) is called a thoracic aortic aneurysm (TAA).

TAAs don't always cause symptoms, even when they're large. Only half of all people who have TAAs notice any symptoms. TAAs are found more often now than in the past because of chest CT scans done for other medical problems.

With a common type of TAA, the walls of the aorta weaken and a section close to the heart enlarges. As a result, the valve between the heart and the aorta can't close properly. This allows blood to leak back into the heart.

A less common type of TAA can develop in the upper back, away from the heart. A TAA in this location may result from an injury to the chest, such as from a car crash.

Other Types of Aneurysms

Brain Aneurysms

Aneurysms in the arteries of the brain are called cerebral aneurysms or brain aneurysms. Brain aneurysms also are called berry aneurysms because they're often the size of a small berry.

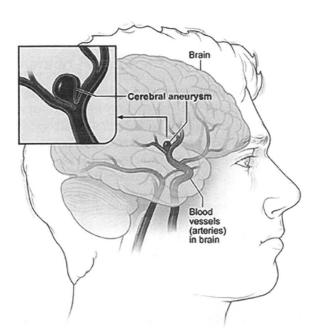

Figure 38.2. *Brain Aneurysm*

The illustration shows a typical location of a brain aneurysm in the arteries that supply blood to the brain. The inset image shows a closeup view of the sac-like aneurysm.

Most brain aneurysms cause no symptoms until they become large, begin to leak blood, or rupture (burst). A ruptured brain aneurysm can cause a stroke.

Peripheral Aneurysms

Aneurysms that occur in arteries other than the aorta and the brain arteries are called peripheral aneurysms. Common locations for peripheral aneurysms include the popliteal, femoral, and carotid arteries.

The popliteal arteries run down the back of the thighs, behind the knees. The femoral arteries are the main arteries in the groin. The carotid arteries are the two main arteries on each side of your neck.

Peripheral aneurysms aren't as likely to rupture or dissect as aortic aneurysms. However, blood clots can form in peripheral aneurysms. If a blood clot breaks away from the aneurysm, it can block blood flow through the artery.

If a peripheral aneurysm is large, it can press on a nearby nerve or vein and cause pain, numbness, or swelling.

Other Names for Aneurysm

- Abdominal aortic aneurysm

- Aortic aneurysm

- Berry aneurysm

- Brain aneurysm

- Cerebral aneurysm

- Peripheral aneurysm

- Thoracic aortic aneurysm

What Causes an Aneurysm?

The force of blood pushing against the walls of an artery combined with damage or injury to the artery's walls can cause an aneurysm.

Many conditions and factors can damage and weaken the walls of the aorta and cause aortic aneurysms. Examples include aging, smoking, high blood pressure, and atherosclerosis. Atherosclerosis is the hardening and narrowing of the arteries due to the buildup of a waxy substance called plaque.

Rarely, infections—such as untreated syphilis (a sexually transmitted infection)—can cause aortic aneurysms. Aortic aneurysms also can occur as a result of diseases that inflame the blood vessels, such as vasculitis.

A family history of aneurysms also may play a role in causing aortic aneurysms.

In addition to the factors above, certain genetic conditions may cause thoracic aortic aneurysms (TAAs). Examples of these conditions include Marfan syndrome, Loeys-Dietz syndrome, Ehlers-Danlos syndrome (the vascular type), and Turner syndrome.

These genetic conditions can weaken the body's connective tissues and damage the aorta. People who have these conditions tend to develop aneurysms at a younger age than other people. They're also at higher risk for rupture and dissection.

Trauma, such as a car accident, also can damage the walls of the aorta and lead to TAAs.

Researchers continue to look for other causes of aortic aneurysms. For example, they're looking for genetic mutations (changes in the genes) that may contribute to or cause aneurysms.

Who Is at Risk for an Aneurysm?

Certain factors put you at higher risk for an aortic aneurysm. These factors include:

- Male gender. Men are more likely than women to have aortic aneurysms.

- Age. The risk for abdominal aortic aneurysms increases as you get older. These aneurysms are more likely to occur in people who are aged 65 or older.

- Smoking. Smoking can damage and weaken the walls of the aorta.

- A family history of aortic aneurysms. People who have family histories of aortic aneurysms are at higher risk for the condition, and they may have aneurysms before the age of 65.

- A history of aneurysms in the arteries of the legs.

- Certain diseases and conditions that weaken the walls of the aorta. Examples include high blood pressure and atherosclerosis.

Having a bicuspid aortic valve can raise the risk of having a thoracic aortic aneurysm. A bicuspid aortic valve has two leaflets instead of the typical three.

Car accidents or trauma also can injure the arteries and increase the risk for aneurysms.

If you have any of these risk factors, talk with your doctor about whether you need screening for aneurysms.

What Are the Signs and Symptoms of an Aneurysm?

The signs and symptoms of an aortic aneurysm depend on the type and location of the aneurysm. Signs and symptoms also depend on whether the aneurysm has ruptured (burst) or is affecting other parts of the body.

Aneurysms can develop and grow for years without causing any signs or symptoms. They often don't cause signs or symptoms until they rupture, grow large enough to press on nearby body parts, or block blood flow.

Abdominal Aortic Aneurysms

Most abdominal aortic aneurysms (AAAs) develop slowly over years. They often don't cause signs or symptoms unless they rupture. If you have an AAA, your doctor may feel a throbbing mass while checking your abdomen.

When symptoms are present, they can include:

- A throbbing feeling in the abdomen

- Deep pain in your back or the side of your abdomen

- Steady, gnawing pain in your abdomen that lasts for hours or days

If an AAA ruptures, symptoms may include sudden, severe pain in your lower abdomen and back; nausea (feeling sick to your stomach) and vomiting; constipation and problems with urination; clammy, sweaty skin; light-headedness; and a rapid heart rate when standing up.

Internal bleeding from a ruptured AAA can send you into shock. Shock is a life-threatening condition in which blood pressure drops so low that the brain, kidneys, and other vital organs can't get enough blood to work well. Shock can be fatal if it's not treated right away.

Thoracic Aortic Aneurysms

A thoracic aortic aneurysm (TAA) may not cause symptoms until it dissects or grows large.

If you have symptoms, they may include:

- pain in your jaw, neck, back, or chest

- coughing and/or hoarseness

- shortness of breath and/or trouble breathing or swallowing

A dissection is a split in one or more layers of the artery wall. The split causes bleeding into and along the layers of the artery wall.

If a TAA ruptures or dissects, you may feel sudden, severe, sharp or stabbing pain starting in your upper back and moving down into your abdomen. You may have pain in your chest and arms, and you can quickly go into shock.

If you have any symptoms of TAA or aortic dissection, call 9–1–1. If left untreated, these conditions may lead to organ damage or death.

How Is an Aneurysm Diagnosed?

If you have an aortic aneurysm but no symptoms, your doctor may find it by chance during a routine physical exam. More often, doctors find aneurysms during tests done for other reasons, such as chest or abdominal pain.

If you have an abdominal aortic aneurysm (AAA), your doctor may feel a throbbing mass in your abdomen. A rapidly growing aneurysm about to rupture (burst) can be tender and very painful when pressed. If you're overweight or obese, it may be hard for your doctor to feel even a large AAA.

If you have an AAA, your doctor may hear rushing blood flow instead of the normal whooshing sound when listening to your abdomen with a stethoscope.

Diagnostic Tests and Procedures

To diagnose and study an aneurysm, your doctor may recommend one or more of the following tests.

Ultrasound and Echocardiography

Ultrasound and echocardiography (echo) are simple, painless tests that use sound waves to create pictures of the structures inside your body. These tests can show the size of an aortic aneurysm, if one is found.

417

Computed Tomography Scan

A computed tomography scan, or CT scan, is a painless test that uses X-rays to take clear, detailed pictures of your organs.

During the test, your doctor will inject dye into a vein in your arm. The dye makes your arteries, including your aorta, visible on the CT scan pictures.

Your doctor may recommend this test if he or she thinks you have an AAA or a thoracic aortic aneurysm (TAA). A CT scan can show the size and shape of an aneurysm. This test provides more detailed pictures than an ultrasound or echo.

Magnetic Resonance Imaging

Magnetic resonance imaging (MRI) uses magnets and radio waves to create pictures of the organs and structures in your body. This test works well for detecting aneurysms and pinpointing their size and exact location.

Angiography

Angiography is a test that uses dye and special X-rays to show the insides of your arteries. This test shows the amount of damage and blockage in blood vessels.

Aortic angiography shows the inside of your aorta. The test may show the location and size of an aortic aneurysm.

How Is an Aneurysm Treated?

Aortic aneurysms are treated with medicines and surgery. Small aneurysms that are found early and aren't causing symptoms may not need treatment. Other aneurysms need to be treated.

The goals of treatment may include:

- Preventing the aneurysm from growing

- Preventing or reversing damage to other body structures

- Preventing or treating a rupture or dissection

- Allowing you to continue doing your normal daily activities

Treatment for an aortic aneurysm is based on its size. Your doctor may recommend routine testing to make sure an aneurysm isn't getting bigger. This method usually is used for aneurysms that are smaller than 5 centimeters (about 2 inches) across.

How often you need testing (for example, every few months or every year) is based on the size of the aneurysm and how fast it's growing. The larger it is and the faster it's growing, the more often you may need to be checked.

Medicines

If you have an aortic aneurysm, your doctor may prescribe medicines before surgery or instead of surgery. Medicines are used to lower blood pressure, relax blood vessels, and lower the risk that the aneurysm will rupture (burst). Beta blockers and calcium channel blockers are the medicines most commonly used.

Surgery

Your doctor may recommend surgery if your aneurysm is growing quickly or is at risk of rupture or dissection.

The two main types of surgery to repair aortic aneurysms are open abdominal or open chest repair and endovascular repair.

Open Abdominal or Open Chest Repair

The standard and most common type of surgery for aortic aneurysms is open abdominal or open chest repair. This surgery involves a major incision (cut) in the abdomen or chest.

General anesthesia is used during this procedure. The term "anesthesia" refers to a loss of feeling and awareness. General anesthesia temporarily puts you to sleep.

During the surgery, the aneurysm is removed. Then, the section of aorta is replaced with a graft made of material such as Dacron® or Teflon®. The surgery takes 3 to 6 hours; you'll remain in the hospital for 5 to 8 days.

If needed, repair of the aortic heart valve also may be done during open abdominal or open chest surgery.

It often takes a month to recover from open abdominal or open chest surgery and return to full activity. Most patients make a full recovery.

Endovascular Repair

In endovascular repair, the aneurysm isn't removed. Instead, a graft is inserted into the aorta to strengthen it. Surgeons do this type of surgery using catheters (tubes) inserted into the arteries; it doesn't require surgically opening the chest or abdomen. General anesthesia is used during this procedure.

The surgeon first inserts a catheter into an artery in the groin (upper thigh) and threads it to the aneurysm. Then, using an X-ray to see the artery, the surgeon threads the graft (also called a stent graft) into the aorta to the aneurysm.

The graft is then expanded inside the aorta and fastened in place to form a stable channel for blood flow. The graft reinforces the weakened section of the aorta. This helps prevent the aneurysm from rupturing.

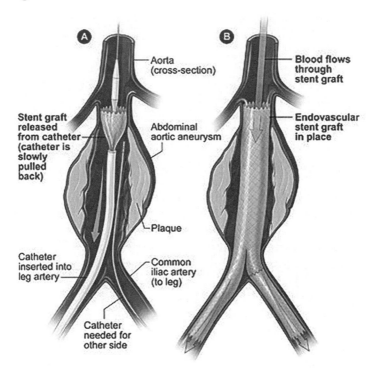

Figure 38.3. *Endovascular Repair*

The illustration shows the placement of a stent graft in an aortic aneurysm. In figure A, a catheter is inserted into an artery in the groin (upper thigh). The catheter is threaded to the abdominal aorta, and the stent graft is released from the catheter. In figure B, the stent graft allows blood to flow through the aneurysm.

The recovery time for endovascular repair is less than the recovery time for open abdominal or open chest repair. However, doctors can't repair all aortic aneurysms with endovascular repair. The location or size of an aneurysm may prevent the use of a stent graft.

How Can an Aneurysm Be Prevented?

The best way to prevent an aortic aneurysm is to avoid the factors that put you at higher risk for one. You can't control all aortic aneurysm risk factors, but lifestyle changes can help you lower some risks.

For example, if you smoke, try to quit. Talk with your doctor about programs and products that can help you quit smoking. Also, try to avoid secondhand smoke. Another important lifestyle change is following a healthy diet. A healthy diet includes a variety of fruits, vegetables, and whole grains. It also includes lean meats, poultry, fish, beans, and fat-free or low-fat milk or milk products. A healthy diet is low in saturated fat, trans fat, cholesterol, sodium (salt), and added sugar.

Be as physically active as you can. Talk with your doctor about the amounts and types of physical activity that are safe for you.

Work with your doctor to control medical conditions such as high blood pressure and high blood cholesterol. Follow your treatment plans and take all of your medicines as your doctor prescribes.

Screening for Aneurysms

Although you may not be able to prevent an aneurysm, early diagnosis and treatment can help prevent rupture and dissection.

Aneurysms can develop and grow large before causing any signs or symptoms. Thus, people who are at high risk for aneurysms may benefit from early, routine screening.

Your doctor may recommend routine screening if you're:

- A man between the ages of 65 and 75 who has ever smoked

- A man or woman between the ages of 65 and 75 who has a family history of aneurysms

If you're at risk, but not in one of these high-risk groups, ask your doctor whether screening will benefit you.

Living with an Aneurysm

If you have an aortic aneurysm, following your treatment plan and having ongoing medical care are important. Early diagnosis and treatment can help prevent rupture and dissection.

Your doctor may advise you to avoid heavy lifting or physical exertion. If your job requires heavy lifting, you may be advised to change jobs.

Also, try to avoid emotional crises. Strong emotions can cause blood pressure to rise, which increases the risk of rupture or dissection. Call your doctor if an emotional crisis occurs.

Your doctor may prescribe medicines to treat your aneurysm. Medicines can lower your blood pressure, relax your blood vessels, and lower the risk that the aneurysm will rupture (burst). Take all of your medicines exactly as your doctor prescribes.

If you have a small aneurysm that isn't causing pain, you may not need treatment. However, aneurysms can develop and grow large before causing any symptoms. Thus, people who are at high risk for aneurysms may benefit from early, routine screening.

Chapter 39

Arteritis

Chapter Contents

Section 39.1

Takayasu Arteritis

This section includes text excerpted from "Takayasu Arteritis," Genetic and Rare Diseases Information Center (GARD), National Center for Advancing Translational Sciences (NCATS), November 3, 2013.

What Is Takayasu Arteritis?

Takayasu arteritis is a condition that causes inflammation of the main blood vessel that carries blood from the heart to the rest of the body (aorta) and its associated branched blood vessels. As a result of the inflammation, the blood vessel walls become thick and make it difficult for blood to flow. Over time, impaired blood flow causes damage to the heart and various other organs of the body. Although the cause remains unknown, Takayasu arteritis appears to be an autoimmune condition, in which cells that fight infection and disease are wrongly targeted against the body's own tissues.

What Are the Signs and Symptoms of Takayasu Arteritis?

- abnormal pattern of respiration
- abnormality of temperature regulation
- abnormality of the aortic valve
- abnormality of the endocardium
- amaurosis fugax
- anemia
- aneurysm
- anorexia

- arteritis
- arthralgia
- arthritis
- cerebral ischemia
- chest pain
- coronary artery disease
- dilatation of the ascending aorta
- gangrene
- gastrointestinal infarctions

- hemoptysis
- hyperhidrosis
- hypertensive crisis
- hypertrophic cardiomyopathy
- inflammatory abnormality of the eye
- migraine
- muscle weakness
- myalgia
- neurological speech impairment
- pulmonary hypertension
- reduced consciousness/confusion
- retinopathy
- seizures
- skin ulcer
- vasculitis
- visual impairment
- weight loss

How Might Takayasu Arteritis Be Treated?

The treatment of Takayasu arteritis is focused on controlling both the inflammatory process and hypertension. Treatment options might include: corticosteroids, medications that block the activity of interkeukin-6 (iL-6 receptor inhibitors), medications that impair the activity of B-lymphocyets (B-cell depletion), medications that are toxic to cells (cytotoxic agents), medications that block the activity of tumor necrosis factor (anti-tumor necrosis factor agents), and antihypertensive agents. Lifestyle modification including exercise and diet might additionally be recommended.

Section 39.2

Giant Cell Arteritis

This section includes text excerpted from "Giant Cell Arteritis,"
Genetic and Rare Diseases Information Center (GARD), National
Center for Advancing Translational Sciences (NCATS), April 5, 2016.

What Is Giant Cell Arteritis?

Giant cell arteritis (GCA) is a form of vasculitis, a group of disorders that cause inflammation of blood vessels. In GCA, the vessels of the head are most involved (especially the temporal arteries, located on each side of the head), but other blood vessels can also become inflamed. The inflammation causes the arteries to narrow, resulting in poor blood flow.

What Are the Signs and Symptoms of Giant Cell Arteritis?

- abdominal pain
- abnormality of temperature regulation
- abnormality of the pericardium
- abnormality of the pleura
- abnormality of thrombocytes
- acrocyanosis
- alopecia
- amaurosis fugax
- anorexia
- aortic dissection
- arterial thrombosis
- arthralgia
- arthritis
- autosomal dominant inheritance
- behavioral abnormality
- blindness
- cerebral ischemia
- conductive hearing impairment
- coronary artery disease
- diabetes insipidus
- dilatation of the ascending aorta
- diplopia

- elevated erythrocyte sedimentation rate
- epistaxis
- gangrene
- gastrointestinal infarctions
- glossitis
- hematuria
- hepatic failure
- hyperhidrosis
- incoordination
- limitation of joint mobility
- mediastinal lymphadenopathy
- meningitis
- migraine
- muscle weakness
- myalgia
- nystagmus
- ophthalmoparesis
- optic atrophy
- paresthesia
- ptosis
- recurrent pharyngitis
- renal insufficiency
- retinal arteritis
- skin ulcer
- sudden cardiac death
- vasculitis
- vertigo
- visual impairment
- weight loss

What Causes Giant Cell Arteritis?

While the exact cause of giant cell arteritis (GCA) is unknown, studies have linked genetic factors, infectious agents, high doses of antibiotics, and a prior history of cardiovascular disease to the development of GCA. These associations have implicated an abnormal immune response.

The genetic factors currently linked to the development of GCA are not thought to directly cause GCA, but they may cause a genetic predisposition to the condition. This means that a person may carry a gene (or more than one gene) that predisposes him/her to developing GCA, but it may not develop unless something in the environment triggers its onset. Familial cases of GCA have been reported.

Recent studies have confirmed a strong association of GCA with the human leukocyte antigen (HLA) gene family, a cluster of genes on chromosome 6. The HLA gene family gives the body instructions to make a group of proteins known as the HLA complex. This complex helps the immune system distinguish between the body's own proteins and those made by foreign invaders such as viruses and bacteria. More specifically, GCA has been associated with HLA class I and class II genes. HLA class I genes give the body instructions to make proteins that occur on the surface of almost all cells. HLA class II genes give instructions to make proteins that occur almost exclusively on the surface of certain immune system cells.

Other genes, which are not part of the HLA gene family, have also been associated with an increased risk to develop GCA. These include the *PTPN22, NLRP1, IL17A, IL33, and LRRC32* genes. Outside of the HLA-related genes, PTPN22 seems to be the most strongly associated with GCA. This gene has already been established as a common susceptibility gene in autoimmunity and has been consistently associated with many autoimmune diseases.

Despite the exact cause of GCA being unknown, several additional factors are known to increase a person's risk to develop GCA. These include:

- age – GCA affects older adults almost exclusively

- being a woman – women are about two times more likely than men to develop GCA

- being of Northern European (especially Scandinavian) descent – people born in Northern European countries appear to have higher rates of GCA

- having polymyalgia rheumatica – about 15 percent of people with polymyalgia rheumatica also have GCA

How Might Giant Cell Arteritis Be Treated?

Giant cell arteritis (GCA) is typically treated with high doses of corticosteroids. Corticosteroids should be started promptly (perhaps even before the diagnosis is confirmed with a biopsy). If not treated promptly, the condition carries a small risk of blindness. The symptoms of GCA usually quickly disappear with treatment, but high doses of corticosteroids are typically maintained for 1 month. Once symptoms are gone and the sed rate is normal, there is much less risk of blindness and the corticosteroid dose may be gradually reduced. Other medications that suppress the immune system are sometimes also needed.

What Is the Long-Term Outlook for People with Giant Cell Arteritis?

People with giant cell arteritis (GCA) who have prompt, adequate therapy typically have a full recovery. Symptoms generally improve within days of starting treatment, and blindness is now a rare complication. However, the course of the condition until full recovery can vary considerably. While the average duration of treatment is 2 years, some people need treatment for 5 years or more. The effects of steroid therapy are often worse than the symptoms of the condition itself. When GCA is properly treated, it rarely recurs. However, people with GCA carry a lifelong risk for the development of large vessel disease, particularly aortic aneurysms. Therefore, long-term followup is extremely important.

The outlook for people who are not treated is extremely poor. Complications may include blindness or other eye and vision problems, or death from myocardial infarction (heart attack), stroke, or dissecting aortic aneurysm. Vision damage that occurs before starting therapy is often irreversible.

Chapter 40

Atherosclerosis

What Is Atherosclerosis?

Atherosclerosis is a disease in which plaque builds up inside your arteries. Arteries are blood vessels that carry oxygen-rich blood to your heart and other parts of your body.

Plaque is made up of fat, cholesterol, calcium, and other substances found in the blood. Over time, plaque hardens and narrows your arteries. This limits the flow of oxygen-rich blood to your organs and other parts of your body.

Atherosclerosis can lead to serious problems, including heart attack, stroke, or even death.

Atherosclerosis-Related Diseases

Atherosclerosis can affect any artery in the body, including arteries in the heart, brain, arms, legs, pelvis, and kidneys. As a result, different diseases may develop based on which arteries are affected.

Coronary Heart Disease

Coronary heart disease (CHD), also called coronary artery disease, occurs when plaque builds up in the coronary arteries. These arteries supply oxygen-rich blood to your heart.

This chapter includes text excerpted from "Atherosclerosis," National Heart, Lung, and Blood Institute (NHLBI), June 22, 2016.

Plaque narrows the coronary arteries and reduces blood flow to your heart muscle. Plaque buildup also makes it more likely that blood clots will form in your arteries. Blood clots can partially or completely block blood flow.

If blood flow to your heart muscle is reduced or blocked, you may have angina (chest pain or discomfort) or a heart attack.

Plaque also can form in the heart's smallest arteries. This disease is called coronary microvascular disease (MVD). In coronary MVD, plaque doesn't cause blockages in the arteries as it does in CHD.

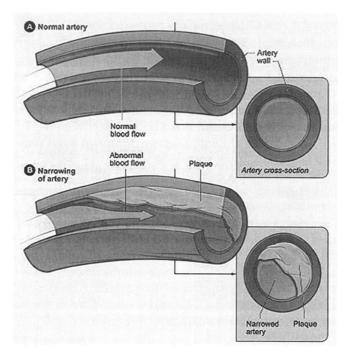

Figure 40.1. *Atherosclerosis*

Figure A shows a normal artery with normal blood flow. The inset image shows a cross-section of a normal artery. Figure B shows an artery with plaque buildup. The inset image shows a cross-section of an artery with plaque buildup.

Carotid Artery Disease

Carotid artery disease occurs if plaque builds up in the arteries on each side of your neck (the carotid arteries). These arteries supply oxygen-rich blood to your brain. If blood flow to your brain is reduced or blocked, you may have a stroke.

Chronic Kidney Disease

Chronic kidney disease can occur if plaque builds up in the renal arteries. These arteries supply oxygen-rich blood to your kidneys.

Over time, chronic kidney disease causes a slow loss of kidney function. The main function of the kidneys is to remove waste and extra water from the body.

Other Names for Atherosclerosis

- Arteriosclerosis
- Hardening of the arteries

What Causes Atherosclerosis?

The exact cause of atherosclerosis isn't known. However, studies show that atherosclerosis is a slow, complex disease that may start in childhood. It develops faster as you age.

Atherosclerosis may start when certain factors damage the inner layers of the arteries. These factors include:

- smoking
- high amounts of certain fats and cholesterol in the blood
- high blood pressure
- high amounts of sugar in the blood due to insulin resistance or diabetes

Plaque may begin to build up where the arteries are damaged. Over time, plaque hardens and narrows the arteries. Eventually, an area of plaque can rupture (break open).

When this happens, blood cell fragments called platelets stick to the site of the injury. They may clump together to form blood clots. Clots narrow the arteries even more, limiting the flow of oxygen-rich blood to your body.

Depending on which arteries are affected, blood clots can worsen angina (chest pain) or cause a heart attack or stroke.

Researchers continue to look for the causes of atherosclerosis. They hope to find answers to questions such as:

- Why and how do the arteries become damaged?
- How does plaque develop and change over time?
- Why does plaque rupture and lead to blood clots?

Who Is at Risk for Atherosclerosis?

The exact cause of atherosclerosis isn't known. However, certain traits, conditions, or habits may raise your risk for the disease. These conditions are known as risk factors. The more risk factors you have, the more likely it is that you'll develop atherosclerosis.

You can control most risk factors and help prevent or delay atherosclerosis. Other risk factors can't be controlled.

Major Risk Factors

- unhealthy blood cholesterol levels
- high blood pressure
- smoking
- insulin resistance
- diabetes
- overweight or obesity
- lack of physical activity
- unhealthy diet
- older age
- family history of early heart disease

Although age and a family history of early heart disease are risk factors, it doesn't mean that you'll develop atherosclerosis if you have one or both. Controlling other risk factors often can lessen genetic influences and prevent atherosclerosis, even in older adults.

Studies show that an increasing number of children and youth are at risk for atherosclerosis. This is due to a number of causes, including rising childhood obesity rates.

Emerging Risk Factors

Scientists continue to study other possible risk factors for atherosclerosis.

High levels of a protein called C-reactive protein (CRP) in the blood may raise the risk for atherosclerosis and heart attack. High levels of CRP are a sign of inflammation in the body.

Inflammation is the body's response to injury or infection. Damage to the arteries' inner walls seems to trigger inflammation and help plaque grow.

People who have low CRP levels may develop atherosclerosis at a slower rate than people who have high CRP levels. Research is under way to find out whether reducing inflammation and lowering CRP levels also can reduce the risk for atherosclerosis.

High levels of triglycerides in the blood also may raise the risk for atherosclerosis, especially in women. Triglycerides are a type of fat.

Studies are under way to find out whether genetics may play a role in atherosclerosis risk.

Other Factors That Affect Atherosclerosis

Other factors also may raise your risk for atherosclerosis, such as:

- **Sleep apnea.** Sleep apnea is a disorder that causes one or more pauses in breathing or shallow breaths while you sleep. Untreated sleep apnea can raise your risk for high blood pressure, diabetes, and even a heart attack or stroke.

- **Stress.** Research shows that the most commonly reported "trigger" for a heart attack is an emotionally upsetting event, especially one involving anger.

- **Alcohol.** Heavy drinking can damage the heart muscle and worsen other risk factors for atherosclerosis. Men should have no more than two drinks containing alcohol a day. Women should have no more than one drink containing alcohol a day.

What Are the Signs and Symptoms of Atherosclerosis?

Atherosclerosis usually doesn't cause signs and symptoms until it severely narrows or totally blocks an artery. Many people don't know they have the disease until they have a medical emergency, such as a heart attack or stroke.

Some people may have signs and symptoms of the disease. Signs and symptoms will depend on which arteries are affected.

Coronary Arteries

The coronary arteries supply oxygen-rich blood to your heart. If plaque narrows or blocks these arteries (a disease called coronary heart disease, or CHD), a common symptom is angina. Angina is chest pain or discomfort that occurs when your heart muscle doesn't get enough oxygen-rich blood.

Angina may feel like pressure or squeezing in your chest. You also may feel it in your shoulders, arms, neck, jaw, or back. Angina pain may even feel like indigestion. The pain tends to get worse with activity and goes away with rest. Emotional stress also can trigger the pain.

Other symptoms of CHD are shortness of breath and arrhythmias. Arrhythmias are problems with the rate or rhythm of the heartbeat.

Plaque also can form in the heart's smallest arteries. This disease is called coronary microvascular disease (MVD). Symptoms of coronary MVD include angina, shortness of breath, sleep problems, fatigue (tiredness), and lack of energy.

Carotid Arteries

The carotid arteries supply oxygen-rich blood to your brain. If plaque narrows or blocks these arteries (a disease called carotid artery disease), you may have symptoms of a stroke. These symptoms may include:

- sudden weakness

- paralysis (an inability to move) or numbness of the face, arms, or legs, especially on one side of the body

- confusion

- trouble speaking or understanding speech

- trouble seeing in one or both eyes

- problems breathing

- dizziness, trouble walking, loss of balance or coordination, and unexplained falls

- loss of consciousness

- sudden and severe headache

Peripheral Arteries

Plaque also can build up in the major arteries that supply oxygen-rich blood to the legs, arms, and pelvis (a disease called peripheral artery disease).

If these major arteries are narrowed or blocked, you may have numbness, pain, and, sometimes, dangerous infections.

Renal Arteries

The renal arteries supply oxygen-rich blood to your kidneys. If plaque builds up in these arteries, you may develop chronic kidney disease. Over time, chronic kidney disease causes a slow loss of kidney function.

Early kidney disease often has no signs or symptoms. As the disease gets worse it can cause tiredness, changes in how you urinate (more often or less often), loss of appetite, nausea (feeling sick to the stomach), swelling in the hands or feet, itchiness or numbness, and trouble concentrating.

How Is Atherosclerosis Diagnosed?

Your doctor will diagnose atherosclerosis based on your medical and family histories, a physical exam, and test results.

Physical Exam

During the physical exam, your doctor may listen to your arteries for an abnormal whooshing sound called a bruit. Your doctor can hear a bruit when placing a stethoscope over an affected artery. A bruit may indicate poor blood flow due to plaque buildup.

Your doctor also may check to see whether any of your pulses (for example, in the leg or foot) are weak or absent. A weak or absent pulse can be a sign of a blocked artery.

Diagnostic Tests

Your doctor may recommend one or more tests to diagnose atherosclerosis. These tests also can help your doctor learn the extent of your disease and plan the best treatment.

- Blood Tests
- Electrocardiogram (EKG)
- Chest X-Ray
- Ankle/Brachial Index
- Echocardiography
- Computed Tomography Scan
- Stress Testing
- Angiography

How Is Atherosclerosis Treated?

Treatments for atherosclerosis may include heart-healthy lifestyle changes, medicines, and medical procedures or surgery. The goals of treatment include:

- lowering the risk of blood clots forming

- preventing atherosclerosis-related diseases

- reducing risk factors in an effort to slow or stop the buildup of plaque

- relieving symptoms

- widening or bypassing plaque-clogged arteries

Heart-Healthy Lifestyle Changes

Your doctor may recommend heart-healthy lifestyle changes if you have atherosclerosis. Heart-healthy lifestyle changes include heart-healthy eating, aiming for a healthy weight, managing stress, physical activity and quitting smoking.

Medicines

Sometimes lifestyle changes alone aren't enough to control your cholesterol levels. For example, you also may need statin medications to control or lower your cholesterol. By lowering your blood cholesterol level, you can decrease your chance of having a heart attack or stroke. Doctors usually prescribe statins for people who have:

- coronary heart disease, peripheral artery disease, or had a prior stroke

- diabetes

- high LDL cholesterol levels

Doctors may discuss beginning statin treatment with people who have an elevated risk for developing heart disease or having a stroke. Your doctor also may prescribe other medications to:

- lower your blood pressure

- lower your blood sugar levels

- prevent blood clots, which can lead to heart attack and stroke

- prevent inflammation

Take all medicines regularly, as your doctor prescribes. Don't change the amount of your medicine or skip a dose unless your doctor tells you to. You should still follow a heart healthy lifestyle, even if you take medicines to treat your atherosclerosis.

Medical Procedures and Surgery

If you have severe atherosclerosis, your doctor may recommend a medical procedure or surgery.

Percutaneous coronary intervention (PCI), also known as coronary angioplasty, is a procedure that's used to open blocked or narrowed coronary (heart) arteries. PCI can improve blood flow to the heart and relieve chest pain. Sometimes a small mesh tube called a stent is placed in the artery to keep it open after the procedure.

Coronary artery bypass grafting (CABG) is a type of surgery. In CABG, arteries or veins from other areas in your body are used to bypass or go around your narrowed coronary arteries. CABG can improve blood flow to your heart, relieve chest pain, and possibly prevent a heart attack.

Bypass grafting also can be used for leg arteries. For this surgery, a healthy blood vessel is used to bypass a narrowed or blocked artery in one of the legs. The healthy blood vessel redirects blood around the blocked artery, improving blood flow to the leg.

Carotid endarterectomy is a type of surgery to remove plaque buildup from the carotid arteries in the neck. This procedure restores blood flow to the brain, which can help prevent a stroke.

How Can Atherosclerosis Be Prevented or Delayed?

Taking action to control your risk factors can help prevent or delay atherosclerosis and its related diseases. Your risk for atherosclerosis increases with the number of risk factors you have.

One step you can take is to adopt a healthy lifestyle, which can include:

- heart-healthy eating
- physical activity
- quit smoking
- weight control

Other steps that can prevent or delay atherosclerosis include knowing your family history of atherosclerosis. If you or someone in your family has an atherosclerosis-related disease, be sure to tell your doctor.

If lifestyle changes aren't enough, your doctor may prescribe medicines to control your atherosclerosis risk factors. Take all of your medicines as your doctor advises.

Living with Atherosclerosis

Improved treatments have reduced the number of deaths from atherosclerosis-related diseases. These treatments also have improved the quality of life for people who have these diseases.

Adopting a healthy lifestyle may help you prevent or delay atherosclerosis and the problems it can cause. This, along with ongoing medical care, can help you avoid the problems of atherosclerosis and live a long, healthy life.

Researchers continue to look for ways to improve the health of people who have atherosclerosis or may develop it.

Ongoing Care

If you have atherosclerosis, work closely with your doctor and other healthcare providers to avoid serious problems, such as heart attack and stroke.

Follow your treatment plan and take all of your medicines as your doctor prescribes. Your doctor will let you know how often you should schedule office visits or blood tests. Be sure to let your doctor know if you have new or worsening symptoms.

Chapter 41

Blood Pressure Disorders

Chapter Contents

Section 41.1

Hypertension (High Blood Pressure)

This section includes text excerpted from "High Blood Pressure,"
National Institute on Aging (NIA), National Institutes of
Health (NIH), May 3, 2016.

You can have high blood pressure, or hypertension, and still feel just fine. That's because high blood pressure often does not cause signs of illness that you can see or feel. But, high blood pressure, sometimes called "the silent killer," is very common in older people and a major health problem. If high blood pressure isn't controlled with lifestyle changes and medicine, it can lead to stroke, heart disease, eye problems, kidney failure, and other health problems. High blood pressure can also cause shortness of breath during light physical activity or exercise.

What Is Blood Pressure?

Blood pressure is the force of blood pushing against the walls of arteries. When the doctor measures your blood pressure, the results are given in two numbers. The first number, called systolic blood pressure, is the pressure caused by your heart pushing out blood. The second number, called diastolic blood pressure, is the pressure when your heart fills with blood. The safest range, often called normal blood pressure, is a systolic blood pressure of less than 120 and a diastolic blood pressure of less than 80. This is stated as 120/80.

Do You Have High Blood Pressure?

One reason to have regular visits to the doctor is to have your blood pressure checked. The doctor will say your blood pressure is high when it measures 140/90 or higher at two or more checkups. He or she may ask you to check your blood pressure at home at different times of the day. If the pressure stays high, even when you are relaxed, the doctor may suggest exercise, changes in your diet, and medications.

The term "prehypertension" describes people whose blood pressure is slightly higher than normal—for example, the first number (systolic) is between 120 and 139, or the second number (diastolic) is between 80 and 89. Prehypertension can put you at risk for developing high blood pressure. Your doctor will probably want you to make changes in your day-to-day habits to try to lower your blood pressure.

Table 41.1. Blood Pressure: What Do the Numbers Mean?

Condition	Systolic (first number)	Diastolic (second number)
Normal Blood Pressure	Less than 120	Less than 80
Prehypertension	Between 120–139	Between 80–89
High Blood Pressure	140 or more	90 or more
Isolated Systolic Hypertension	140 or more	Less than 90

What if Just the First Number Is High?

For older people, the first number (systolic) often is 140 or greater, but the second number (diastolic) is less than 90. This problem is called isolated systolic hypertension. It is the most common form of high blood pressure in older people and can lead to serious health problems. Isolated systolic hypertension is treated in the same way as regular high blood pressure but often requires more than one type of blood pressure medication. If your systolic pressure is 140 or higher, ask your doctor how you can lower it.

What if Your Blood Pressure Is Low?

If your systolic blood pressure is less than 90, you may have low blood pressure. You may feel lightheaded, dizzy, or even faint. Low blood pressure, or hypotension, can be caused by not drinking enough liquids (dehydration), blood loss, or too much medication.

Some Risks You Can't Change

Anyone can get high blood pressure. But, some people have a greater chance of having it because of things they can't change. These are:

- **Age.** The chance of having high blood pressure increases as you get older.

- **Gender.** Before age 55, men have a greater chance of having high blood pressure. Women are more likely to have high blood pressure after menopause.

- **Family history.** High blood pressure tends to run in some families.

- **Race.** African-Americans are at increased risk for high blood pressure.

How Can I Control My Blood Pressure?

High blood pressure is very common in older people—over time most people find that aging causes changes to their heart. This is true even for people who have heart healthy habits. The good news is that blood pressure can be controlled in most people.

There are many lifestyle changes you can make to lower your risk of high blood pressure, including:

- keep a healthy weight

- exercise every day

- eat a healthy diet

- cut down on salt

- drink less alcohol

- don't smoke

- get a good night's sleep

If these lifestyle changes don't lower your blood pressure enough to a safe level, your doctor will also prescribe medicine. You may try several kinds or combinations of medicines before finding a plan that works best for you. Medicine can control your blood pressure, but it can't cure it. You will likely need to take medicine for the rest of your life. Plan with your doctor how to manage your blood pressure.

High Blood Pressure Facts

High blood pressure is serious because it can lead to major health problems. Make a point of learning what blood pressure should be. And, remember:

- High blood pressure may not make you feel sick, but it is serious. See a doctor to treat it.

- You can lower your blood pressure by changing your day-to-day habits and by taking medicine, if needed.

- If you take high blood pressure medicine, making some lifestyle changes may help lower the dose you need.

- If you take blood pressure medicine and your blood pressure is 120 or less, that's good. It means medicine and lifestyle changes are working. If another doctor asks if you have high blood pressure, the answer is, "Yes, but it is being treated."

- Tell your doctor about all the drugs you take. Don't forget to mention over-the-counter drugs, vitamins, and dietary supplements. They may affect your blood pressure. They also can change how well your blood pressure medicine works.

- Blood pressure pills should be taken at the same time each day. For example, take your medicine in the morning with breakfast or in the evening after brushing your teeth. If you miss a dose, do not double the dose the next day.

- Don't take more of your blood pressure medicine than your doctor prescribes. Do not stop taking your high blood pressure medicine unless your doctor tells you to stop. Don't skip a day or take half a pill. Remember to refill your medicine before you run out of pills.

- Before having surgery, ask your doctor if you should take your blood pressure medicine on that day.

- Get up slowly from a seated or lying position and stand for a bit. This lets your blood pressure adjust before walking to prevent dizziness, fainting, or a fall.

If your doctor asks you to take your blood pressure at home, keep in mind:

- There are many blood pressure home monitors for sale. Ask your doctor, nurse, or pharmacist to see which monitor you need and to show you how to use it. Have your monitor checked at the doctor's office to make sure it works correctly.

- Avoid smoking, exercise, and caffeine 30 minutes before taking your blood pressure.

- Make sure you are sitting with your feet on the floor and your back is against something.

- Relax quietly for 5 minutes before checking your blood pressure.

- Keep a list of your blood pressure numbers to share with your doctor, physician's assistant, or nurse.

Section 41.2

Portal Hypertension

This section contains text excerpted from the following sources: Text beginning with the heading "Cirrhosis" is excerpted from "Cirrhosis," National Institute of Diabetes and Digestive and Kidney Diseases (NIDDK), April 2014; Text under the heading "Complications" is excerpted from "Chapter 13: Complications of Liver Disease, Action Plan for Liver Disease Research," National Institute of Diabetes and Digestive and Kidney Diseases (NIDDK), 2014.

Cirrhosis

Cirrhosis is a condition in which the liver slowly deteriorates and is unable to function normally due to chronic, or long lasting, injury. Scar tissue replaces healthy liver tissue and partially blocks the flow of blood through the liver.

A healthy liver is necessary for survival. The liver can regenerate most of its own cells when they become damaged. However, if injury to the liver is too severe or long lasting, regeneration is incomplete, and the liver creates scar tissue. Scarring of the liver, also called fibrosis, may lead to cirrhosis.

The buildup of scar tissue that causes cirrhosis is usually a slow and gradual process. In the early stages of cirrhosis, the liver continues to function. However, as cirrhosis gets worse and scar tissue replaces more healthy tissue, the liver will begin to fail. Chronic liver failure, which is also called end-stage liver disease, progresses over months, years, or even decades. With end-stage liver disease, the liver can no longer perform important functions or effectively replace damaged cells.

Cirrhosis and Portal Hypertension

The portal vein carries blood from the stomach, intestines, spleen, gallbladder, and pancreas to the liver. In cirrhosis, scar tissue partially blocks the normal flow of blood, which increases the pressure in the portal vein. This condition is called portal hypertension. Portal hypertension is a common complication of cirrhosis. This condition may lead to other complications, such as

- fluid buildup leading to edema and ascites

- enlarged blood vessels, called varices, in the esophagus, stomach, or both

- an enlarged spleen, called splenomegaly

- mental confusion due to a buildup of toxins that are ordinarily removed by the liver, a condition called hepatic encephalopathy

Section 41.3

Preeclampsia and Eclampsia

This section includes text excerpted from "Preeclampsia and Eclampsia," Eunice Kennedy Shriver National Institute of Child Health and Human Development (NICHD), June 18, 2013.

What Are Preeclampsia and Eclampsia?

Preeclampsia and eclampsia are part of the spectrum of high blood pressure, or hypertensive disorders that can occur during pregnancy. At the mild end of the spectrum is **gestational hypertension**, which occurs when a woman who previously had normal blood pressure develops high blood pressure when she is more than 20 weeks pregnant. This problem occurs without other symptoms. Typically, gestational hypertension does not harm the mother or fetus and resolves after delivery. However, about 15% to 25% of women with gestational hypertension will go on to develop preeclampsia.

Preeclampsia is a condition that develops in women with previously normal blood pressure at 20 weeks of pregnancy or greater and includes increased blood pressure (levels greater than 140/90), increased swelling, and protein in the urine. The condition can be serious, and, if it is severe enough to affect brain function, causing seizures or coma, it is called **eclampsia**.

One of the serious complications of hypertensive disorders in pregnancy is **HELLP syndrome**, when a pregnant woman with preeclampsia or eclampsia sustains damage to the liver and blood cells. The letters in the name HELLP stand for the following problems:

H – **H**emolysis, in which oxygen-carrying red blood cells break down

EL – **E**levated **L**iver enzymes, showing damage to the liver

LP – **L**ow **P**latelet count, in which the cells responsible for stopping bleeding are low

What Causes Preeclampsia and Eclampsia?

The causes of preeclampsia and eclampsia are not known. These disorders previously were believed to be caused by a toxin in the blood (referred to as toxemia), but healthcare providers now know that is not true.

To learn more about preeclampsia and eclampsia, scientists are investigating many factors that could contribute to the development and progression of these diseases, including:

- placental abnormalities, such as insufficient blood flow
- genetic factors
- environmental exposures
- nutritional factors
- maternal immunology and autoimmune disorders
- cardiovascular and inflammatory changes
- hormonal imbalances

What Are the Risks of Preeclampsia and Eclampsia to the Mother?

Risks during Pregnancy

Preeclampsia during pregnancy is mild in 75 percent of cases. However, a woman can progress from mild to severe preeclampsia or full eclampsia very quickly—even in a matter of days—especially if she is not treated. Both preeclampsia and eclampsia can cause serious health problems for the mother and infant.

Preeclampsia affects the placenta as well as the mother's kidneys, liver, brain, and other organ and blood systems. The condition could lead to a separation of the placenta from the uterus (referred to as placental abruption), preterm delivery, and pregnancy loss. In some cases, preeclampsia can lead to organ failure or stroke. In severe cases, preeclampsia can develop into eclampsia, which can lead to seizures. Seizures in eclampsia cause a woman to lose consciousness, fall to the ground, and twitch uncontrollably. If not treated, these conditions can cause the death of the mother and/or the fetus.

Expecting mothers rarely die from preeclampsia in the developed world, but it is still a major cause of illness and death globally. According to the World Health Organization (WHO), preeclampsia and eclampsia cause 14 percent of maternal deaths each year, or about 50,000 to 75,000 women worldwide.

Risks after Pregnancy

In uncomplicated preeclampsia, the mother's high blood pressure and increased protein in the urine usually resolve within 6 weeks of the infant's birth. Studies, however, have shown that women who have had preeclampsia are four times more likely to develop hypertension and twice as likely to develop ischemic heart disease (reduced blood supply to the heart muscle, which can cause heart attacks), a blood clot in a vein, and stroke.

Less commonly, mothers who had preeclampsia during pregnancy could experience permanent damage to their organs. Preeclampsia could lead to kidney and liver damage or fluid in the lungs.

What Are the Risks to the Fetus?

Preeclampsia affects the flow of blood to the placenta. Risks to the fetus include:

- Lack of oxygen and nutrients, leading to poor fetal growth due to preeclampsia itself or if the placenta separates from the uterus before birth (placental abruption)

- Preterm birth

- Stillbirth if placental abruption leads to heavy bleeding in the mother

449

According to the Preeclampsia Foundation, each year, about 10,500 infants in the United States and about half a million worldwide die due to preeclampsia. Stillbirths are more likely to occur when the mother has a more severe form of preeclampsia, including HELLP syndrome.

Preeclampsia also can raise the risk of some long-term health issues related to preterm birth, including learning disorders, cerebral palsy, epilepsy, deafness, and blindness. Infants born preterm also risk extended hospitalization and small size. Infants who experienced poor growth in the uterus may later be at a higher risk of diabetes, congestive heart failure, and hypertension.

How Many Women Are Affected by or at Risk of Preeclampsia?

The exact number of women who develop preeclampsia is not known. Some scientists and healthcare providers estimate that preeclampsia affects 5% to 10% of all pregnancies globally. The rates are lower in the United States (about 3% to 5% of women), but it is estimated to account for 40% to 60% of maternal deaths in developing countries. Disorders related to high blood pressure are the second leading cause of stillbirths and early neonatal deaths in developing nations.

In addition, HELLP syndrome occurs in about 10% to 20% of all women with severe preeclampsia or eclampsia.

Risk Factors for Preeclampsia

Preeclampsia occurs primarily in first pregnancies. Other factors that can increase a woman's risk include:

- Chronic high blood pressure or kidney disease before pregnancy

- High blood pressure or preeclampsia in an earlier pregnancy

- Obesity

- Women who are younger than age 20 or older than 35

- Women who are pregnant with more than one fetus

- Being African American

- Having a family history of preeclampsia

According to the World Health Organization, among women who have had preeclampsia, about 20% to 40% of their daughters and 11% to 37% of their sisters also will get the disorder.

Preeclampsia is more common among women who have histories of certain health conditions, such as migraine headaches, diabetes, rheumatoid arthritis, lupus, scleroderma, urinary tract infection, gum disease, polycystic ovary syndrome, multiple sclerosis, gestational diabetes, and sickle cell disease.

Preeclampsia is also more common in pregnancies resulting from egg donation, donor insemination, or *in vitro* fertilization.

What Are the Symptoms of Preeclampsia, Eclampsia, and HELLP Syndrome?

Preeclampsia

Possible symptoms of preeclampsia include:

- High blood pressure
- Too much protein in the urine
- Swelling in a woman's face and hands (a woman's feet might swell too, but swollen feet are common during pregnancy and may not signal a problem)
- Systemic problems, such as headache, blurred vision, and right upper quadrant abdominal pain

Eclampsia

Women with preeclampsia can develop seizures. The following symptoms are cause for immediate concern:

- Severe headache
- Vision problems, such as temporary blindness
- Abdominal pain, especially in the upper right area of the belly
- Nausea and vomiting
- Smaller urine output or not urinating very often

HELLP Syndrome

HELLP syndrome can lead to serious complications, including liver failure and death.

A pregnant woman with HELLP syndrome might bleed or bruise easily and/or experience abdominal pain, nausea or vomiting, headache, or extreme fatigue. Although most women who develop HELLP syndrome already have high blood pressure and preeclampsia, sometimes the syndrome is the first sign. In addition, HELLP syndrome can occur without a woman having either high blood pressure or protein in her urine.

How Do Healthcare Providers Diagnose Preeclampsia, Eclampsia, and HELLP Syndrome

A healthcare provider should check a pregnant woman's blood pressure and urine during each prenatal visit. If the blood pressure reading is considered high (140/90 or higher), especially after the 20th week of pregnancy, the healthcare provider will likely perform more extensive lab tests to look for extra protein in the urine (called proteinuria) as well as other abnormalities.

Gestational hypertension is diagnosed if the woman has high blood pressure but no protein in the urine. Gestational hypertension occurs when women with normal blood pressure levels before pregnancy develop high blood pressure after 20 weeks of pregnancy. Gestational hypertension can develop into preeclampsia.

Mild preeclampsia is diagnosed when a pregnant woman has:

- Systolic blood pressure (top number) of 140 mmHg or higher or diastolic blood pressure (bottom number) of 90 mmHg or higher
- Urine with 0.3 or more grams of protein in a 24-hour specimen (a collection of every drop of urine within 24 hours)

Severe preeclampsia occurs when a pregnant woman has:

- Systolic blood pressure of 160 mmHg or higher or diastolic blood pressure of 110 mmHg or higher on two occasions at least 6 hours apart
- Urine with 5 or more grams of protein in a 24-hour specimen or 3 or more grams of protein on 2 random urine samples collected at least 4 hours apart
- Test results suggesting blood or liver damage—for example, blood tests that reveal low numbers of red blood cells, low numbers of platelets, or high liver enzymes
- Symptoms that include severe weight gain, difficulty breathing, or fluid buildup

Eclampsia occurs when women with preeclampsia develop seizures.

A healthcare provider may do other tests to assess the health of the mother and fetus, including:

- Blood tests to see how well the mother's liver and kidneys are working

- Blood tests to check blood platelet levels to see how well the mother's blood is clotting

- Blood tests to count the total number of red blood cells in the mother's blood

- A maternal weight check

- An ultrasound to assess the fetus's size

- A check of the fetus's heart rate

- A physical exam to look for swelling in the mother's face, hands, or legs as well as abdominal tenderness or an enlarged liver

HELLP syndrome is diagnosed when laboratory tests show hemolysis, elevated liver enzymes, and low platelets. There also may or may not be extra protein in the urine.

What Are the Treatments for Preeclampsia, Eclampsia, and HELLP Syndrome?

Preeclampsia

The only cure for preeclampsia when it occurs during pregnancy is delivering the fetus. Treatment decisions need to take into account the severity of the condition and the potential for maternal complications, how far along the pregnancy is, and the potential risks to the fetus. Ideally, the healthcare provider will minimize risks to the mother while giving the fetus as much time as possible to mature before delivery.

If the fetus is at 37 weeks or later, the healthcare provider will usually want to deliver it to avoid further complications.

If the fetus is younger than 37 weeks, however, the woman and her healthcare provider may want to consider other options that give the fetus more time to develop, depending on how severe the condition is. A healthcare provider may consider the following treatment options:

- If the preeclampsia is mild, it may be possible to wait to deliver the infant. To help prevent further complications, the healthcare provider may ask the woman to go on bed rest (to try to lower blood pressure and increase the blood flow to the placenta).

- Close monitoring of the woman and her fetus will be needed. Tests for the mother might include blood and urine tests to see if the preeclampsia is progressing (such as tests to assess platelet counts, liver enzymes, kidney function, and urinary protein levels). Tests for the fetus might include ultrasound, heart rate monitoring, assessment of fetal growth, and amniotic fluid assessment.

- Anticonvulsive medication, such as magnesium sulfate, might be used to prevent a seizure.

- In some cases, such as with severe preeclampsia, the woman will be admitted to the hospital so she can be monitored closely. Treatment in the hospital might include intravenous medication to control blood pressure and prevent seizures or other complications as well as steroid injections to help speed up the development of the fetus's lungs.

When a woman has severe preeclampsia, the doctor will probably want to deliver the fetus as soon as possible. Delivery usually is suggested if the pregnancy has lasted more than 34 weeks. If the fetus is less than 34 weeks, the doctor will probably prescribe corticosteroids to help speed up the maturation of the lungs.

In some cases, the doctor must deliver the fetus prematurely, even if that means likely complications for the infant because of the risk of severe maternal complications. The symptoms of preeclampsia usually go away within 6 weeks of delivery.

Eclampsia

Eclampsia—the onset of seizures in a woman with preeclampsia—is considered a medical emergency. Immediate treatment, usually in a hospital, is needed to stop the mother's seizures; treat blood pressure levels that are too high; and deliver the infant.

Magnesium sulfate (a type of mineral) may be given to treat active seizures and prevent future seizures. Antihypertensive medications may be given to lower the blood pressure.

The only cure for gestational eclampsia is to deliver the fetus.

HELLP Syndrome

HELLP syndrome, a special type of severe preeclampsia, can lead to serious complications for the mother, including liver failure and death, as well as the fetus.

The healthcare provider may consider the following treatments after a diagnosis of HELLP syndrome:

- Delivery, particularly if the pregnancy is 34 weeks or later.

- Hospitalization to provide intravenous medication to control blood pressure and prevent seizures or other complications as well as steroid injections to help speed up the development of the fetus's lungs.

Preeclampsia and Eclampsia: Other FAQs

If I Have High Blood Pressure, Can I Take Steps to Prevent Problems Like Preeclampsia during Pregnancy?

There is no known way to prevent preeclampsia. However, you can take steps to lower your risk.

If you currently have chronic hypertension (high blood pressure not due to pregnancy), you may be at higher-than-average risk for getting preeclampsia during pregnancy. Your risk is also higher if you had gestational hypertension (high blood pressure that occurs only during pregnancy) or preeclampsia with a previous pregnancy, if you are obese, or if you have other risk factors.

Talk with your healthcare provider about how hypertension might affect your pregnancy and what you can do to lower your risk of complications.

Before You get Pregnant

Visit your healthcare provider for a preconception visit to discuss what you can do to lower your risk. Your healthcare provider may recommend ways to control your blood pressure, if needed, by limiting your salt intake, exercising regularly, and losing weight if you are overweight.

If you take medication to control your blood pressure, ask your healthcare provider if you should change it. Some medications should not be used during pregnancy. Your healthcare provider may be able to recommend safer alternatives.

While You are Pregnant

Be sure to get regular prenatal care, including regular blood pressure checks, urine tests for protein, as well as regular weight checks.

Avoid alcohol and tobacco.

Talk with your doctor about any drugs or supplements, including vitamins and herbs, that you take or are thinking of taking.

If I Had Preeclampsia with a Previous Pregnancy, Will I Have It Again in Later Pregnancies?

If you had preeclampsia during your first pregnancy, your risk of developing preeclampsia again is about 15 percent. Your risk is even higher if you delivered your first child before 28 weeks of pregnancy or if you are overweight or obese.

Your risk of having preeclampsia again is also higher if you developed preeclampsia early in your previous pregnancy, if you developed chronic hypertension or diabetes after the first pregnancy, or if you had *in vitro* fertilization or are carrying more than one fetus. Having severe preeclampsia or HELLP syndrome during the first pregnancy also raises your risk.

If you had HELLP syndrome during a pregnancy, you have about a 25 percent chance of getting it again.

Section 41.4

Hypotension (Low Blood Pressure)

This section includes text excerpted from "Hypotension," National Heart, Lung, and Blood Institute (NHLBI), November 1, 2010. Reviewed July 2016.

What Is Hypotension?

Hypotension is abnormally low blood pressure. Blood pressure is the force of blood pushing against the walls of the arteries as the heart pumps out blood.

Blood pressure is measured as systolic and diastolic pressures. "Systolic" refers to blood pressure when the heart beats while pumping blood. "Diastolic" refers to blood pressure when the heart is at rest between beats.

You most often will see blood pressure numbers written with the systolic number above or before the diastolic number, such as 120/80 mmHg. (The mmHg is millimeters of mercury—the units used to measure blood pressure.)

Normal blood pressure in adults is lower than 120/80 mmHg. Hypotension is blood pressure that's lower than 90/60 mmHg.

Types of Hypotension

There are several types of hypotension. People who always have low blood pressure have chronic asymptomatic hypotension. They usually have no signs or symptoms and need no treatment. Their low blood pressure is normal for them.

Other types of hypotension occur if blood pressure suddenly drops too low. The signs and symptoms range from mild to severe.

The three main types of this kind of hypotension are orthostatic hypotension, neurally mediated hypotension, and severe hypotension linked to shock.

Orthostatic Hypotension

This type of hypotension occurs when standing up from a sitting or lying down position. You may feel dizzy or light-headed, or you may even faint.

Orthostatic hypotension occurs if your body isn't able to adjust blood pressure and blood flow fast enough for the change in position. The drop in blood pressure usually lasts only for a few seconds or minutes after you stand up. You may need to sit or lie down for a short time while your blood pressure returns to normal.

Orthostatic hypotension can occur in all age groups. However, it's more common in older adults, especially those who are frail or in poor health. This type of hypotension can be a symptom of another medical condition. Thus, treatment often focuses on treating underlying conditions.

Some people have orthostatic hypotension, but also have high blood pressure when lying down.

A form of orthostatic hypotension called postprandial hypotension is a sudden drop in blood pressure after a meal. This type of hypotension mostly affects older adults. People who have high blood pressure or a central nervous system disorder, such as Parkinson's disease, also are at increased risk for postprandial hypotension.

Neurally Mediated Hypotension

With neurally mediated hypotension (NMH), blood pressure drops after you've been standing for a long time. You may feel dizzy, faint, or sick to the stomach as a result. NMH also can occur as the result of an unpleasant, upsetting, or scary situation.

NMH affects children and young adults more often than people in other age groups. Children often outgrow NMH.

Severe Hypotension Linked to Shock

Shock is a life-threatening condition in which blood pressure drops so low that the brain, kidneys, and other vital organs can't get enough blood to work well. Blood pressure drops much lower in shock than in other types of hypotension.

Many factors can cause shock. Examples include major blood loss, certain severe infections, severe burns and allergic reactions, and poisoning. Shock can be fatal if it's not treated right away.

Other Names for Hypotension

- low blood pressure
- neurally mediated hypotension
- neurogenic orthostatic hypotension
- orthostatic hypotension
- postprandial hypotension
- postural hypotension
- shock

What Causes Hypotension?

Conditions or factors that disrupt the body's ability to control blood pressure cause hypotension. The different types of hypotension have different causes.

Orthostatic Hypotension

Orthostatic hypotension has many causes. Sometimes two or more factors combine to cause this type of low blood pressure.

Dehydration is the most common cause of orthostatic hypotension. Dehydration occurs if the body loses more water than it takes in.

You may become dehydrated if you don't drink enough fluids or if you sweat a lot during physical activity. Fever, vomiting, and severe diarrhea also can cause dehydration.

Orthostatic hypotension also may occur during pregnancy, but it usually goes away after birth.

Because an older body doesn't manage changes in blood pressure as well as a younger body, getting older also can lead to this type of hypotension.

Postprandial hypotension (a type of orthostatic hypotension) mostly affects older adults. Postprandial hypotension is a sudden drop in blood pressure after a meal.

Certain medical conditions can raise your risk of orthostatic hypotension, including:

- Heart conditions, such as heart attack, heart valve disease, bradycardia (a very low heart rate), and heart failure. These conditions prevent the heart from pumping enough blood to the body

- Anemia

- Severe infections

- Endocrine conditions, such as thyroid disorders, Addison disease, low blood sugar, and diabetes

- Central nervous system disorders, such as Parkinson disease

- Pulmonary embolism

Some medicines for high blood pressure and heart disease can raise your risk of orthostatic hypotension. These medicines include:

- Diuretics, also called "water pills"

- Calcium channel blockers

- Angiotensin-converting enzyme (ACE) inhibitors

- Angiotensin II receptor blockers

- Nitrates

- Beta blockers

Medicines for conditions such as anxiety, depression, erectile dysfunction, and central nervous system disorders also can increase your risk of orthostatic hypotension.

Other substances, when taken with high blood pressure medicines, also can lead to orthostatic hypotension. These substances include alcohol, barbiturates, and some prescription and over-the-counter medicines.

Finally, other factors or conditions that can trigger orthostatic hypotension include being out in the heat or being immobile for a long time. "Immobile" means you can't move around very much.

Neurally Mediated Hypotension

Neurally mediated hypotension (NMH) occurs when the brain and heart don't communicate with each other properly.

For example, when you stand for a long time, blood begins to pool in your legs. This causes your blood pressure to drop. In NMH, the body mistakenly tells the brain that blood pressure is high. In response, the brain slows the heart rate. This makes blood pressure drop even more, causing dizziness and other symptoms.

Severe Hypotension Linked to Shock

Many factors and conditions can cause severe hypotension linked to shock. Some of these factors also can cause orthostatic hypotension. In shock, though, blood pressure drops very low and doesn't return to normal on its own.

Some severe infections can cause shock. This is known as septic shock. It can occur if bacteria enters the bloodstream. The bacteria release a toxin (poison) that leads to a dangerous drop in blood pressure.

A severe loss of blood or fluids from the body also can cause shock. This is known as hypovolemic shock. Hypovolemic shock can happen as a result of:

- major external bleeding (for example, from a severe cut or injury)

- major internal bleeding (for example, from a ruptured blood vessel or injury that causes bleeding inside the body)

- major loss of body fluids from severe burns

- severe swelling of the pancreas (an organ that produces enzymes and hormones, such as insulin)

- severe diarrhea

- severe kidney disease

- overuse of diuretics

A major decrease in the heart's ability to pump blood also can cause shock. This is known as cardiogenic shock.

A heart attack, pulmonary embolism, or an ongoing arrhythmia that disrupts heart function can cause this type of shock.

A sudden and extreme relaxation of the arteries linked to a drop in blood pressure also can cause shock. This is known as vasodilatory shock. It can occur due to:

- a severe head injury
- a reaction to certain medicines
- liver failure
- poisoning
- a severe allergic reaction (called anaphylactic shock)

Who Is at Risk for Hypotension?

Hypotension can affect people of all ages. However, people in certain age groups are more likely to have certain types of hypotension.

Older adults are more likely to have orthostatic and postprandial hypotension. Children and young adults are more likely to have neurally mediated hypotension.

People who take certain medicines—such as diuretics ("water pills") or other high blood pressure medicines—are at increased risk for hypotension. Certain conditions also increase the risk for hypotension. Examples include central nervous system disorders (such as Parkinson disease) and some heart conditions.

Other risk factors for hypotension include being immobile (not being able to move around very much) for long periods, being out in the heat for a long time, and pregnancy. Hypotension during pregnancy is normal and usually goes away after birth.

What Are the Signs and Symptoms of Hypotension?

Orthostatic Hypotension and Neurally Mediated Hypotension

The signs and symptoms of orthostatic hypotension and neurally mediated hypotension (NMH) are similar. They include:

- dizziness or light-headedness
- blurry vision

- confusion

- weakness

- fatigue (feeling tired)

- nausea (feeling sick to your stomach)

Orthostatic hypotension may happen within a few seconds or minutes of standing up after you've been sitting or lying down.

You may feel that you're going to faint, or you may actually faint. These signs and symptoms go away if you sit or lie down for a few minutes until your blood pressure adjusts to normal.

The signs and symptoms of NMH occur after standing for a long time or in response to an unpleasant, upsetting, or scary situation. The drop in blood pressure with NMH doesn't last long and often goes away after sitting down.

Severe Hypotension Linked to Shock

In shock, not enough blood and oxygen flow to the body's major organs, including the brain. The early signs and symptoms of reduced blood flow to the brain include light-headedness, sleepiness, and confusion.

In the earliest stages of shock, it may be hard to detect any signs or symptoms. In older people, the first symptom may only be confusion.

Over time, as shock worsens, a person won't be able to sit up without passing out. If the shock continues, the person will lose consciousness. Shock often is fatal if not treated right away.

Other signs and symptoms of shock vary, depending on what's causing the shock. When low blood volume (from major blood loss, for example) or poor pumping action in the heart (from heart failure, for example) causes shock:

- The skin becomes cold and sweaty. It often looks blue or pale. If pressed, the color returns to normal more slowly than usual. A bluish network of lines appears under the skin.

- The pulse becomes weak and rapid.

- The person begins to breathe very quickly.

When extreme relaxation of blood vessels causes shock (such as in vasodilatory shock), a person feels warm and flushed at first. Later, the skin becomes cold and sweaty, and the person feels very sleepy.

How Is Hypotension Diagnosed?

Hypotension is diagnosed based on your medical history, a physical exam, and test results. Your doctor will want to know:

- The type of hypotension you have and how severe it is.
- Whether an underlying condition is causing the hypotension.

Diagnostic Tests

Shock is a life-threatening condition that requires emergency treatment. For other types of hypotension, your doctor may recommend tests to find out how your blood pressure responds in certain situations.

The test results will help your doctor understand why you're fainting or having other symptoms.

- blood tests
- electrocardiogram (EKG)
- holter and event monitors
- echocardiography
- stress test
- valsalva maneuver
- tilt table test

How Is Hypotension Treated?

Treatment depends on the type of hypotension you have and the severity of your signs and symptoms. The goal of treatment is to bring blood pressure back to normal to relieve signs and symptoms. Another goal is to manage any underlying condition causing the hypotension.

Your response to treatment depends on your age, overall health, and strength. It also depends on how easily you can stop, start, or change medicines.

In a healthy person, low blood pressure without signs or symptoms usually isn't a problem and needs no treatment.

If you have signs or symptoms of hypotension, you should sit or lie down right away. Put your feet above the level of your heart. If your signs or symptoms don't go away quickly, you should seek medical care.

Orthostatic Hypotension

Many treatments are available for orthostatic hypotension. If you have this condition, your doctor may advise making lifestyle changes, such as:

- Drinking plenty of fluids, such as water or sports drinks that contain nutrients like sodium and potassium.

- Drinking little or no alcohol.

- Standing up slowly.

- Not crossing your legs while sitting.

- Slowly increasing the amount of time you sit up if you've been immobile for a long time because of a medical condition. The term "immobile" refers to not being able to move around very much.

- Eating small, low-carbohydrate meals if you have postprandial hypotension (a form of orthostatic hypotension).

Talk with your doctor about using compression stockings. These stockings apply pressure to your lower legs. The pressure helps move blood throughout your body.

If medicine is causing your low blood pressure, your doctor may change the medicine or adjust the dose you take.

Several medicines are used to treat orthostatic hypotension. These medicines, which raise blood pressure, include fludrocortisone and midodrine.

Neurally Mediated Hypotension

If you have neurally mediated hypotension (NMH), you may need to make lifestyle changes. These may include:

- Avoiding situations that trigger symptoms, such as standing for long periods. Unpleasant, upsetting, or scary situations also can trigger symptoms.

- Drinking plenty of fluids, such as water or sports drinks that contain nutrients like sodium and potassium.

- Increasing your salt intake (as your doctor advises).

- Learning to recognize symptoms that occur before fainting and taking action to raise your blood pressure. For example, sitting down and putting your head between your knees or lying down can help raise blood pressure.

If medicine is causing your hypotension, your doctor may change the medicine or adjust the dose you take. He or she also may prescribe medicine to treat NMH.

Children who have NHM often outgrow it.

Severe Hypotension Linked to Shock

Shock is a life-threatening emergency. People who have shock need prompt treatment from medical personnel.

The goals of treating shock are to:

- Restore blood flow to the organs as quickly as possible to prevent organ damage

- Find and reverse the cause of shock

Blood or special fluids are put into the bloodstream to restore blood flow to the organs. Medicines can help raise blood pressure or make the heartbeat stronger. Depending on the cause of the shock, other treatments—such as antibiotics or surgery—may be needed.

Living with Hypotension

Doctors can successfully treat hypotension. Many people who had the condition and were successfully treated live normal, healthy lives.

If you have hypotension, you can take steps to prevent or limit symptoms, such as dizzy spells and fainting.

If you have orthostatic hypotension, get up slowly after sitting or lying down, or move your legs before changing your position. Eat small, low-carbohydrate meals if you have postprandial hypotension (a form of orthostatic hypotension).

If you have neurally mediated hypotension, try not to stand for long periods. If you do have to stand for a long time, move around and wear compression stockings. These stockings apply pressure to your lower legs. The pressure helps move blood throughout your body.

Drink plenty of fluids, such as water or sports drinks that contain nutrients like sodium and potassium. Also, try to avoid unpleasant, upsetting, or scary situations. Learn to recognize symptoms and take action to raise your blood pressure. Children who have NMH often outgrow it.

Other lifestyle changes also can help you control hypotension.

Ask your doctor about learning how to measure your own blood pressure. This will help you find out what a normal blood pressure reading is for you. Keeping a record of blood pressure readings done by health providers also can help you learn more about your blood pressure.

Severe hypotension linked to shock is an emergency. Shock can lead to death if it's not treated right away.

Signs and symptoms of shock include light-headedness, sleepiness, and confusion. Over time, as shock worsens, a person won't be able to sit up without passing out. If the shock continues, the person can lose consciousness.

Other signs and symptoms of shock include cold and sweaty skin, a weak and rapid pulse, and rapid breathing.

Section 41.5

Cardiogenic Shock

This section includes text excerpted from "Cardiogenic Shock," National Heart, Lung, and Blood Institute (NHLBI), July 1, 2011. Reviewed July 2016.

What Is Cardiogenic Shock?

Cardiogenic shock is a condition in which a suddenly weakened heart isn't able to pump enough blood to meet the body's needs. The condition is a medical emergency and is fatal if not treated right away.

The most common cause of cardiogenic shock is damage to the heart muscle from a severe heart attack. However, not everyone who has a heart attack has cardiogenic shock. In fact, on average, only about 7 percent of people who have heart attacks develop the condition.

If cardiogenic shock does occur, it's very dangerous. When people die from heart attacks in hospitals, cardiogenic shock is the most common cause of death.

What Is Shock?

The medical term "shock" refers to a state in which not enough blood and oxygen reach important organs in the body, such as the brain and kidneys. Shock causes very low blood pressure and may be life threatening.

Shock can have many causes. Cardiogenic shock is only one type of shock. Other types of shock include hypovolemic shock and vasodilatory shock.

Hypovolemic shock is a condition in which the heart can't pump enough blood to the body because of severe blood loss.

In vasodilatory shock, the blood vessels suddenly relax. When the blood vessels are too relaxed, blood pressure drops and blood flow becomes very low. Without enough blood pressure, blood and oxygen don't reach the body's organs.

A bacterial infection in the bloodstream, a severe allergic reaction, or damage to the nervous system (brain and nerves) may cause vasodilatory shock.

When a person is in shock (from any cause), not enough blood and oxygen are reaching the body's organs. If shock lasts more than a few minutes, the lack of oxygen starts to damage the body's organs. If shock isn't treated quickly, it can cause permanent organ damage or death.

Some of the signs and symptoms of shock include:

- confusion or lack of alertness
- loss of consciousness
- a sudden and ongoing rapid heartbeat
- sweating
- pale skin
- a weak pulse
- rapid breathing
- decreased or no urine output
- cool hands and feet

What Causes Cardiogenic Shock?

Immediate Causes

Cardiogenic shock occurs if the heart suddenly can't pump enough oxygen-rich blood to the body. The most common cause of cardiogenic shock is damage to the heart muscle from a severe heart attack.

This damage prevents the heart's main pumping chamber, the left ventricle, from working well. As a result, the heart can't pump enough oxygen-rich blood to the rest of the body.

In about 3 percent of cardiogenic shock cases, the heart's lower right chamber, the right ventricle, doesn't work well. This means the heart can't properly pump blood to the lungs, where it picks up oxygen to bring back to the heart and the rest of the body.

Without enough oxygen-rich blood reaching the body's major organs, many problems can occur. For example:

- Cardiogenic shock can cause death if the flow of oxygen-rich blood to the organs isn't restored quickly. This is why emergency medical treatment is required.

- If organs don't get enough oxygen-rich blood, they won't work well. Cells in the organs die, and the organs may never work well again.

- As some organs stop working, they may cause problems with other bodily functions. This, in turn, can worsen shock. For example:

  - If the kidneys aren't working well, the levels of important chemicals in the body change. This may cause the heart and other muscles to become even weaker, limiting blood flow even more.

  - If the liver isn't working well, the body stops making proteins that help the blood clot. This can lead to more bleeding if the shock is due to blood loss.

How well the brain, kidneys, and other organs recover will depend on how long a person is in shock. The less time a person is in shock, the less damage will occur to the organs. This is another reason why emergency treatment is so important.

Underlying Causes

The underlying causes of cardiogenic shock are conditions that weaken the heart and prevent it from pumping enough oxygen-rich blood to the body.

Heart Attack

Most heart attacks occur as a result of coronary heart disease (CHD). CHD is a condition in which a waxy substance called plaque narrows or blocks the coronary (heart) arteries.

Plaque reduces blood flow to your heart muscle. It also makes it more likely that blood clots will form in your arteries. Blood clots can partially or completely block blood flow.

Conditions Caused by Heart Attack

Heart attacks can cause some serious heart conditions that can lead to cardiogenic shock. One example is ventricular septal rupture. This condition occurs if the wall that separates the ventricles (the heart's two lower chambers) breaks down.

The breakdown happens because cells in the wall have died due to a heart attack. Without the wall to separate them, the ventricles can't pump properly.

Heart attacks also can cause papillary muscle infarction or rupture. This condition occurs if the muscles that help anchor the heart valves stop working or break because a heart attack cuts off their blood supply. If this happens, blood doesn't flow correctly between the heart's chambers. This prevents the heart from pumping properly.

Other Heart Conditions

Serious heart conditions that may occur with or without a heart attack can cause cardiogenic shock. Examples include:

- **Myocarditis.** This is inflammation of the heart muscle.

- **Endocarditis.** This is an infection of the inner lining of the heart chambers and valves.

- **Life-threatening arrhythmias.** These are problems with the rate or rhythm of the heartbeat.

- **Pericardial tamponade.** This is too much fluid or blood around the heart. The fluid squeezes the heart muscle so it can't pump properly.

Pulmonary Embolism

Pulmonary embolism (PE) is a sudden blockage in a lung artery. This condition usually is caused by a blood clot that travels to the lung from a vein in the leg. PE can damage your heart and other organs in your body.

Who Is at Risk for Cardiogenic Shock?

The most common risk factor for cardiogenic shock is having a heart attack. If you've had a heart attack, the following factors can further increase your risk for cardiogenic shock:

- older age

- a history of heart attacks or heart failure

- coronary heart disease that affects all of the heart's major blood vessels

- high blood pressure

- diabetes

Women who have heart attacks are at higher risk for cardiogenic shock than men who have heart attacks.

What Are the Signs and Symptoms of Cardiogenic Shock?

A lack of oxygen-rich blood reaching the brain, kidneys, skin, and other parts of the body causes the signs and symptoms of cardiogenic shock.

Some of the typical signs and symptoms of shock usually include at least two or more of the following:

- confusion or lack of alertness

- loss of consciousness

- a sudden and ongoing rapid heartbeat

- sweating

- pale skin

- a weak pulse

- rapid breathing

- decreased or no urine output

- cool hands and feet

Any of these alone is unlikely to be a sign or symptom of shock.

How Is Cardiogenic Shock Diagnosed?

The first step in diagnosing cardiogenic shock is to identify that a person is in shock. At that point, emergency treatment should begin.

Once emergency treatment starts, doctors can look for the specific cause of the shock. If the reason for the shock is that the heart isn't pumping strongly enough, then the diagnosis is cardiogenic shock.

Tests and Procedures to Diagnose Shock and Its Underlying Causes

- blood pressure test
- electrocardiogram (EKG)
- echocardiography
- chest X-ray
- cardiac enzyme test

- coronary angiography
- pulmonary artery catheterization
- blood tests

How Is Cardiogenic Shock Treated?

Cardiogenic shock is life threatening and requires emergency medical treatment. The condition usually is diagnosed after a person has been admitted to a hospital for a heart attack. If the person isn't already in a hospital, emergency treatment can start as soon as medical personnel arrive.

The first goal of emergency treatment for cardiogenic shock is to improve the flow of blood and oxygen to the body's organs.

Sometimes both the shock and its cause are treated at the same time. For example, doctors may quickly open a blocked blood vessel that's damaging the heart. Often, this can get the patient out of shock with little or no additional treatment.

Emergency Life Support

Emergency life support treatment is needed for any type of shock. This treatment helps get oxygen-rich blood flowing to the brain, kidneys, and other organs.

Restoring blood flow to the organs keeps the patient alive and may prevent long-term damage to the organs. Emergency life support treatment includes:

- Giving the patient extra oxygen to breathe so that more oxygen reaches the lungs, the heart, and the rest of the body.

- Providing breathing support if needed. A ventilator might be used to protect the airway and provide the patient with extra oxygen. A ventilator is a machine that supports breathing.

- Giving the patient fluids, including blood and blood products, through a needle inserted in a vein (when the shock is due to blood loss). This can help get more blood to major organs and the rest of the body. This treatment usually isn't used for

471

cardiogenic shock because the heart can't pump the blood that's already in the body. Also, too much fluid is in the lungs, making it hard to breathe.

Medicines

During and after emergency life support treatment, doctors will try to find out what's causing the shock. If the reason for the shock is that the heart isn't pumping strongly enough, then the diagnosis is cardiogenic shock.

Treatment for cardiogenic shock will depend on its cause. Doctors may prescribe medicines to:

- prevent blood clots from forming

- increase the force with which the heart muscle contracts

- treat a heart attack

Medical Devices

Medical devices can help the heart pump and improve blood flow. Devices used to treat cardiogenic shock may include:

- **An intra-aortic balloon pump**. This device is placed in the aorta, the main blood vessel that carries blood from the heart to the body. A balloon at the tip of the device is inflated and deflated in a rhythm that matches the heart's pumping rhythm. This allows the weakened heart muscle to pump as much blood as it can, which helps get more blood to vital organs, such as the brain and kidneys.

- **A left ventricular assist device (LVAD)**. This device is a battery-operated pump that takes over part of the heart's pumping action. An LVAD helps the heart pump blood to the body. This device may be used if damage to the left ventricle, the heart's main pumping chamber, is causing shock.

Medical Procedures and Surgery

Sometimes medicines and medical devices aren't enough to treat cardiogenic shock.

Medical procedures and surgery can restore blood flow to the heart and the rest of the body, repair heart damage, and help keep a patient alive while he or she recovers from shock.

Surgery also can improve the chances of long-term survival. Surgery done within 6 hours of the onset of shock symptoms has the greatest chance of improving survival.

The types of procedures and surgery used to treat underlying causes of cardiogenic shock include:

- Percutaneous coronary intervention (PCI) and stents. PCI, also known as coronary angioplasty, is a procedure used to open narrowed or blocked coronary (heart) arteries and treat an ongoing heart attack. A stent is a small mesh tube that's placed in a coronary artery during PCI to help keep it open.

- Coronary artery bypass grafting. For this surgery, arteries or veins from other parts of the body are used to bypass (that is, go around) narrowed coronary arteries. This creates a new passage for oxygen-rich blood to reach the heart.

- Surgery to repair damaged heart valves.

- Surgery to repair a break in the wall that separates the heart's chambers. This break is called a septal rupture.

- Heart transplant. This type of surgery rarely is done during an emergency situation like cardiogenic shock because of other available options. Also, doctors need to do very careful testing to make sure a patient will benefit from a heart transplant and to find a matching heart from a donor. Still, in some cases, doctors may recommend a transplant if they feel it's the best way to improve a patient's chances of long-term survival.

How Can Cardiogenic Shock Be Prevented?

The best way to prevent cardiogenic shock is to lower your risk for coronary heart disease (CHD) and heart attack.

If you already have CHD, it's important to get ongoing treatment from a doctor who has experience treating heart problems.

If you have a heart attack, you should get treatment right away to try to prevent cardiogenic shock and other possible complications.

Section 41.6

Syncope (Fainting)

This section includes text excerpted from "Syncope," National
Institute of Neurological Disorders and Stroke (NINDS),
October 4, 2011. Reviewed July 2016.

What Is Syncope?

Syncope is a medical term used to describe a temporary loss of
consciousness due to the sudden decline of blood flow to the brain.
Syncope is commonly called fainting or "passing out." If an individual
is about to faint, he or she will feel dizzy, lightheaded, or nauseous
and their field of vision may "white out" or "blackout." The skin may
be cold and clammy. The person drops to the floor as he or she loses
consciousness. After fainting, an individual may be unconscious for a
minute or two, but will revive and slowly return to normal. Syncope
can occur in otherwise healthy people and affects all age groups, but
occurs more often in the elderly.

There are several types of syncope.

- *Vasovagal syncope* usually has an easily identified triggering
  event such as emotional stress, trauma, pain, the sight of blood,
  or prolonged standing.

- *Carotid sinus syncope* happens because of constriction of the
  carotid artery in the neck and can occur after turning the head,
  while shaving, or when wearing a tight collar.

- *Situational syncope* happens during urination, defecation,
  coughing, or as a result of gastrointestinal stimulation.

Syncope can also be a symptom of heart disease or abnormalities
that create an uneven heart rate or rhythm that temporarily affect
blood volume and its distribution in the body. Syncope isn't normally a
primary sign of a neurological disorder, but it may indicate an increased
risk for neurologic disorders such as Parkinson disease, postural orthostatic tachycardia syndrome (POTS), diabetic neuropathy, and other
types of neuropathy. Certain classes of drugs are associated with an

increased risk of syncope, including diuretics, calcium antagonists, ACE inhibitors, nitrates, antipsychotics, antihistamines, levodopa, narcotics, and alcohol.

Is There Any Treatment?

The immediate treatment for an individual who has fainted involves checking first to see if their airway is open and they are breathing. The person should remain lying down for at least 10–15 minutes, preferably in a cool and quiet space. If this isn't possible, have the individual sit forward and lower their head below their shoulders and between their knees. Ice or cold water in a cup is refreshing. For individuals who have problems with chronic fainting spells, therapy should focus on recognizing the triggers and learning techniques to keep from fainting. At the appearance of warning signs such as lightheadedness, nausea, or cold and clammy skin, counter-pressure maneuvers that involve gripping fingers into a fist, tensing the arms, and crossing the legs or squeezing the thighs together can be used to ward off a fainting spell. If fainting spells occur often without a triggering event, syncope may be a sign of an underlying heart disease.

What Is the Prognosis?

Syncope is a dramatic event and can be life-threatening if not treated properly. Generally, however, people recover completely within minutes to hours. If syncope is symptomatic of an underlying condition, then the prognosis will reflect the course of the disorder.

Chapter 42

Carotid Artery Disease

What Is Carotid Artery Disease?

Carotid artery disease is a disease in which a waxy substance called plaque builds up inside the carotid arteries. You have two common carotid arteries, one on each side of your neck. They each divide into internal and external carotid arteries.

The internal carotid arteries supply oxygen-rich blood to your brain. The external carotid arteries supply oxygen-rich blood to your face, scalp, and neck.

Carotid artery disease is serious because it can cause a stroke, also called a "brain attack." A stroke occurs if blood flow to your brain is cut off.

If blood flow is cut off for more than a few minutes, the cells in your brain start to die. This impairs the parts of the body that the brain cells control. A stroke can cause lasting brain damage; long-term disability, such as vision or speech problems or paralysis (an inability to move); or death.

What Causes Carotid Artery Disease?

Carotid artery disease seems to start when damage occurs to the inner layers of the carotid arteries.

Major factors that contribute to damage include:

- smoking

This chapter includes text excerpted from "Carotid Artery Disease," National Heart, Lung, and Blood Institute (NIILBI), June 22, 2016.

- high levels of certain fats and cholesterol in the blood

- high blood pressure

- high levels of sugar in the blood due to insulin resistance or diabetes

When damage occurs, your body starts a healing process. The healing may cause plaque to build up where the arteries are damaged.

The plaque in an artery can crack or rupture. If this happens, blood cell fragments called platelets will stick to the site of the injury and may clump together to form blood clots.

The buildup of plaque or blood clots can severely narrow or block the carotid arteries. This limits the flow of oxygen-rich blood to your brain, which can cause a stroke.

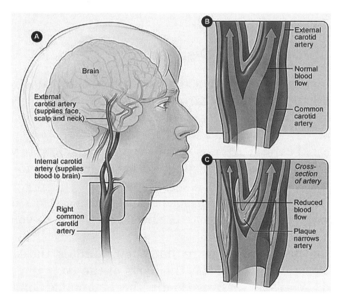

Figure 42.1. *Carotid Arteries*

Figure A shows the location of the right carotid artery in the head and neck. Figure B shows the inside of a normal carotid artery that has normal blood flow. Figure C show the inside of a carotid artery that has plaque buildup and reduced blood flow.

Who Is at Risk for Carotid Artery Disease?

The major risk factors for carotid artery disease, listed below, also are the major risk factors for coronary heart disease (also called coronary artery disease) and peripheral artery disease.

- diabetes

- family history of atherosclerosis

- high blood pressure (Hypertension)

- lack of physical activity

- metabolic syndrome

- older age

- overweight or obesity

- smoking

- unhealthy blood cholesterol levels

- unhealthy diet

Having any of these risk factors does not guarantee that you'll develop carotid artery disease. However, if you know that you have one or more risk factors, you can take steps to help prevent or delay the disease.

If you have plaque buildup in your carotid arteries, you also may have plaque buildup in other arteries. People who have carotid artery disease also are at increased risk for coronary heart disease.

What Are the Signs and Symptoms of Carotid Artery Disease?

Carotid artery disease may not cause signs or symptoms until it severely narrows or blocks a carotid artery. Signs and symptoms may include a bruit, a transient ischemic attack (TIA), or a stroke.

Bruit

During a physical exam, your doctor may listen to your carotid arteries with a stethoscope. He or she may hear a whooshing sound called a bruit. This sound may suggest changed or reduced blood flow due to plaque buildup. To find out more, your doctor may recommend tests.

Not all people who have carotid artery disease have bruits.

Transient Ischemic Attack (Mini-Stroke)

For some people, having a transient ischemic attack (TIA), or "mini-stroke," is the first sign of carotid artery disease. During a mini-stroke, you may have some or all of the symptoms of a stroke. However, the symptoms usually go away on their own within 24 hours.

Stroke and mini-stroke symptoms may include:

- a sudden, severe headache with no known cause

- dizziness or loss of balance

- inability to move one or more of your limbs

- sudden trouble seeing in one or both eyes

- sudden weakness or numbness in the face or limbs, often on just one side of the body

- trouble speaking or understanding speech

Even if the symptoms stop quickly, **call 9–1–1 for emergency help.** Do not drive yourself to the hospital. It's important to get checked and to get treatment started as soon as possible.

A mini-stroke is a warning sign that you're at high risk of having a stroke. You shouldn't ignore these symptoms. Getting medical care can help find possible causes of a mini-stroke and help you manage risk factors. These actions might prevent a future stroke.

Although a mini-stroke may warn of a stroke, it doesn't predict when a stroke will happen. A stroke may occur days, weeks, or even months after a mini-stroke.

Stroke

The symptoms of a stroke are the same as those of a mini-stroke, but the results are not. A stroke can cause lasting brain damage; long-term disability, such as vision or speech problems or paralysis (an inability to move); or death. Most people who have strokes have not previously had warning mini-strokes.

Getting treatment for a stroke right away is very important. You have the best chance for full recovery if treatment to open a blocked artery is given within 4 hours of symptom onset. The sooner treatment occurs, the better your chances of recovery.

Learning the signs and symptoms of a stroke will allow you to help yourself or someone close to you lower the risk of brain damage or death due to a stroke.

How Is Carotid Artery Disease Diagnosed?

Your doctor will diagnose carotid artery disease based on your medical history, a physical exam, and test results.

Medical History

Your doctor will find out whether you have any of the major risk factors for carotid artery disease. He or she also will ask whether you've had any signs or symptoms of a mini-stroke or stroke.

Physical Exam

To check your carotid arteries, your doctor will listen to them with a stethoscope. He or she will listen for a whooshing sound called a bruit. This sound may indicate changed or reduced blood flow due to plaque buildup. To find out more, your doctor may recommend tests.

Diagnostic Tests

The following tests are common for diagnosing carotid artery disease. If you have symptoms of a mini-stroke or stroke, your doctor may use other tests as well.

- carotid ultrasound
- carotid angiography
- magnetic resonance angiography
- computed tomography angiography

How Is Carotid Artery Disease Treated?

Treatments for carotid artery disease may include heart-healthy lifestyle changes, medicines, and medical procedures. The goals of treatment are to stop the disease from getting worse and to prevent a stroke. Your treatment will depend on your symptoms, how severe the disease is, and your age and overall health.

Heart-Healthy Lifestyle Changes

Your doctor may recommend heart-healthy lifestyle changes if you have carotid artery disease. Heart-healthy lifestyle changes include:

- heart-healthy eating
- aiming for a healthy weight
- managing stress
- physical activity
- quitting smoking

Medicines

If you have a stroke caused by a blood clot, you may be given a clot-dissolving, or clot-busting, medication. This type of medication must be given within 4 hours of symptom onset. The sooner treatment occurs, the better your chances of recovery.

Medicines to prevent blood clots are the mainstay treatment for people who have carotid artery disease. They prevent platelets from clumping together and forming blood clots in your carotid arteries, which can lead to a stroke. Two common medications are:

- Aspirin
- Clopidogrel

Sometimes lifestyle changes alone aren't enough to control your cholesterol levels. For example, you also may need statin medications to control or lower your cholesterol. By lowering your blood cholesterol level, you can decrease your chance of having a heart attack or stroke. Doctors usually prescribe statins for people who have:

- diabetes
- heart disease or have had a stroke
- high LDL cholesterol levels

Doctors may discuss beginning statin treatment with those who have an elevated risk for developing heart disease or having a stroke.

You may need other medications to treat diseases and conditions that damage the carotid arteries. Your doctor also may prescribe medications to:

- lower your blood pressure
- lower your blood sugar level
- prevent blood clots from forming, which can lead to stroke
- prevent or reduce inflammation

Take all medicines regularly, as your doctor prescribes. Don't change the amount of your medicine or skip a dose unless your doctor tells you to. Your healthcare team will help find a treatment plan that's right for you.

Medical Procedures

You may need a medical procedure if you have symptoms caused by the narrowing of the carotid artery. Doctors use one of two methods to open narrowed or blocked carotid arteries: carotid endarterectomy and carotid artery angioplasty and stenting.

Carotid Endarterectomy

Carotid endarterectomy is mainly for people whose carotid arteries are blocked 50 percent or more.

For the procedure, a surgeon will make a cut in your neck to reach the narrowed or blocked carotid artery. Next, he or she will make a cut in the blocked part of the artery and remove the artery's inner lining that is blocking the blood flow.

Finally, your surgeon will close the artery with stitches and stop any bleeding. He or she will then close the cut in your neck.

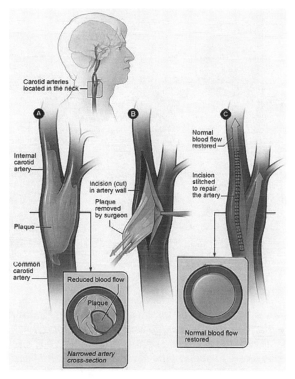

Figure 42.2. *Carotid Endarterectomy*

The illustration shows the process of carotid endarterectomy. Figure A shows a carotid artery with plaque buildup. The inset image shows a cross-section of the narrowed carotid artery. Figure B shows how the carotid artery is cut and how the plaque is removed. Figure C shows the artery stitched up and normal blood flow restored. The inset image shows a cross-section of the artery with plaque removed and normal blood flow restored.

Carotid Artery Angioplasty and Stenting

Doctors use a procedure called angioplasty to widen the carotid arteries and restore blood flow to the brain.

A thin tube with a deflated balloon on the end is threaded through a blood vessel in your neck to the narrowed or blocked carotid artery. Once in place, the balloon is inflated to push the plaque outward against the wall of the artery.

A stent (a small mesh tube) is then put in the artery to support the inner artery wall. The stent also helps prevent the artery from becoming narrowed or blocked again.

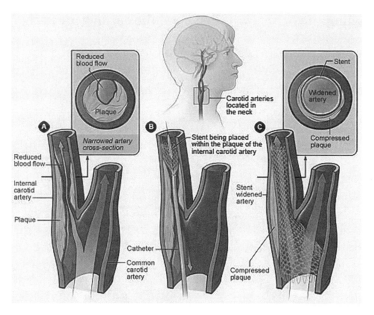

Figure 42.3. *Carotid Artery Stenting*

The illustration shows the process of carotid artery stenting. Figure A shows an internal carotid artery that has plaque buildup and reduced blood flow. The inset image shows a cross-section of the narrowed carotid artery. Figure B shows a stent being placed in the carotid artery to support the inner artery wall and keep the artery open. Figure C shows normal blood flow restored in the stent-widened artery. The inset image shows a cross-section of the stent-widened artery.

How Can Carotid Artery Disease Be Prevented?

Taking action to control your risk factors can help prevent or delay carotid artery disease and stroke. Your risk for carotid artery disease increases with the number of risk factors you have.

One step you can take is to make heart-healthy lifestyle changes, which can include:

- heart-healthy eating
- aiming for a healthy weight
- physical activity
- quit smoking

Other steps that can prevent or delay carotid artery disease include knowing your family history of carotid artery disease. If you or someone in your family has carotid artery disease, be sure to tell your doctor.

If lifestyle changes aren't enough, your doctor may prescribe medicines to control your carotid artery disease risk factors. Take all of your medicines as your doctor advises.

Living with Carotid Artery Disease

If you have carotid artery disease, you can take steps to manage the condition, reduce risk factors, and prevent complications. These steps include making heart-healthy lifestyle changes, following your treatment plan, and getting ongoing care.

Having carotid artery disease raises your risk of having a stroke. Know the warning signs of a stroke—such as weakness and trouble speaking—and what to do if they occur.

Treatment Plan

Following your treatment plan may help prevent your carotid artery disease from getting worse. It also can lower your risk for stroke and other health problems.

You may need to take medicines to control certain risk factors and to prevent blood clots that could cause a stroke. Taking prescribed medicines and following a healthy lifestyle can help control carotid artery disease. However, they don't cure the disease. You'll likely have to stick with your treatment plan for life.

Ongoing Care

If you have carotid artery disease, having ongoing medical care is important.

Most people who have the disease will need to have their blood pressure checked regularly and their blood sugar and blood cholesterol levels tested one or more times a year. If you have diabetes, you'll need routine blood sugar tests and other tests.

Testing shows whether these conditions are under control, or whether your doctor needs to adjust your treatment for better results.

If you've had a stroke or procedures to restore blood flow in your carotid arteries, you'll likely need a yearly carotid Doppler ultrasound test. This test shows how well blood flows through your carotid arteries.

Repeating this test over time will show whether the narrowing in your carotid arteries is getting worse. Results also can show how well procedures to treat your arteries have worked.

Follow up with your doctor regularly. The sooner your doctor spots problems, the sooner he or she can prescribe treatment.

Stroke Warning Signs

The signs and symptoms of stroke may include:

- Sudden weakness or numbness in the face or limbs, often on only one side of the body.

- The inability to move one or more of your limbs.

- Trouble speaking or understanding speech.

- Sudden trouble seeing in one or both eyes.

- Dizziness or loss of balance.

- A sudden, severe headache with no known cause.

If you're a candidate for clot-busting therapy, you have the best chance for full recovery if treatment to open a blocked artery is given within 4 hours of symptom onset. The sooner treatment occurs, the better your chances of recovery.

Make those close to you aware of stroke symptoms and the need for urgent action. Learning the signs and symptoms of a stroke will allow you to help yourself or someone close to you lower the risk of damage or death due to a stroke.

Chapter 43

Coronary Artery and Heart Disease

Chapter Contents

Section 43.1

Coronary Artery Disease

This section includes text excerpted from "Coronary Heart Disease," National Heart, Lung, and Blood Institute (NHLBI), June 22, 2016.

What Is Coronary Heart Disease?

Coronary heart disease (CHD) is a disease in which a waxy substance called plaque builds up inside the coronary arteries. These arteries supply oxygen-rich blood to your heart muscle.

When plaque builds up in the arteries, the condition is called atherosclerosis. The buildup of plaque occurs over many years.

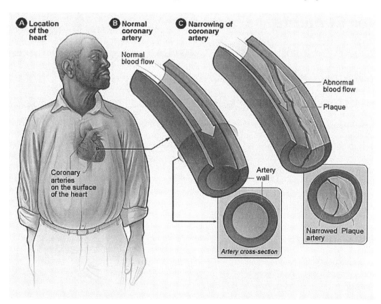

Figure 43.1. *Atherosclerosis*

Figure A shows the location of the heart in the body. Figure B shows a normal coronary artery with normal blood flow. The inset image shows a cross-section of a normal coronary artery. Figure C shows a coronary artery narrowed by plaque. The buildup of plaque limits the flow of oxygen-rich blood through the artery. The inset image shows a cross-section of the plaque-narrowed artery.

Over time, plaque can harden or rupture (break open). Hardened plaque narrows the coronary arteries and reduces the flow of oxygen-rich blood to the heart.

If the plaque ruptures, a blood clot can form on its surface. A large blood clot can mostly or completely block blood flow through a coronary artery. Over time, ruptured plaque also hardens and narrows the coronary arteries.

Other Names for Coronary Heart Disease

- Atherosclerosis
- Coronary artery disease
- Hardening of the arteries
- Heart disease
- Ischemic heart disease
- Narrowing of the arteries

What Causes Coronary Heart Disease?

Research suggests that coronary heart disease (CHD) starts when certain factors damage the inner layers of the coronary arteries. These factors include:

- smoking
- high levels of certain fats and cholesterol in the blood
- high blood pressure
- high levels of sugar in the blood due to insulin resistance or diabetes
- blood vessel inflammation

Plaque might begin to build up where the arteries are damaged. The buildup of plaque in the coronary arteries may start in childhood.

Over time, plaque can harden or rupture (break open). Hardened plaque narrows the coronary arteries and reduces the flow of oxygen-rich blood to the heart. This can cause angina (chest pain or discomfort).

If the plaque ruptures, blood cell fragments called platelets stick to the site of the injury. They may clump together to form blood clots.

Blood clots can further narrow the coronary arteries and worsen angina. If a clot becomes large enough, it can mostly or completely block a coronary artery and cause a heart attack.

Who Is at Risk for Coronary Heart Disease?

In the United States, coronary heart disease (CHD) is a leading cause of death for both men and women. Each year, about 370,000 Americans die from coronary heart disease.

Certain traits, conditions, or habits may raise your risk for CHD. The more risk factors you have, the more likely you are to develop the disease.

You can control many risk factors, which may help prevent or delay CHD.

Major Risk Factors

- unhealthy blood cholesterol levels
- high blood pressure
- smoking
- insulin resistance
- diabetes
- overweight or obesity
- metabolic syndrome
- lack of physical activity
- unhealthy diet
- older age
- a family history of early coronary heart disease

Although older age and a family history of early heart disease are risk factors, it doesn't mean that you'll develop CHD if you have one or both. Controlling other risk factors often can lessen genetic influences and help prevent CHD, even in older adults.

Emerging Risk Factors

Researchers continue to study other possible risk factors for CHD.

High levels of a protein called C-reactive protein (CRP) in the blood may raise the risk of CHD and heart attack. High levels of CRP are a sign of inflammation in the body.

Inflammation is the body's response to injury or infection. Damage to the arteries' inner walls may trigger inflammation and help plaque grow.

Research is under way to find out whether reducing inflammation and lowering CRP levels also can reduce the risk of CHD and heart attack.

High levels of triglycerides in the blood also may raise the risk of CHD, especially in women. Triglycerides are a type of fat.

Other Risks Related to Coronary Heart Disease

Other conditions and factors also may contribute to CHD, including:

- sleep apnea
- alcohol
- stress
- preeclampsia

What Are the Signs and Symptoms of Coronary Heart Disease?

A common symptom of coronary heart disease (CHD) is angina. Angina is chest pain or discomfort that occurs if an area of your heart muscle doesn't get enough oxygen-rich blood.

Angina may feel like pressure or squeezing in your chest. You also may feel it in your shoulders, arms, neck, jaw, or back. Angina pain may even feel like indigestion. The pain tends to get worse with activity and go away with rest. Emotional stress also can trigger the pain.

Another common symptom of CHD is shortness of breath. This symptom occurs if CHD causes heart failure. When you have heart failure, your heart can't pump enough blood to meet your body's needs. Fluid builds up in your lungs, making it hard to breathe.

The severity of these symptoms varies. They may get more severe as the buildup of plaque continues to narrow the coronary arteries.

Signs and Symptoms of Heart Problems Related to Coronary Heart Disease

Some people who have CHD have no signs or symptoms—a condition called silent CHD. The disease might not be diagnosed until a person has signs or symptoms of a heart attack, heart failure, or an arrhythmia (an irregular heartbeat).

Heart Attack

A heart attack occurs if the flow of oxygen-rich blood to a section of heart muscle is cut off. This can happen if an area of plaque in a coronary artery ruptures (breaks open).

Blood cell fragments called platelets stick to the site of the injury and may clump together to form blood clots. If a clot becomes large enough, it can mostly or completely block blood flow through a coronary artery.

If the blockage isn't treated quickly, the portion of heart muscle fed by the artery begins to die. Healthy heart tissue is replaced with scar tissue. This heart damage may not be obvious, or it may cause severe or long-lasting problems.

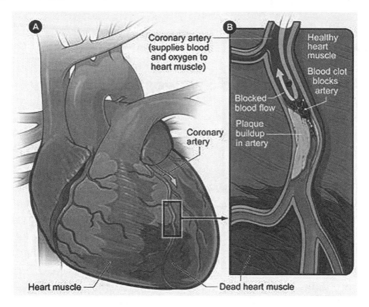

Figure 43.2. *Heart with Muscle Damage and a Blocked Artery*

Figure A is an overview of a heart and coronary artery showing damage (dead heart muscle) caused by a heart attack. Figure B is a cross-section of the coronary artery with plaque buildup and a blood clot.

The most common heart attack symptom is chest pain or discomfort. Most heart attacks involve discomfort in the center or left side of the chest that often lasts for more than a few minutes or goes away and comes back.

The discomfort can feel like uncomfortable pressure, squeezing, fullness, or pain. The feeling can be mild or severe. Heart attack pain sometimes feels like indigestion or heartburn.

The symptoms of angina can be similar to the symptoms of a heart attack. Angina pain usually lasts for only a few minutes and goes away with rest.

Chest pain or discomfort that doesn't go away or changes from its usual pattern (for example, occurs more often or while you're resting) might be a sign of a heart attack. If you don't know whether your chest pain is angina or a heart attack, call 9–1–1.

All chest pain should be checked by a doctor.

Other common signs and symptoms of a heart attack include:

- Upper body discomfort in one or both arms, the back, neck, jaw, or upper part of the stomach

- Shortness of breath, which may occur with or before chest discomfort

- Nausea (feeling sick to your stomach), vomiting, light-headedness or fainting, or breaking out in a cold sweat

- Sleep problems, fatigue (tiredness), or lack of energy

Heart Failure

Heart failure is a condition in which your heart can't pump enough blood to meet your body's needs. Heart failure doesn't mean that your heart has stopped or is about to stop working.

The most common signs and symptoms of heart failure are shortness of breath or trouble breathing; fatigue; and swelling in the ankles, feet, legs, stomach, and veins in the neck.

All of these symptoms are the result of fluid buildup in your body. When symptoms start, you may feel tired and short of breath after routine physical effort, like climbing stairs.

Arrhythmia

An arrhythmia is a problem with the rate or rhythm of the heartbeat. When you have an arrhythmia, you may notice that your heart is skipping beats or beating too fast.

Some people describe arrhythmias as a fluttering feeling in the chest. These feelings are called palpitations.

Some arrhythmias can cause your heart to suddenly stop beating. This condition is called sudden cardiac arrest (SCA). SCA usually causes death if it's not treated within minutes.

How Is Coronary Heart Disease Diagnosed?

Your doctor will diagnose coronary heart disease (CHD) based on your medical and family histories, your risk factors for CHD, a physical exam, and the results from tests and procedures.

No single test can diagnose CHD. If your doctor thinks you have CHD, he or she may recommend one or more of the following tests.

- electrocardiogram (EKG)
- stress testing
- echocardiography
- chest X-ray
- blood tests
- coronary angiography and cardiac catheterization

How Is Coronary Heart Disease Treated?

Treatments for coronary heart disease include heart-healthy lifestyle changes, medicines, medical procedures and surgery, and cardiac rehabilitation. Treatment goals may include:

- Lowering the risk of blood clots forming (blood clots can cause a heart attack)
- Preventing complications of coronary heart disease
- Reducing risk factors in an effort to slow, stop, or reverse the buildup of plaque
- Relieving symptoms
- Widening or bypassing clogged arteries

Heart-Healthy Lifestyle Changes

Your doctor may recommend heart-healthy lifestyle changes if you have coronary heart disease. Heart-healthy lifestyle changes include:

- heart-healthy eating
- physical activity
- maintaining a healthy weight
- quitting smoking
- managing stress

Medicines

Sometimes lifestyle changes aren't enough to control your blood cholesterol levels. For example, you may need statin medications to control or lower your cholesterol. By lowering your cholesterol level, you can decrease your chance of having a heart attack or stroke. Doctors usually prescribe statins for people who have:

- coronary heart disease, peripheral artery disease, or had a stroke
- diabetes
- high LDL cholesterol levels

Doctors may discuss beginning statin treatment with those who have an elevated risk for developing heart disease or having a stroke. Your doctor also may prescribe other medications to:

- Decrease your chance of having a heart attack or dying suddenly.

- Lower your blood pressure.
- Prevent blood clots, which can lead to heart attack or stroke.
- Prevent or delay the need for a stent or percutaneous coronary intervention (PCI) or surgery, such as coronary artery bypass grafting (CABG).
- Reduce your heart's workload and relieve coronary heart disease symptoms.

Take all medicines regularly, as your doctor prescribes. Don't change the amount of your medicine or skip a dose unless your doctor tells you to. You should still follow a heart healthy lifestyle, even if you take medicines to treat your coronary heart disease.

Medical Procedures and Surgery

You may need a procedure or surgery to treat coronary heart disease. Both PCI and CABG are used to treat blocked coronary arteries. You and your doctor can discuss which treatment is right for you.

Percutaneous Coronary Intervention

Percutaneous coronary intervention, commonly known as angioplasty, is a nonsurgical procedure that opens blocked or narrowed coronary arteries. A thin, flexible tube with a balloon or other device on the end is threaded through a blood vessel to the narrowed or blocked coronary artery. Once in place, the balloon is inflated to compress the plaque against the wall of the artery. This restores blood flow through the artery.

During the procedure, the doctor may put a small mesh tube called a stent in the artery. The stent helps prevent blockages in the artery in the months or years after angioplasty.

Coronary Artery Bypass Grafting

CABG is a type of surgery in which arteries or veins from other areas in your body are used to bypass (that is, go around) your narrowed coronary arteries. CABG can improve blood flow to your heart, relieve chest pain, and possibly prevent a heart attack.

Cardiac Rehabilitation

Your doctor may prescribe cardiac rehabilitation (rehab) for angina or after CABG, angioplasty, or a heart attack. Nearly everyone who has coronary heart disease can benefit from cardiac rehab. Cardiac rehab is a medically supervised program that may help improve the health and well-being of people who have heart problems.

Rehab has two parts:

- education, counseling, and training
- exercise training

How Can Coronary Heart Disease Be Prevented or Delayed?

You can prevent and control coronary heart disease (CHD) by taking action to control your risk factors with heart-healthy lifestyle changes and medicines. Examples of risk factors you can control include high blood cholesterol, high blood pressure, and overweight and obesity. Only a few risk factors—such as age, gender, and family history—can't be controlled.

Your risk for CHD increases with the number of risk factors you have. To reduce your risk of CHD and heart attack, try to control each risk factor you have by adopting the following heart-healthy lifestyles:

- heart-healthy eating
- maintaining a healthy weight
- managing stress
- physical activity
- quitting smoking

Know your family history of health problems related to CHD. If you or someone in your family has CHD, be sure to tell your doctor. If lifestyle changes aren't enough, you also may need medicines to control your CHD risk factors.

Living with Coronary Heart Disease

Coronary heart disease (CHD) can cause serious complications. However, if you follow your doctor's advice and adopt healthy lifestyle habits, you can prevent or reduce the risk of:

- dying suddenly from heart problems
- having a heart attack and damaging your heart muscle
- damaging your heart because of reduced oxygen supply
- having arrhythmias (irregular heartbeats)

Ongoing Care

Work closely with your doctor to control your blood pressure and manage your blood cholesterol and blood sugar levels.

A blood test called a lipoprotein panel will measure your cholesterol and triglyceride levels. A fasting blood glucose test will check your blood sugar level and show whether you're at risk for or have diabetes.

These tests show whether your risk factors are controlled, or whether your doctor needs to adjust your treatment for better results.

Talk with your doctor about how often you should schedule office visits or blood tests. Between those visits, call your doctor if you have any new symptoms or if your symptoms worsen.

Heart Attack Warning Signs

CHD raises your risk for a heart attack. Learn the signs and symptoms of a heart attack, and call 9–1–1 if you have any of these symptoms:

- Chest pain or discomfort. This involves uncomfortable pressure, squeezing, fullness, or pain in the center or left side of the chest that can be mild or strong. This pain or discomfort often lasts more than a few minutes or goes away and comes back.

- Upper body discomfort in one or both arms, the back, neck, jaw, or upper part of the stomach.

- Shortness of breath, which may occur with or before chest discomfort.

- Nausea (feeling sick to your stomach), vomiting, light-headedness or fainting, or breaking out in a cold sweat.

Symptoms also may include sleep problems, fatigue (tiredness), and lack of energy.

The symptoms of angina can be similar to the symptoms of a heart attack. Angina pain usually lasts for only a few minutes and goes away with rest.

Chest pain or discomfort that doesn't go away or changes from its usual pattern (for example, occurs more often or while you're resting) can be a sign of a heart attack. If you don't know whether your chest pain is angina or a heart attack, call 9–1–1.

Let the people you see regularly know you're at risk for a heart attack. They can seek emergency care for you if you suddenly faint, collapse, or have other severe symptoms.

Section 43.2

Angina

This section includes text excerpted from "Angina,"
National Heart, Lung, and Blood Institute (NHLBI),
June 1, 2011. Reviewed July 2016.

What Is Angina?

Angina is chest pain or discomfort that occurs if an area of your heart muscle doesn't get enough oxygen-rich blood.

Angina may feel like pressure or squeezing in your chest. The pain also can occur in your shoulders, arms, neck, jaw, or back. Angina pain may even feel like indigestion.

Angina isn't a disease; it's a symptom of an underlying heart problem. Angina usually is a symptom of coronary heart disease (CHD).

CHD is the most common type of heart disease in adults. It occurs if a waxy substance called plaque builds up on the inner walls of your coronary arteries. These arteries carry oxygen-rich blood to your heart.

Plaque narrows and stiffens the coronary arteries. This reduces the flow of oxygen-rich blood to the heart muscle, causing chest pain. Plaque buildup also makes it more likely that blood clots will form in your arteries. Blood clots can partially or completely block blood flow, which can cause a heart attack.

Angina also can be a symptom of coronary microvascular disease (MVD). This is heart disease that affects the heart's smallest coronary arteries. In coronary MVD, plaque doesn't create blockages in the arteries like it does in CHD.

Studies have shown that coronary MVD is more likely to affect women than men. Coronary MVD also is called cardiac syndrome X and nonobstructive CHD.

Types of Angina

The major types of angina are stable, unstable, variant (Prinzmetal), and microvascular. Knowing how the types differ is important. This is because they have different symptoms and require different treatments.

498

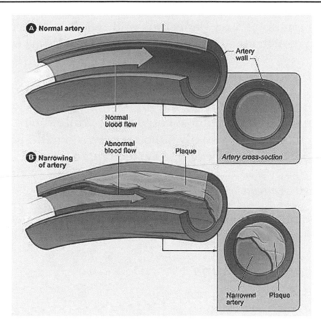

Figure 43.3. *Plaque Buildup in an Artery*

Figure A shows a normal artery with normal blood flow. The inset image shows a cross-section of a normal artery. Figure B shows an artery with plaque buildup. The inset image shows a cross-section of an artery with plaque buildup.

Stable Angina

Stable angina is the most common type of angina. It occurs when the heart is working harder than usual. Stable angina has a regular pattern. ("Pattern" refers to how often the angina occurs, how severe it is, and what factors trigger it.)

If you have stable angina, you can learn its pattern and predict when the pain will occur. The pain usually goes away a few minutes after you rest or take your angina medicine.

Stable angina isn't a heart attack, but it suggests that a heart attack is more likely to happen in the future.

Unstable Angina

Unstable angina doesn't follow a pattern. It may occur more often and be more severe than stable angina. Unstable angina also can occur with or without physical exertion, and rest or medicine may not relieve the pain.

Unstable angina is very dangerous and requires emergency treatment. This type of angina is a sign that a heart attack may happen soon.

Variant (Prinzmetal) Angina

Variant angina is rare. A spasm in a coronary artery causes this type of angina. Variant angina usually occurs while you're at rest, and the pain can be severe. It usually happens between midnight and early morning. Medicine can relieve this type of angina.

Microvascular Angina

Microvascular angina can be more severe and last longer than other types of angina. Medicine may not relieve this type of angina.

Other Names for Angina

- acute coronary syndrome
- angina pectoris
- chest pain
- coronary artery spasms
- microvascular angina
- Prinzmetal angina
- stable or common angina
- unstable angina
- variant angina

What Causes Angina?

Underlying Causes

Angina usually is a symptom of coronary heart disease (CHD). This means that the underlying causes of angina generally are the same as the underlying causes of CHD.

Research suggests that CHD starts when certain factors damage the inner layers of the coronary arteries. These factors include:

- smoking
- high amounts of certain fats and cholesterol in the blood

- high blood pressure

- high amounts of sugar in the blood due to insulin resistance or diabetes

Plaque may begin to build up where the arteries are damaged. When plaque builds up in the arteries, the condition is called atherosclerosis.

Plaque narrows or blocks the arteries, reducing blood flow to the heart muscle. Some plaque is hard and stable and causes the arteries to become narrow and stiff. This can greatly reduce blood flow to the heart and cause angina.

Other plaque is soft and more likely to rupture (break open) and cause blood clots. Blood clots can partially or totally block the coronary arteries and cause angina or a heart attack.

Immediate Causes

Many factors can trigger angina pain, depending on the type of angina you have.

Stable Angina

Physical exertion is the most common trigger of stable angina. Severely narrowed arteries may allow enough blood to reach the heart when the demand for oxygen is low, such as when you're sitting.

However, with physical exertion—like walking up a hill or climbing stairs—the heart works harder and needs more oxygen.

Other triggers of stable angina include:

- emotional stress

- exposure to very hot or cold temperatures

- heavy meals

- smoking

Unstable Angina

Blood clots that partially or totally block an artery cause unstable angina.

If plaque in an artery ruptures, blood clots may form. This creates a blockage. A clot may grow large enough to completely block the artery and cause a heart attack.

Blood clots may form, partially dissolve, and later form again. Angina can occur each time a clot blocks an artery.

Variant Angina

A spasm in a coronary artery causes variant angina. The spasm causes the walls of the artery to tighten and narrow. Blood flow to the heart slows or stops. Variant angina can occur in people who have CHD and in those who don't.

The coronary arteries can spasm as a result of:

- exposure to cold
- emotional stress
- medicines that tighten or narrow blood vessels
- smoking
- cocaine use

Microvascular Angina

This type of angina may be a symptom of coronary microvascular disease (MVD). Coronary MVD is heart disease that affects the heart's smallest coronary arteries.

Reduced blood flow in the small coronary arteries may cause microvascular angina. Plaque in the arteries, artery spasms, or damaged or diseased artery walls can reduce blood flow through the small coronary arteries.

Who Is at Risk for Angina?

Angina is a symptom of an underlying heart problem. It's usually a symptom of coronary heart disease (CHD), but it also can be a symptom of coronary microvascular disease (MVD). So, if you're at risk for CHD or coronary MVD, you're also at risk for angina.

The major risk factors for CHD and coronary MVD include:

- unhealthy cholesterol levels
- high blood pressure
- smoking
- insulin resistance or diabetes
- overweight or obesity
- metabolic syndrome
- lack of physical activity
- unhealthy diet

- older age. (The risk increases for men after 45 years of age and for women after 55 years of age.)

- family history of early heart disease

People sometimes think that because men have more heart attacks than women, men also suffer from angina more often. In fact, overall, angina occurs equally among men and women.

Microvascular angina, however, occurs more often in women. About 70 percent of the cases of microvascular angina occur in women around the time of menopause.

Unstable angina occurs more often in older adults. Variant angina is rare; it accounts for only about 2 out of 100 cases of angina. People who have variant angina often are younger than those who have other forms of angina.

What Are the Signs and Symptoms of Angina?

Pain and discomfort are the main symptoms of angina. Angina often is described as pressure, squeezing, burning, or tightness in the chest. The pain or discomfort usually starts behind the breastbone.

Pain from angina also can occur in the arms, shoulders, neck, jaw, throat, or back. The pain may feel like indigestion. Some people say that angina pain is hard to describe or that they can't tell exactly where the pain is coming from.

Signs and symptoms such as nausea (feeling sick to your stomach), fatigue (tiredness), shortness of breath, sweating, light-headedness, and weakness also may occur.

Women are more likely to feel discomfort in the neck, jaw, throat, abdomen, or back. Shortness of breath is more common in older people and those who have diabetes. Weakness, dizziness, and confusion can mask the signs and symptoms of angina in elderly people.

Symptoms also vary based on the type of angina you have.

Because angina has so many possible symptoms and causes, all chest pain should be checked by a doctor. Chest pain that lasts longer than a few minutes and isn't relieved by rest or angina medicine may be a sign of a heart attack.

Stable Angina

The pain or discomfort:

- occurs when the heart must work harder, usually during physical exertion

- doesn't come as a surprise, and episodes of pain tend to be alike
- usually lasts a short time (5 minutes or less)
- is relieved by rest or medicine
- may feel like gas or indigestion
- may feel like chest pain that spreads to the arms, back, or other areas

Unstable Angina

The pain or discomfort:

- often occurs at rest, while sleeping at night, or with little physical exertion
- comes as a surprise
- is more severe and lasts longer than stable angina (as long as 30 minutes)
- usually isn't relieved by rest or medicine
- may get worse over time
- may mean that a heart attack will happen soon

Variant Angina

The pain or discomfort:

- usually occurs at rest and during the night or early morning hours
- tends to be severe
- is relieved by medicine

Microvascular Angina

The pain or discomfort:

- may be more severe and last longer than other types of angina pain
- may occur with shortness of breath, sleep problems, fatigue, and lack of energy
- often is first noticed during routine daily activities and times of mental stress

How Is Angina Diagnosed?

The most important issues to address when you go to the doctor with chest pain are:

- What's causing the chest pain

- Whether you're having or are about to have a heart attack

Angina is a symptom of an underlying heart problem, usually coronary heart disease (CHD). The type of angina pain you have can be a sign of how severe the CHD is and whether it's likely to cause a heart attack.

If you have chest pain, your doctor will want to find out whether it's angina. He or she also will want to know whether the angina is stable or unstable. If it's unstable, you may need emergency medical treatment to try to prevent a heart attack.

To diagnose chest pain as stable or unstable angina, your doctor will do a physical exam, ask about your symptoms, and ask about your risk factors for and your family history of CHD or other heart diseases.

Your doctor also may ask questions about your symptoms, such as:

- What brings on the pain or discomfort and what relieves it?

- What does the pain or discomfort feel like (for example, heaviness or tightness)?

- How often does the pain occur?

- Where do you feel the pain or discomfort?

- How severe is the pain or discomfort?

- How long does the pain or discomfort last?

Diagnostic Tests and Procedures

If your doctor thinks that you have unstable angina or that your angina is related to a serious heart condition, he or she may recommend one or more tests.

- electrocardiogram (EKG)

- stress testing

- chest X-ray

- coronary angiography and cardiac catheterization

- computed tomography angiography
- blood tests

How Is Angina Treated?

Treatments for angina include lifestyle changes, medicines, medical procedures, cardiac rehabilitation (rehab), and other therapies. The main goals of treatment are to:

- Reduce pain and discomfort and how often it occurs

- Prevent or lower your risk for heart attack and death by treating your underlying heart condition

Lifestyle changes and medicines may be the only treatments needed if your symptoms are mild and aren't getting worse. If lifestyle changes and medicines don't control angina, you may need medical procedures or cardiac rehab.

Unstable angina is an emergency condition that requires treatment in a hospital.

Lifestyle Changes

Making lifestyle changes can help prevent episodes of angina. You can:

- Slow down or take rest breaks if physical exertion triggers angina.

- Avoid large meals and rich foods that leave you feeling stuffed if heavy meals trigger angina.

- Try to avoid situations that make you upset or stressed if emotional stress triggers angina. Learn ways to handle stress that can't be avoided.

You also can make lifestyle changes that help lower your risk for coronary heart disease. One of the most important changes is to quit smoking. Following a healthy diet is another important lifestyle change.

Other important lifestyle changes include:

- Being physically active.

- Maintaining a healthy weight.

- Taking all medicines as your doctor prescribes, especially if you have diabetes.

Medicines

Nitrates are the medicines most commonly used to treat angina. They relax and widen blood vessels. This allows more blood to flow to the heart, while reducing the heart's workload.

Nitroglycerin is the most commonly used nitrate for angina. Nitroglycerin that dissolves under your tongue or between your cheek and gum is used to relieve angina episodes.

Nitroglycerin pills and skin patches are used to prevent angina episodes. However, pills and skin patches act too slowly to relieve pain during an angina attack.

Other medicines also are used to treat angina, such as beta blockers, calcium channel blockers, ACE inhibitors, oral antiplatelet medicines, or anticoagulants (blood thinners). These medicines can help:

- lower blood pressure and cholesterol levels

- slow the heart rate

- relax blood vessels

- reduce strain on the heart

- prevent blood clots from forming

People who have stable angina may be advised to get annual flu shots.

Medical Procedures

If lifestyle changes and medicines don't control angina, you may need a medical procedure to treat the underlying heart disease. Both angioplasty and coronary artery bypass grafting (CABG) are commonly used to treat heart disease.

Angioplasty opens blocked or narrowed coronary arteries. During angioplasty, a thin tube with a balloon or other device on the end is threaded through a blood vessel to the narrowed or blocked coronary artery.

Once in place, the balloon is inflated to push the plaque outward against the wall of the artery. This widens the artery and restores blood flow.

Angioplasty can improve blood flow to your heart and relieve chest pain. A small mesh tube called a stent usually is placed in the artery to help keep it open after the procedure.

During CABG, healthy arteries or veins taken from other areas in your body are used to bypass (that is, go around) your narrowed coronary arteries. Bypass surgery can improve blood flow to your heart, relieve chest pain, and possibly prevent a heart attack.

Cardiac Rehabilitation

Your doctor may recommend cardiac rehab for angina or after angioplasty, CABG, or a heart attack. Cardiac rehab is a medically supervised program that can help improve the health and well-being of people who have heart problems.

Rehab has two parts:

- exercise training

- education, counseling, and training

Enhanced External Counterpulsation Therapy

Enhanced external counterpulsation (EECP) therapy is helpful for some people who have angina. Large cuffs, similar to blood pressure cuffs, are put on your legs. The cuffs are inflated and deflated in sync with your heartbeat.

EECP therapy improves the flow of oxygen-rich blood to your heart muscle and helps relieve angina. You typically get 35 1-hour treatments over 7 weeks.

How Can Angina Be Prevented?

You can prevent or lower your risk for angina and heart disease by making lifestyle changes and treating related conditions.

Making Lifestyle Changes

Healthy lifestyle choices can help prevent or delay angina and heart disease. To adopt a healthy lifestyle, you can:

- quit smoking and avoid secondhand smoke

- avoid angina triggers

- follow a healthy diet

- be physically active

- maintain a healthy weight

- learn ways to handle stress and relax

- take your medicines as your doctor prescribes

Treating Related Conditions

You also can help prevent or delay angina and heart disease by treating related conditions, such as high blood cholesterol, high blood pressure, diabetes, and overweight or obesity.

If you have one or more of these conditions, talk with your doctor about how to control them. Follow your treatment plan and take all of your medicines as your doctor prescribes.

Living with Angina

Angina isn't a heart attack, but it does increase your risk of having a heart attack. The risk is even higher if you have unstable angina.

For these reasons, it's important that you know:

- The usual pattern of your angina, if you have it.

- What medicines you take (keep a list) and how to take them. Make sure your medicines are readily available.

- How to control your angina.

- The limits of your physical activity.

- How and when to seek medical attention.

Know the Pattern of Your Angina

Stable angina usually occurs in a pattern. You should know:

- what causes the pain to occur

- what the pain feels like

- how long the pain usually lasts

- whether rest or medicine relieves the pain

After several episodes, you'll learn the pattern of your angina. You'll want to pay attention to whether the pattern changes. Pattern changes may include angina that occurs more often, lasts longer, is more severe, occurs without physical exertion, or doesn't go away with rest or medicines.

These changes may be a sign that your symptoms are getting worse or becoming unstable. You should seek medical help. Unstable angina suggests that you're at high risk for a heart attack very soon.

Know Your Medicines

You should know what medicines you're taking, the purpose of each, how and when to take them, and possible side effects. Know exactly when and how to take fast-acting nitroglycerin or other nitrates to relieve chest pain.

Correctly storing your angina medicines and knowing when to replace them also is important. Your doctor can advise you about this.

If you have side effects from your medicines, let your doctor know. You should never stop taking your medicines without your doctor's approval.

Talk with your doctor if you have any questions or concerns about taking your angina medicines. Tell him or her about any other medicines you're taking. Some medicines can cause serious problems if they're taken with nitrates or other angina medicines.

Know How to Control Your Angina

After several angina episodes, you'll know the level of activity, stress, and other factors that trigger your angina. By knowing this, you can take steps to prevent or lessen the severity of episodes.

Physical Exertion

Know what level of physical exertion triggers your angina and try to stop and rest before chest pain starts. For example, if walking up a flight of stairs leads to chest pain, stop halfway and rest before continuing.

If chest pain occurs during physical exertion, stop and rest or take your angina medicine. The pain should go away in a few minutes.

Emotional Stress

Anger, arguing, and worrying are examples of emotional stress that can trigger angina. Try to avoid or limit situations that cause these emotions.

Exercise and relaxation can help relieve stress. Alcohol and drug use play a part in causing stress and don't relieve it. If stress is a problem for you, talk with your doctor about getting help for it.

Eating Large Meals

If large meals lead to chest pain, eat smaller meals. Also, avoid eating rich foods.

Know the Limits of Your Physical Activity

Most people who have stable angina can continue their normal activities. This includes work, hobbies, and sexual relations. However, if you do very strenuous activities or have a stressful job, talk with your doctor.

Know How and When to Seek Medical Attention

Angina increases your risk for a heart attack. It's important that you and your family know how and when to seek medical attention.

Talk with your doctor about making an emergency action plan. The plan should include making sure you and your family members know:

- the signs and symptoms of a heart attack

- how to use aspirin and nitroglycerin when needed

- how to access emergency medical services in your community

- the location of the nearest hospital that offers 24-hour emergency heart care

Discuss your emergency plan with your family members. Take action quickly if your chest pain becomes severe, lasts longer than a few minutes, or isn't relieved by rest or medicine.

Section 43.3

Heart Attack

This section includes text excerpted from "Heart Attack," National Heart, Lung, and Blood Institute (NHLBI), June 22, 2015.

What Is a Heart Attack?

A heart attack happens when the flow of oxygen-rich blood to a section of heart muscle suddenly becomes blocked and the heart can't get oxygen. If blood flow isn't restored quickly, the section of heart muscle begins to die.

Heart attack treatment works best when it's given right after symptoms occur.

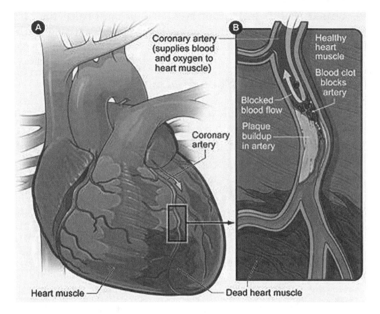

Figure 43.4. *Heart with Muscle Damage and a Blocked Artery*

Other Names for a Heart Attack

- Myocardial infarction (MI)
- Acute myocardial infarction (AMI)
- Acute coronary syndrome
- Coronary thrombosis
- Coronary occlusion

What Causes a Heart Attack?

Coronary Heart Disease

A heart attack happens if the flow of oxygen-rich blood to a section of heart muscle suddenly becomes blocked and the heart can't get oxygen. Most heart attacks occur as a result of coronary heart disease (CHD).

CHD is a condition in which a waxy substance called plaque builds up inside of the coronary arteries. These arteries supply oxygen-rich blood to your heart.

When plaque builds up in the arteries, the condition is called atherosclerosis. The buildup of plaque occurs over many years.

Eventually, an area of plaque can rupture (break open) inside of an artery. This causes a blood clot to form on the plaque's surface. If the clot becomes large enough, it can mostly or completely block blood flow through a coronary artery.

If the blockage isn't treated quickly, the portion of heart muscle fed by the artery begins to die. Healthy heart tissue is replaced with scar tissue. This heart damage may not be obvious, or it may cause severe or long-lasting problems.

Coronary Artery Spasm

A less common cause of heart attack is a severe spasm (tightening) of a coronary artery. The spasm cuts off blood flow through the artery. Spasms can occur in coronary arteries that aren't affected by atherosclerosis.

What causes a coronary artery to spasm isn't always clear. A spasm may be related to:

- taking certain drugs, such as cocaine

- emotional stress or pain

- exposure to extreme cold

- cigarette smoking

Who Is at Risk for a Heart Attack?

Certain risk factors make it more likely that you'll develop coronary heart disease (CHD) and have a heart attack. You can control many of these risk factors.

Risk Factors You Can Control

The major risk factors for a heart attack that you can control include:

- smoking

- high blood pressure

- high blood cholesterol

- overweight and obesity

- an unhealthy diet (for example, a diet high in saturated fat, trans fat, cholesterol, and sodium)

- lack of routine physical activity

- high blood sugar due to insulin resistance or diabetes

Some of these risk factors—such as obesity, high blood pressure, and high blood sugar—tend to occur together. When they do, it's called metabolic syndrome.

In general, a person who has metabolic syndrome is twice as likely to develop heart disease and five times as likely to develop diabetes as someone who doesn't have metabolic syndrome.

Risk Factors You Can't Control

Risk factors that you can't control include:

- age

- family history of early heart disease

- preeclampsia

What Are the Symptoms of a Heart Attack?

Not all heart attacks begin with the sudden, crushing chest pain that often is shown on TV or in the movies. In one study, for example, one-third of the patients who had heart attacks had no chest pain. These patients were more likely to be older, female, or diabetic.

The symptoms of a heart attack can vary from person to person. Some people can have few symptoms and are surprised to learn they've had a heart attack. If you've already had a heart attack, your symptoms may not be the same for another one. It is important for you to know the most common symptoms of a heart attack and also remember these facts:

- Heart attacks can start slowly and cause only mild pain or discomfort. Symptoms can be mild or more intense and sudden. Symptoms also may come and go over several hours.

- People who have high blood sugar (diabetes) may have no symptoms or very mild ones.

- The most common symptom, in both men and women, is chest pain or discomfort.

- Women are somewhat more likely to have shortness of breath, nausea and vomiting, unusual tiredness (sometimes for days), and pain in the back, shoulders, and jaw.

Some people don't have symptoms at all. Heart attacks that occur without any symptoms or with very mild symptoms are called silent heart attacks.

Most Common Symptoms

The most common warning symptoms of a heart attack for both men and women are:

- Chest pain or discomfort

- Upper body discomfort

- Shortness of breath

The symptoms of angina can be similar to the symptoms of a heart attack. Angina is chest pain that occurs in people who have coronary heart disease, usually when they're active. Angina pain usually lasts for only a few minutes and goes away with rest.

Chest pain or discomfort that doesn't go away or changes from its usual pattern (for example, occurs more often or while you're resting) can be a sign of a heart attack.

All chest pain should be checked by a doctor.

Other Common Signs and Symptoms

Pay attention to these other possible symptoms of a heart attack:

- Breaking out in a cold sweat

- Feeling unusually tired for no reason, sometimes for days (especially if you are a woman)

- Nausea (feeling sick to the stomach) and vomiting

- Light-headedness or sudden dizziness

- Any sudden, new symptoms or a change in the pattern of symptoms you already have (for example, if your symptoms become stronger or last longer than usual)

Not everyone having a heart attack has typical symptoms. If you've already had a heart attack, your symptoms may not be the same for another one. However, some people may have a pattern of symptoms that recur.

The more signs and symptoms you have, the more likely it is that you're having a heart attack.

Quick Action Can Save Your Life: Call 9–1–1

The signs and symptoms of a heart attack can develop suddenly. However, they also can develop slowly—sometimes within hours, days, or weeks of a heart attack.

Any time you think you might be having heart attack symptoms or a heart attack, don't ignore it or feel embarrassed to call for help. Call 9–1–1 for emergency medical care, even if you are not sure whether you're having a heart attack. Here's why:

- Acting fast can save your life.

- An ambulance is the best and safest way to get to the hospital. Emergency medical services (EMS) personnel can check how you are doing and start life-saving medicines and other treatments right away. People who arrive by ambulance often receive faster treatment at the hospital.

- The 9–1–1 operator or EMS technician can give you advice. You might be told to crush or chew an aspirin if you're not allergic, unless there is a medical reason for you not to take one. Aspirin taken during a heart attack can limit the damage to your heart and save your life.

Every minute matters. Never delay calling 9–1–1 to take aspirin or do anything else you think might help.

How Is a Heart Attack Diagnosed?

Your doctor will diagnose a heart attack based on your signs and symptoms, your medical and family histories, and test results.

Diagnostic Tests

- electrocardiogram (EKG)
- blood tests
- coronary angiography

How Is a Heart Attack Treated?

Early treatment for a heart attack can prevent or limit damage to the heart muscle. Acting fast, **by calling 9–1–1** at the first symptoms of a heart attack, can save your life. Medical personnel can begin diagnosis and treatment even before you get to the hospital.

Immediate Treatment

Certain treatments usually are started right away if a heart attack is suspected, even before the diagnosis is confirmed. These include:

- Aspirin to prevent further blood clotting
- Nitroglycerin to reduce your heart's workload and improve blood flow through the coronary arteries
- Oxygen therapy
- Treatment for chest pain

Once the diagnosis of a heart attack is confirmed or strongly suspected, doctors start treatments promptly to try to restore blood flow through the blood vessels supplying the heart. The two main treatments are clot-busting medicines and percutaneous coronary intervention, also known as coronary angioplasty, a procedure used to open blocked coronary arteries.

Clot-Busting Medicines

Thrombolytic medicines, also called clot busters, are used to dissolve blood clots that are blocking the coronary arteries. To work best, these medicines must be given within several hours of the start of heart attack symptoms. Ideally, the medicine should be given as soon as possible.

Percutaneous Coronary Intervention

Percutaneous coronary intervention is a nonsurgical procedure that opens blocked or narrowed coronary arteries. A thin, flexible tube (catheter) with a balloon or other device on the end is threaded through a blood vessel, usually in the groin (upper thigh), to the narrowed or blocked coronary artery. Once in place, the balloon located at the tip of the catheter is inflated to compress the plaque and related clot against the wall of the artery. This restores blood flow through the artery. During the procedure, the doctor may put a small mesh tube called a stent in the artery. The stent helps to keep the blood vessel open to prevent blockages in the artery in the months or years after the procedure.

Other Treatments for Heart Attack

Other treatments for heart attack include.

- medicines

- medical procedures
- heart-healthy lifestyle changes
- cardiac rehabilitation

Medicines

Your doctor may prescribe one or more of the following medicines.

- **ACE inhibitors.** ACE inhibitors lower blood pressure and reduce strain on your heart. They also help slow down further weakening of the heart muscle.

- **Anticlotting medicines.** Anticlotting medicines stop platelets from clumping together and forming unwanted blood clots. Examples of anticlotting medicines include aspirin and clopidogrel.

- **Anticoagulants.** Anticoagulants, or blood thinners, prevent blood clots from forming in your arteries. These medicines also keep existing clots from getting larger.

- **Beta blockers.** Beta blockers decrease your heart's workload. These medicines also are used to relieve chest pain and discomfort and to help prevent another heart attack. Beta blockers also are used to treat arrhythmias (irregular heartbeats).

- **Statin medicines.** Statins control or lower your blood cholesterol. By lowering your blood cholesterol level, you can decrease your chance of having another heart attack or stroke.

You also may be given medicines to relieve pain and anxiety, and treat arrhythmias. Take all medicines regularly, as your doctor prescribes. Don't change the amount of your medicine or skip a dose unless your doctor tells you to.

Medical Procedures

Coronary artery bypass grafting also may be used to treat a heart attack. During coronary artery bypass grafting, a surgeon removes a healthy artery or vein from your body. The artery or vein is then connected, or grafted, to bypass the blocked section of the coronary artery. The grafted artery or vein bypasses (that is, goes around) the blocked portion of the coronary artery. This provides a new route for blood to flow to the heart muscle.

Heart-Healthy Lifestyle Changes

Treatment for a heart attack usually includes making heart-healthy lifestyle changes. Your doctor also may recommend:

- heart-healthy eating
- physical activity
- aiming for healthy weight
- quitting smoking
- managing stress

Taking these steps can lower your chances of having another heart attack.

Cardiac Rehabilitation

Your doctor may recommend cardiac rehabilitation (cardiac rehab) to help you recover from a heart attack and to help prevent another heart attack. Nearly everyone who has had a heart attack can benefit from rehab. Cardiac rehab is a medically supervised program that may help improve the health and well-being of people who have heart problems.

Rehab has two parts:

- education, counseling, and training
- exercise training

How Can a Heart Attack Be Prevented?

Lowering your risk factors for coronary heart disease can help you prevent a heart attack. Even if you already have coronary heart disease, you still can take steps to lower your risk for a heart attack. These steps involve making heart-healthy lifestyle changes and getting ongoing medical care.

Heart-Healthy Lifestyle Changes

A heart-healthy lifestyle can help prevent a heart attack and includes heart-healthy eating, being physically active, quitting smoking, managing stress, and managing your weight.

Ongoing Care

Treat Related Conditions

Treating conditions that make a heart attack more likely also can help lower your risk for a heart attack.

These conditions may include:

- Diabetes (high blood sugar)
- High blood cholesterol
- High blood pressure

Have an Emergency Action Plan

Make sure that you have an emergency action plan in case you or someone in your family has a heart attack. This is very important if you're at high risk for, or have already had, a heart attack.

Write down a list of medicines you are taking, medicines you are allergic to, your healthcare provider's phone numbers (both during and after office hours), and contact information for a friend or relative. Keep the list in a handy place to share in a medical emergency.

Life after a Heart Attack

Many people survive heart attacks and live active, full lives. If you get help quickly, treatment can limit damage to your heart muscle. Less heart damage improves your chances for a better quality of life after a heart attack.

Medical Followup

After a heart attack, you'll need treatment for coronary heart disease (CHD). This will help prevent another heart attack. Your doctor may recommend:

- Lifestyle changes, such as following a healthy diet, being physically active, maintaining a healthy weight, and quitting smoking
- Medicines to control chest pain or discomfort, high blood cholesterol, high blood pressure, and your heart's workload
- A cardiac rehabilitation program

If you find it hard to get your medicines or take them, talk with your doctor. Don't stop taking medicines that can help you prevent another heart attack.

Returning to Normal Activities

After a heart attack, most people who don't have chest pain or discomfort or other problems can safely return to most of their normal activities within a few weeks. Most can begin walking right away.

Sexual activity also can begin within a few weeks for most patients. Talk with your doctor about a safe schedule for returning to your normal routine.

If allowed by State law, driving usually can begin within a week for most patients who don't have chest pain or discomfort or other problems. Each State has rules about driving a motor vehicle following a serious illness. People who have complications shouldn't drive until their symptoms have been stable for a few weeks.

Risk of a Repeat Heart Attack

Once you've had a heart attack, you're at higher risk for another one. Knowing the difference between angina and a heart attack is important. Angina is chest pain that occurs in people who have CHD.

The pain from angina usually occurs after physical exertion and goes away in a few minutes when you rest or take medicine as directed.

The pain from a heart attack usually is more severe than the pain from angina. Heart attack pain doesn't go away when you rest or take medicine.

The symptoms of a second heart attack may not be the same as those of a first heart attack. Don't take a chance if you're in doubt. Always call 9–1–1 right away if you or someone else has heart attack symptoms.

Unfortunately, most heart attack victims wait 2 hours or more after their symptoms start before they seek medical help. This delay can result in lasting heart damage or death.

Chapter 44

Fibromuscular Dysplasia

What Is Fibromuscular Dysplasia?

Fibromuscular dysplasia (FMD) is the abnormal development or growth of cells in the walls of arteries that can cause the vessels to narrow or bulge. The carotid arteries, which pass through the neck and supply blood to the brain, are commonly affected. Arteries within the brain and kidneys can also be affected. A characteristic "string of beads" pattern caused by the alternating narrowing and enlarging of the artery can block or reduce blood flow to the brain, causing a stroke or mini-stroke. Some patients experience no symptoms of the disease while others may have high blood pressure, dizziness or vertigo, chronic headache, intracranial aneurysm, ringing in the ears, weakness or numbness in the face, neck pain, or changes in vision. FMD is most often seen in persons age 25 to 50 years and affects women more often than men. More than one family member may be affected by the disease. The cause of FMD is unknown. An angiogram can detect the degree of narrowing or obstruction of the artery and identify changes such as a tear (dissection) or weak area (aneurysm) in the vessel wall. FMD can also be diagnosed using computed tomography, magnetic resonance imaging, or ultrasound.

This chapter includes text excerpted from "Fibromuscular Dysplasia," National Institute of Neurological Disorders and Stroke (NINDS), June 23, 2011. Reviewed July 2016.

Is There Any Treatment?

There is no standard protocol to treat FMD. Any treatment to improve blood flow is based on the arteries affected and the progression and severity of the disease. The carotid arteries should be tested if FMD is found elsewhere in the body since carotid involvement is linked to an increased risk of stroke. Patients with minimal narrowing may take a daily antiplatelet such as an aspirin or an anticoagulant to thin the blood and reduce the chances that a clot might form. Medications such as aspirin can also be taken for headache and neck pain, symptoms that can come from FMD. Patients with arterial disease who smoke should be encouraged to quit as smoking worsens the disease. Further treatment may include angioplasty, in which a small balloon is inserted through a catheter and inflated to open the artery. Small tubes called stents may be inserted to keep arteries open. Surgery may be needed to treat aneurysms that have the potential to rupture and cause bleeding within the brain.

What Is the Prognosis?

Currently there is no cure for FMD. Medicines and angioplasty can reduce the risk of initial or recurrent stroke. In rare cases, FMD-related aneurysms can burst and bleed into the brain, causing stroke, permanent nerve damage, or death.

Chapter 45

Klippel–Trénaunay Syndrome

What Is Klippel–Trénaunay syndrome?

Klippel–Trénaunay syndrome (KTS) is a condition that affects the development of blood vessels, soft tissues, and bones. This condition has three characteristic features: a red birthmark called a port-wine stain; overgrowth of soft tissues and bones; and vein malformations such as varicose veins or malformations of deep veins in the limbs. The overgrowth of bones and soft tissues usually begins in infancy and is most often limited to one leg. However, it can also affect the arms or, rarely, the torso. The overgrowth can cause pain, a feeling of heaviness, and reduced movement in the affected area. The exact cause of KTS is unclear. It is thought to occur sporadically (in people with no family history of the condition), however several recent studies have found KTS may be caused by mutations in the *PIK3CA* gene. Treatment is symptomatic and supportive.

What Are the Signs and Symptoms of Klippel–Trénaunay Syndrome?

The Human Phenotype Ontology (HPO) provides the following list of signs and symptoms for Klippel–Trénaunay syndrome.

- abnormality of blood and blood-forming tissues
- abnormality of coagulation

This chapter includes text excerpted from "Klippel–Trénaunay Syndrome," Genetic and Rare Diseases Information Center (GARD), February 9, 2015.

- abnormality of the menstrual cycle
- abnormality of the pulmonary artery
- abnormality of the skin
- abnormality of the tricuspid valve
- arteriovenous fistula
- ascites
- atria septal defect
- bone pain
- cataract
- cavernous hemangioma
- cellulitis
- cognitive impairment
- congestive heart failure
- cutis marmorata
- facial asymmetry
- finger syndactyly
- gastrointestinal hemorrhage
- glaucoma
- hand polydactyly
- hemangioma
- hematuria
- hemihypertrophy
- hepatomegaly
- hydrops fetalis
- hypercoagulability
- hyperpigmented nevi and streak
- intellectual disability
- large face
- lower limb asymmetry
- lymphangioma
- lymphedema
- macrocephaly
- macrodactyly of finger
- melanocytic nevus
- microcephaly
- microcytic anemia
- multiple lipomas
- oligodactyly (hands)
- patent ductus arteriosus
- peripheral arteriovenous fistula
- pulmonary embolism
- respiratory insufficiency
- scoliosis
- seizures
- skin ulcer
- split hand
- sporadic
- syndactyly
- tall stature
- telangiectasia of the skin
- thrombophlebitis
- venous insufficiency
- visceral angiomatosis

What Causes Klippel–Trénaunay Syndrome?

The underlying cause of Klippel–Trénaunay syndrome (KTS) is currently unknown. There have been many theories about what may cause this condition, including:

- paradominant inheritance—a theory that may explain occasional familial cases of sporadic conditions. This theory proposes that a person may inherit a mutation in one copy of a gene responsible for a condition, but another, acquired mutation (somatic mutation) must occur in the other copy of the gene after conception for a person to develop signs and symptoms.

- somatic mosaicism of an otherwise dominant lethal gene

- disturbance of blood vessel formation (vasculogenesis) in the embryonic period

- defects in the mesoderm (one of three layers of an embryo, which gives rise to structures including connective tissue, muscle, and bone)

- various chromosomal translocations and mutations-there have been case reports of these, but none of them have been proven to have any definite association with the condition.

However recently, medical researchers have found multiple cases of KTS associated with mutations in the *PIK3CA* gene. Some researchers believe all KTS is likely caused by mutations in this gene and when a mutation cannot be found, the affected person may actually have a different condition such as Beckwith-Wiedemann syndrome. More research studies will need to be completed to reach a consensus among medical researchers.

If Klippel–Trénaunay Syndrome (KTS) Is Not Inherited, How Does It Come about?

Studies suggest that KTS may result from gene mutations that are not inherited. These genetic changes, which are called somatic mutations, probably occur very early in development and are present only in certain cells. Somatic mutations could explain why the signs and symptoms of KTS are often limited to specific areas of the body.

Is There a Cure or Treatment for Klippel–Trénaunay Syndrome (KTS)?

There is no cure for KTS. Treatment is symptomatic and supportive. Conservative treatments seem most effective while limiting the chances for undesired side effects. This may include the use of elastic garments and pumps to relieve lymphedema and protect limbs from trauma or orthopedic devices for discrepancies in limb length. Laser therapy may be used to diminish or eliminate some skin lesions (port-wine stains). Surgery may be used for tissue debulking, vein repair, or to correct uneven growth in the limbs.

Chapter 46

Peripheral Vascular Disease

Chapter Contents

Section 46.1

Peripheral Artery Disease

This section includes text excerpted from "Peripheral Artery Disease," National Heart, Lung, and Blood Institute (NHLBI), June 22, 2016.

What Is Peripheral Artery Disease?

Peripheral artery disease (P.A.D.) is a disease in which plaque builds up in the arteries that carry blood to your head, organs, and limbs. Plaque is made up of fat, cholesterol, calcium, fibrous tissue, and other substances in the blood.

When plaque builds up in the body's arteries, the condition is called atherosclerosis. Over time, plaque can harden and narrow the arteries. This limits the flow of oxygen-rich blood to your organs and other parts of your body.

P.A.D. usually affects the arteries in the legs, but it also can affect the arteries that carry blood from your heart to your head, arms, kidneys, and stomach. This section focuses on P.A.D. that affects blood flow to the legs.

Other Names for Peripheral Artery Disease

- Atherosclerotic peripheral arterial disease

- Claudication

- Hardening of the arteries

- Leg cramps from poor circulation

- Peripheral arterial disease

- Peripheral vascular disease

- Poor circulation

- Vascular disease

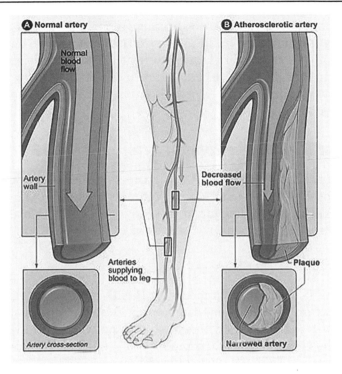

Figure 46.1. *Normal Artery and Artery with Plaque Buildup*

The illustration shows how P.A.D. can affect arteries in the legs. Figure A shows a normal artery with normal blood flow. The inset image shows a cross-section of the normal artery. Figure B shows an artery with plaque buildup that's partially blocking blood flow. The inset image shows a cross-section of the narrowed artery.

What Causes Peripheral Artery Disease?

The most common cause of peripheral artery disease (P.A.D.) is atherosclerosis. Atherosclerosis is a disease in which plaque builds up in your arteries. The exact cause of atherosclerosis isn't known.

The disease may start if certain factors damage the inner layers of the arteries. These factors include:

- smoking

- high amounts of certain fats and cholesterol in the blood

- high blood pressure

- high amounts of sugar in the blood due to insulin resistance or diabetes

When damage occurs, your body starts a healing process. The healing may cause plaque to build up where the arteries are damaged.

Eventually, a section of plaque can rupture (break open), causing a blood clot to form at the site. The buildup of plaque or blood clots can severely narrow or block the arteries and limit the flow of oxygen-rich blood to your body.

Who Is at Risk for Peripheral Artery Disease?

Peripheral artery disease (P.A.D.) affects millions of people in the United States. The disease is more common in blacks than any other racial or ethnic group. The major risk factors for P.A.D. are smoking, older age, and having certain diseases or conditions.

Smoking

Smoking is the main risk factor for P.A.D. and your risk increases if you smoke or have a history of smoking. Quitting smoking slows the progress of P.A.D. People who smoke and people who have diabetes are at highest risk for P.A.D. complications, such as gangrene (tissue death) in the leg from decreased blood flow.

Older Age

Older age also is a risk factor for P.A.D. Plaque builds up in your arteries as you age. Older age combined with other risk factors, such as smoking or diabetes, also puts you at higher risk for P.A.D.

Diseases and Conditions

Many diseases and conditions can raise your risk of P.A.D., including:

- diabetes
- high blood pressure
- high blood cholesterol
- coronary heart disease
- stroke
- metabolic syndrome

What Are the Signs and Symptoms of Peripheral Artery Disease?

Many people who have peripheral artery disease (P.A.D.) don't have any signs or symptoms.

Even if you don't have signs or symptoms, ask your doctor whether you should get checked for P.A.D. if you're:

- aged 70 or older

- aged 50 or older and have a history of smoking or diabetes

- younger than 50 and have diabetes and one or more risk factors for atherosclerosis

Intermittent Claudication

People who have P.A.D. may have symptoms when walking or climbing stairs, which may include pain, numbness, aching, or heaviness in the leg muscles. Symptoms also may include cramping in the affected leg(s) and in the buttocks, thighs, calves, and feet. Symptoms may ease after resting. These symptoms are called intermittent claudication.

Other Signs and Symptoms

Other signs and symptoms of P.A.D. include:

- weak or absent pulses in the legs or feet

- sores or wounds on the toes, feet, or legs that heal slowly, poorly, or not at all

- a pale or bluish color to the skin

- a lower temperature in one leg compared to the other leg

- poor nail growth on the toes and decreased hair growth on the legs

- erectile dysfunction, especially among men who have diabetes

How Is Peripheral Artery Disease Diagnosed?

Peripheral artery disease (P.A.D.) is diagnosed based on your medical and family histories, a physical exam, and test results.

P.A.D. often is diagnosed after symptoms are reported. A correct diagnosis is important because people who have P.A.D. are at higher risk for coronary heart disease (CHD), heart attack, stroke, and transient ischemic attack ("mini-stroke"). If you have P.A.D, your doctor also may want to check for signs of these diseases and conditions.

Medical and Family Histories

Your doctor may ask:

- whether you have any risk factors for P.A.D. For example, he or she may ask whether you smoke or have diabetes.

- about your symptoms, including any symptoms that occur when walking, exercising, sitting, standing, or climbing.

- about your diet.

- about any medicines you take, including prescription and over-the-counter medicines.

- whether anyone in your family has a history of heart or blood vessel diseases.

Physical Exam

During the physical exam, your doctor will look for signs of P.A.D. He or she may check the blood flow in your legs or feet to see whether you have weak or absent pulses.

Your doctor also may check the pulses in your leg arteries for an abnormal whooshing sound called a bruit. He or she can hear this sound with a stethoscope. A bruit may be a warning sign of a narrowed or blocked artery.

Your doctor may compare blood pressure between your limbs to see whether the pressure is lower in the affected limb. He or she also may check for poor wound healing or any changes in your hair, skin, or nails that may be signs of P.A.D.

Diagnostic Tests

Ankle-Brachial Index

A simple test called an ankle-brachial index (ABI) often is used to diagnose P.A.D. The ABI compares blood pressure in your ankle to blood pressure in your arm. This test shows how well blood is flowing in your limbs.

ABI can show whether P.A.D. is affecting your limbs, but it won't show which blood vessels are narrowed or blocked.

A normal ABI result is 1.0 or greater (with a range of 0.90 to 1.30). The test takes about 10 to 15 minutes to measure both arms and both ankles. This test may be done yearly to see whether P.A.D. is getting worse.

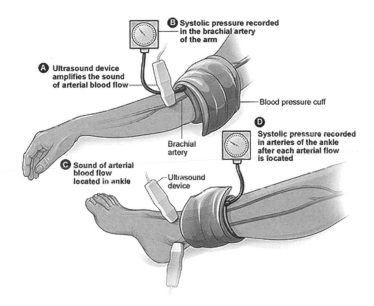

Figure 46.2. *Ankle-Brachial Index*

The illustration shows the ankle-brachial index test. The test compares blood pressure in the ankle to blood pressure in the arm.
As the blood pressure cuff deflates, the blood pressure in the arteries is recorded.

Doppler Ultrasound

A Doppler ultrasound looks at blood flow in the major arteries and veins in the limbs. During this test, a handheld device is placed on your body and passed back and forth over the affected area. A computer converts sound waves into a picture of blood flow in the arteries and veins.

The results of this test can show whether a blood vessel is blocked. The results also can help show the severity of P.A.D.

Treadmill Test

A treadmill test can show the severity of symptoms and the level of exercise that brings them on. You'll walk on a treadmill for this test. This shows whether you have any problems during normal walking.

You may have an ABI test before and after the treadmill test. This will help compare blood flow in your arms and legs before and after exercise.

Magnetic Resonance Angiogram

A magnetic resonance angiogram (MRA) uses magnetic and radio wave energy to take pictures of your blood vessels. This test is a type of magnetic resonance imaging (MRI).

An MRA can show the location and severity of a blocked blood vessel. If you have a pacemaker, man-made joint, stent, surgical clips, mechanical heart valve, or other metallic devices in your body, you might not be able to have an MRA. Ask your doctor whether an MRA is an option for you.

Arteriogram

An arteriogram provides a "road map" of the arteries. Doctors use this test to find the exact location of a blocked artery.

For this test, dye is injected through a needle or catheter (tube) into one of your arteries. This may make you feel mildly flushed. After the dye is injected, an X-ray is taken. The X-ray can show the location, type, and extent of the blockage in the artery.

Some doctors use a newer method of arteriogram that uses tiny ultrasound cameras. These cameras take pictures of the insides of the blood vessels. This method is called intravascular ultrasound.

Blood Tests

Your doctor may recommend blood tests to check for P.A.D. risk factors. For example, blood tests can help diagnose conditions such as diabetes and high blood cholesterol.

How Is Peripheral Artery Disease Treated?

Treatments for peripheral artery disease (P.A.D.) include heart-healthy lifestyle changes, medicines, and surgery or procedures.

The overall goals of treating P.A.D. include reducing risk of heart attack and stroke; reducing symptoms of claudication; improving mobility and overall quality of life; and preventing complications. Treatment is based on your signs and symptoms, risk factors, and the results of physical exams and tests.

Treatment may slow or stop the progression of the disease and reduce the risk of complications. Without treatment, P.A.D. may progress, resulting in serious tissue damage in the form of sores or gangrene (tissue death) due to inadequate blood flow. In extreme cases of P.A.D., also referred to as critical limb ischemia (CLI), removal (amputation) of part of the leg or foot may be necessary.

Heart-Healthy Lifestyle Changes

Treatment often includes making life-long heart-healthy lifestyle changes such as:

- physical activity
- quitting smoking
- heart-healthy eating

Surgery or Procedures

Bypass Grafting

Your doctor may recommend bypass grafting surgery if blood flow in your limb is blocked or nearly blocked. For this surgery, your doctor uses a blood vessel from another part of your body or a synthetic tube to make a graft.

This graft bypasses (that is, goes around) the blocked part of the artery. The bypass allows blood to flow around the blockage. This surgery doesn't cure P.A.D., but it may increase blood flow to the affected limb.

Angioplasty and Stent Placement

Your doctor may recommend angioplasty to restore blood flow through a narrowed or blocked artery.

During this procedure, a catheter (thin tube) with a balloon at the tip is inserted into a blocked artery. The balloon is then inflated, which pushes plaque outward against the artery wall. This widens the artery and restores blood flow.

A stent (a small mesh tube) may be placed in the artery during angioplasty. A stent helps keep the artery open after angioplasty is done. Some stents are coated with medicine to help prevent blockages in the artery.

Atherectomy

Atherectomy is a procedure that removes plaque buildup from an artery. During the procedure, a catheter is used to insert a small cutting device into the blocked artery. The device is used to shave or cut off plaque.

The bits of plaque are removed from the body through the catheter or washed away in the bloodstream (if they're small enough).

Doctors also can perform atherectomy using a special laser that dissolves the blockage.

Other Types of Treatment

Researchers are studying cell and gene therapies to treat P.A.D. However, these treatments aren't yet available outside of clinical trials.

How Can Peripheral Artery Disease Be Prevented?

Taking action to control your risk factors can help prevent or delay peripheral artery disease (P.A.D.) and its complications. Know your family history of health problems related to P.A.D. If you or someone in your family has the disease, be sure to tell your doctor. Controlling risk factors includes the following.

- Be physically active.
- Be screened for P.A.D. A simple office test, called an ankle-brachial index or ABI, can help determine whether you have P.A.D.
- Follow heart-healthy eating.
- If you smoke, quit.
- If you're overweight or obese, work with your doctor to create a reasonable weight-loss plan.

The lifestyle changes described above can reduce your risk of developing P.A.D. These changes also can help prevent and control conditions that can be associated with P.A.D., such as coronary heart disease, diabetes, high blood pressure, high blood cholesterol, and stroke.

Living with Peripheral Artery Disease

If you have peripheral artery disease (P.A.D.), you're more likely to also have coronary heart disease, heart attack, stroke, and transient ischemic attack ("mini-stroke"). However, you can take steps to treat and control P.A.D. and lower your risk for these other conditions.

Living with Peripheral Artery Disease Symptoms

If you have P.A.D., you may feel pain in your calf or thigh muscles after walking. Try to take a break and allow the pain to ease before walking again. Over time, this may increase the distance that you can walk without pain.

Talk with your doctor about taking part in a supervised exercise program. This type of program has been shown to reduce P.A.D. symptoms.

Check your feet and toes regularly for sores or possible infections. Wear comfortable shoes that fit well. Maintain good foot hygiene and have professional medical treatment for corns, bunions, or calluses.

Ongoing Healthcare Needs and Lifestyle Changes

See your doctor for checkups as he or she advises. If you have P.A.D. without symptoms, you still should see your doctor regularly. Take all medicines as your doctor prescribes.

Heart-healthy lifestyle changes can help prevent or delay P.A.D. and other related problems, such as coronary heart disease, heart attack, stroke, and transient ischemic attack. Heart-healthy lifestyle changes include physical activity, quitting smoking, and heart-healthy eating.

Section 46.2

Buerger Disease

This section includes text excerpted from "Buerger Disease," Genetic and Rare Diseases Information Center (GARD), June 16, 2015.

What Is Buerger Disease?

Buerger disease is a disease of the arteries and veins in the arms and legs. The arteries and veins become inflamed which can lead to narrowed and blocked vessels. This reduces blood flow resulting in pain and eventually damage to affected tissues. Buerger disease nearly always occurs in association with cigarette or other tobacco use. Quitting all forms of tobacco is an essential part of treatment.

What Are the Signs and Symptoms of Buerger Disease?

* acrocyanosis
* arterial thrombosis

- arthralgia
- autosomal recessive inheritance
- gangrene
- hyperhidrosis
- insomnia
- limb pain
- paresthesia
- skin ulcer
- vasculitis

What Causes Buerger Disease?

Buerger disease has a strong relationship to cigarette smoking. This association may be due to direct poisioning of cells from some component of tobacco, or by hypersensitivity to the same components. Many people with Buerger disease will show hypersensitivities to injection of tobacco extracts into their skin. There may be a genetic component to susceptibility to Buerger disease as well. It is possible that these genetic influences account for the higher prevalence of Buerger disease in people of Israeli, Indian subcontinent, and Japanese descent. Certain HLA (human leukocyte antigen) haplotypes have also been found in association with Buerger disease.

How Is Buerger Disease Treated?

Currently there is not a cure for Buerger disease, however there are treatments that can help control it. The most essential part of treatment is to avoid all tobacco and nicotine products. Even one cigarette a day can worsen the disease. A doctor can help a person with Buerger disease learn about safe medications and programs to combat smoking/nicotine addiction. Continued smoking is associated with an overall amputation rate of 40 to 50 percent.

The following treatments may also be helpful, but do not replace smoking/nicotine cessation:

- medications to dilate blood vessels and improve blood flow (e.g., intravenous Iloprost)
- medications to dissolve blood clots
- treatment with calcium channel blockers
- walking exercises
- intermittent compression of the arms and legs to increase blood flow to your extremities

- surgical sympathectomy (a controversial surgery to cut the nerves to the affected area to control pain and increase blood flow)

- therapeutic angiogenesis (medications to stimulate growth of new blood vessels)

- spinal cord stimulation

- amputation, if infection or gangrene occurs

Section 46.3

Raynaud Phenomenon

This section includes text excerpted from "Raynaud's Phenomenon," National Institute of Arthritis and Musculoskeletal and Skin Diseases (NIAMS), November 2014.

What Is Raynaud Phenomenon?

Raynaud phenomenon is a disorder that affects blood vessels, mostly in the fingers and toes. It causes the blood vessels to narrow when you are:

- cold

- feeling stressed

Primary Raynaud phenomenon happens on its own. Secondary Raynaud phenomenon happens along with some other health problem.

Who Gets Raynaud Phenomenon?

People of all ages can have Raynaud phenomenon. Raynaud phenomenon may run in families, but more research is needed.

The primary form is the most common. It most often starts between age 15 and 25. It is most common in:

- women

- people living in cold places

The secondary form tends to start after age 35 to 40. It is most common in people with connective tissue diseases, such as scleroderma, Sjögren syndrome, and lupus. Other possible causes include:

- carpal tunnel syndrome, which affects nerves in the wrists
- blood vessel disease
- some medicines used to treat high blood pressure, migraines, or cancer
- some over-the-counter cold medicines
- some narcotics

People with certain jobs may be more likely to get the secondary form:

- workers who are around certain chemicals
- people who use tools that vibrate, such as a jackhammer.

What Are the Symptoms of Raynaud Phenomenon?

The body saves heat when it is cold by slowing the supply of blood to the skin. It does this by making blood vessels more narrow.

With Raynaud phenomenon, the body's reaction to cold or stress is stronger than normal. It makes blood vessels narrow faster and tighter than normal. When this happens, it is called an "attack."

During an attack, the fingers and toes can change colors. They may go from white to blue to red. They may also feel cold and numb from lack of blood flow. As the attack ends and blood flow returns, fingers or toes can throb and tingle. After the cold parts of the body warm up, normal blood flow returns in about 15 minutes.

What Is the Difference between Primary and Secondary Raynaud Phenomenon?

Primary Raynaud phenomenon is often so mild a person never seeks treatment.

Secondary Raynaud phenomenon is more serious and complex. It is caused when diseases reduce blood flow to fingers and toes.

How Does a Doctor Diagnose Raynaud Phenomenon?

It is fairly easy to diagnose Raynaud phenomenon. But it is harder to find out whether a person has the primary or the secondary form of the disorder.

Doctors will diagnose which form it is using a complete history, an exam, and tests. Tests may include:

- blood tests
- looking at fingernail tissue with a microscope

What Is the Treatment for Raynaud Phenomenon?

Treatment aims to:

- reduce how many attacks you have
- make attacks less severe
- prevent tissue damage
- prevent loss of finger and toe tissue

Primary Raynaud phenomenon does not lead to tissue damage, so nondrug treatment is used first. Treatment with medicine is more common with secondary Raynaud.

Severe cases of Raynaud can lead to sores or gangrene (tissue death) in the fingers and toes. These cases can be painful and hard to treat. In severe cases that cause skin ulcers and serious tissue damage, surgery may be used.

Nondrug Treatments and Self-Help Measures

To reduce how long and severe attacks are:

- Keep your hands and feet warm and dry.
- Warm your hands and feet with warm water.
- Avoid air conditioning.
- Wear gloves to touch frozen or cold foods.
- Wear many layers of loose clothing and a hat when it's cold.
- Use chemical warmers, such as small heating pouches that can be placed in pockets, mittens, boots, or shoes.
- Talk to your doctor before exercising outside in cold weather.
- Don't smoke.
- Avoid medicines that make symptoms worse.
- Control stress.

- Exercise regularly.

  See a doctor if:

- You worry about attacks.

- You have questions about self-care.

- Attacks happen on just one side of your body.

- You have sores or ulcers on your fingers or toes.

Treatment with Medications

People with secondary Raynaud phenomenon are often treated with:

- blood pressure medicines

- medicines that relax blood vessels

If blood flow doesn't return and finger loss is a risk, you will need other medicines.

Pregnant woman should not take these medicines. Sometimes Raynaud phenomenon gets better or goes away when a woman is pregnant.

Section 46.4

Erythromelalgia

This section includes text excerpted from "Erythromelalgia," Genetic and Rare Diseases Information Center (GARD), December 11, 2013.

What Is Erythromelalgia?

Erythromelalgia (EM) is a rare condition characterized by episodes of burning pain, warmth, swelling and redness in parts of the body, particularly the hands and feet. This condition may occur spontaneously (primary EM) or secondary to neurological diseases, autoimmune diseases, or myeloproliferative disorders (secondary EM). Episodes may be triggered by increased body temperature, alcohol, and eating spicy foods. About 15 percent of cases are caused by mutations in the *SCN9A* gene and are inherited in an autosomal dominant manner. Other cases may be caused by unidentified genes or by non-genetic factors. Treatment depends on the underlying cause and may include topical and/or oral medications. In some cases, the condition goes away without treatment.

What Are the Signs and Symptoms of Erythromelalgia?

Currently it is very difficult to predict how a person's primary erythromelalgia will affect them overtime. The cause of primary erythromelalgia is not well understood. Much of the literature regarding the long term outlook for people with idiopathic primary erythromelalgia is compiled from individual case reports. Erythromelalgia is usually a chronic or persistent condition, however there have been cases that have fully resolved with time. Many people with primary erythromelalgia have stable symptoms, however cases of progressive disease (symptoms worsening overtime) have also been described. Pain is a characteristic/classic feature of primary erythromelalgia.

Signs and Symptoms

- abnormality of the musculature
- autosomal dominant inheritance
- blurred vision
- constipation
- diarrhea
- dysautonomia
- hyperhidrosis
- juvenile onset
- myalgia
- pain
- palpitations
- xerostomia

What Causes Erythromelalgia?

About 15 percent of cases of erythromelalgia are caused by mutations in the *SCN9A* gene. The *SCN9A* gene gives instructions for making part of a sodium channel which carries sodium into cells and helps them make and transmit electrical signals. These sodium channels are found in nerve cells that transmit pain signals to the spine and brain. Mutations that cause erythromelalgia cause increased transmission of pain signals, leading to the signs and symptoms of the condition. In some of these cases, an affected individual inherits the mutation from an affected parent. In other cases, a new mutation occurs for the first time in an individual with no history of the condition in the family.

In the remainder of cases, the exact underlying cause is not currently known. Evidence suggests that it results from abnormalities in the normal narrowing and widening of certain blood vessels, leading to abnormalities in blood flow to the hands and feet. There may be a variety of non-genetic causes, or mutations in other genes that have not yet been identified.

How Is Erythromelalgia Diagnosed?

Erythromelalgia can be diagnosed through a clinical exam and medical history. Additional tests may include a skin biopsy and thermography to evaluate skin temperature. Blood tests or other studies may be done to rule out other conditions that can cause similar symptoms.

What Treatment Is Available for Erythromelalgia?

There appear to be several subtypes of erythromelalgia and different subtypes respond to different therapies. Treatment consists of trying various approaches until the best therapy is found. Patients respond quite variably to drug therapy and no single therapy has proved consistently effective. Spontaneous remissions have also been known to occur.

Drugs shown to be effective in relieving pain in some individuals include: aspirin, prostaglandins (misoprostol), serotonin-norepinephrine reuptake inhibitors (venlafaxine and sertraline) and selective serotonin reuptake inhibitors (SSRIs), anticonvulsants (gabapentin), sodium channel blockers, carbamazepine, tricyclic antidepressants (amitriptyline and imipramine), calcium antagonists (nifedipine and diltiazem), magnesium, sodium nitroprusside infusion, and cyclosporine. Other treatments include: cooling or elevating the extremity, topical treatment with capsaicin cream, and surgical sympathectomy (a procedure where the sympathetic nerve fibers are selectively cut). Avoidance of triggers (such as warmth, prolonged standing, etc.) may reduce the number or severity of flare ups.

Does Avoiding Triggers Improve the Long-Term Outlook of People with Primary Erythromelalgia?

Avoiding triggers is key to the management of current symptoms, but little is known regarding how this affects the long-term course of an individual's condition.

Chapter 47

Renal Artery Stenosis (RAS)

What Are Renal Artery Stenosis (RAS) and Renovascular Hypertension (RVH)?

Renal artery stenosis is the narrowing of one or both renal arteries. "Renal" means "kidney" and "stenosis" means "narrowing." The renal arteries are blood vessels that carry blood to the kidneys from the aorta—the main blood vessel that carries blood from the heart to arteries throughout the body.

RVH is high blood pressure caused by RAS. Blood pressure is written with two numbers separated by a slash, 120/80, and is said as "120 over 80." The top number is called the systolic pressure and represents the pressure as the heart beats and pushes blood through the blood vessels. The bottom number is called the diastolic pressure and represents the pressure as blood vessels relax between heartbeats. A person's blood pressure is considered normal if it stays at or below 120/80. High blood pressure is a systolic pressure of 140 or above or a diastolic pressure of 90 or above.

What Are the Kidneys and What Do They Do?

The kidneys are two bean-shaped organs, each about the size of a fist. They are located just below the rib cage, one on each side of the

---

This chapter includes text excerpted from "Renal Artery Stenosis (RAS)," National Institute of Diabetes and Digestive and Kidney Diseases (NIDDK), July 2014.

spine. Every day, the two kidneys filter about 120 to 150 quarts of blood to produce about 1 to 2 quarts of urine, composed of wastes and extra fluid.

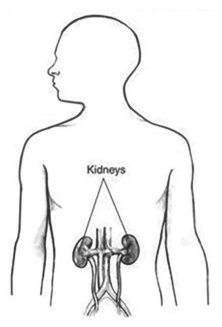

Figure 47.1. *Kidneys*

The kidneys are two bean-shaped organs.

What Causes RAS?

About 90 percent of RAS is caused by atherosclerosis—clogging, narrowing, and hardening of the renal arteries. In these cases, RAS develops when plaque—a sticky substance made up of fat, cholesterol, calcium, and other material found in the blood—builds up on the inner wall of one or both renal arteries. Plaque buildup is what makes the artery wall hard and narrow.

Most other cases of RAS are caused by fibromuscular dysplasia (FMD)—the abnormal development or growth of cells on the renal artery walls—which can cause blood vessels to narrow. Rarely, RAS is caused by other conditions.

Who Is at Risk for RAS?

People at risk for artherosclerosis are also at risk for RAS.

Risk factors for RAS caused by artherosclerosis include:

- high blood cholesterol levels
- high blood pressure
- smoking
- insulin resistance
- diabetes
- being overweight or obese
- lack of physical activity
- a diet high in fat, cholesterol, sodium, and sugar
- being a man older than 45 or a woman older than 55
- a family history of early heart disease

The risk factors for RAS caused by FMD are unknown, but FMD is most common in women and people 25 to 50 years of age. FMD can affect more than one person in a family, indicating that it may be caused by an inherited gene.

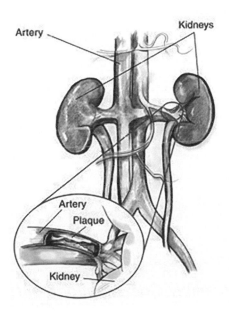

Figure 47.2. *Plaque Build-Up in RAS*

In most cases of RAS, plaque builds up on the inner wall of one or both renal arteries.

What Are the Symptoms of RAS?

In many cases, RAS has no symptoms until it becomes severe.

The signs of RAS are usually either high blood pressure or decreased kidney function, or both, but RAS is often overlooked as a cause of high blood pressure. RAS should be considered as a cause of high blood pressure in people who

- are older than age 50 when they develop high blood pressure or have a marked increase in blood pressure

- have no family history of high blood pressure

- cannot be successfully treated with at least three or more different types of blood pressure medications

Symptoms of a significant decrease in kidney function include

- increase or decrease in urination

- edema—swelling, usually in the legs, feet, or ankles and less often in the hands or face

- drowsiness or tiredness

- generalized itching or numbness

- dry skin

- headaches

- weight loss

- appetite loss

- nausea

- vomiting

- sleep problems

- trouble concentrating

- darkened skin

- muscle cramps

What Are the Possible Complications of RAS?

People with RAS are at increased risk for complications resulting from loss of kidney function or atherosclerosis occurring in other blood vessels, such as

- chronic kidney disease (CKD)—reduced kidney function over a period of time

- coronary artery disease—narrowing and hardening of arteries that supply blood to the heart

- stroke—brain damage caused by lack of blood flow to the brain

- peripheral vascular disease—blockage of blood vessels that restricts flow of blood from the heart to other parts of the body, particularly the legs

RAS can lead to kidney failure, described as end-stage renal disease when treated with blood-filtering treatments called dialysis or a kidney transplant, though this is uncommon in people who receive ongoing treatment for RAS.

How Is RAS. Diagnosed?

A healthcare provider can diagnose RAS by listening to the abdomen with a stethoscope and performing imaging tests. When blood flows through a narrow artery, it sometimes makes a whooshing sound, called a bruit. The healthcare provider may place a stethoscope on the front or the side of the abdomen to listen for this sound. The absence of this sound, however, does not exclude the possibility of RAS.

In some cases, RAS is found when a person has a test for another reason. For example, a healthcare provider may find RAS during a coronary angiogram for diagnosis of heart problems. A coronary angiogram is a procedure that uses a special dye, called contrast medium, and X-rays to see how blood flows through the heart.

The following imaging tests are used to diagnose RAS:

- duplex ultrasound

- catheter angiogram

- computerized tomographic angiography (CTA) scan

- magnetic resonance angiogram (MRA)

How Is RAS Treated?

Treatment for RAS includes lifestyle changes, medications, and surgery and aims to

- prevent RAS from getting worse

- treat RVH

- relieve the blockage of the renal arteries

RAS that has not led to RVH or caused a significant blockage of the artery may not need treatment. RAS that needs to be treated, also called critical RAS, is defined by the American Heart Association (AHA) as a reduction by more than 60 percent in the diameter of the renal artery. However, healthcare providers are not exactly sure what degree of blockage will cause significant problems.

Lifestyle Changes

The first step in treating RAS is making lifestyle changes that promote healthy blood vessels throughout the body, including the renal arteries. The best ways to keep plaque from building up in the arteries are to exercise, maintain a healthy body weight, and choose healthy foods. People who smoke should quit to help protect their kidneys and other internal organs.

Medications

People with RVH may need to take medications that—when taken as prescribed by their healthcare provider—lower blood pressure and can also significantly slow the progression of kidney disease. Two types of blood pressure-lowering medications, angiotensin-converting enzyme (ACE) inhibitors and angiotensin receptor blockers (ARBs), have proven effective in slowing the progression of kidney disease. Many people require two or more medications to control their blood pressure. In addition to an ACE inhibitor or an ARB, a diuretic—a medication that helps the kidneys remove fluid from the blood—may be prescribed. Beta blockers, calcium channel blockers, and other blood pressure medications may also be needed. Some people with RAS cannot take an ACE inhibitor or ARB due to the effects on the kidneys. People with RAS who are prescribed an ACE inhibitor or ARB should have their kidney function checked within a few weeks of starting the medication.

A cholesterol-lowering medication to prevent plaque from building up in the arteries and a blood-thinner, such as aspirin, to help the blood flow more easily through the arteries may also be prescribed.

Surgery

Although surgery has been used in the past for treatment of RAS due to atherosclerosis, recent studies have not shown improved outcomes with surgery compared with medication. However, surgery may be recommended for people with RAS caused by FMD or RAS that does not improve with medication. Different types of surgery for RAS include the following. The procedures are performed in a hospital by a vascular surgeon—a doctor who specializes in repairing blood vessels. Anesthesia is needed.

- angioplasty and stenting
- endarterectomy or bypass surgery

Chapter 48

Sepsis

What Is Sepsis?

Sepsis is a serious medical condition caused by an overwhelming immune response to infection. Immune chemicals released into the blood to combat the infection trigger widespread inflammation, which leads to blood clots and leaky vessels. This results in impaired blood flow, which damages the body's organs by depriving them of nutrients and oxygen.

In severe cases, one or more organs fail. In the worst cases, blood pressure drops, the heart weakens and the patient spirals toward septic shock. Once this happens, multiple organs—lungs, kidneys, liver—may quickly fail and the patient can die.

Sepsis is a major challenge in the intensive care unit, where it's one of the leading causes of death. It arises unpredictably and can progress rapidly.

What Causes Sepsis?

Sepsis does not arise on its own. It stems from another medical condition such as an infection in the lungs, urinary tract, skin, abdomen (such as appendicitis) or other part of the body. Invasive medical procedures like the insertion of a vascular catheter can introduce bacteria into the bloodstream and bring on the condition.

This chapter includes text excerpted from "Sepsis Fact Sheet," National Institute of General Medical Sciences (NIGMS), August 2014.

Many different types of microbes can cause sepsis, including bacteria, fungi and viruses, but bacteria are the most common culprits. Severe cases often result from a body-wide infection that spreads through the bloodstream, but sepsis can also stem from a localized infection.

Who Gets Sepsis?

Anyone can get sepsis, but people with weakened immune systems, children, infants and the elderly are most vulnerable. People with chronic illnesses, such as diabetes, AIDS, cancer and kidney or liver disease, are also at increased risk, as are those who have experienced a severe burn or physical trauma.

How Many People Get Sepsis?

Every year, severe sepsis strikes more than a million Americans. It's been estimated that between 28 and 50 percent of these people die—far more than the number of U.S. deaths from prostate cancer, breast cancer and AIDS combined.

The number of sepsis cases per year has been on the rise in the United States. This is likely due to a combination of factors, including increased awareness and tracking of the condition, an aging population, the increased longevity of people with chronic diseases, the spread of antibiotic-resistant organisms, an upsurge in invasive procedures and broader use of immunosuppressive and chemotherapeutic agents.

What Are the Symptoms of Sepsis?

Common symptoms of sepsis are fever, chills, rapid breathing and heart rate, rash, confusion and disorientation. Many of these symptoms, such as fever and difficulty breathing, mimic other conditions, making sepsis hard to diagnose in its early stages.

How Is Sepsis Diagnosed?

Doctors diagnose sepsis by examining patients for fever, increased heart rate and increased respiratory rate. They often perform a blood test to see if a patient has an abnormal number of white blood cells, a common sign of sepsis; or an elevated lactate level, which correlates with severity of the condition. Doctors may also test blood and other bodily fluids such as urine and sputum for the presence of infectious agents.

In addition, a chest X-ray or a CT scan can help identify the site of infection.

How Is Sepsis Treated?

People with sepsis are usually treated in hospital intensive care units. Doctors try to quell the infection, sustain the vital organs and prevent a drop in blood pressure.

The first step is often treatment with broad-spectrum antibiotics, medicines that kill many types of bacteria. Once lab tests identify the infectious agent, doctors can select medicine that specifically targets the microbe. Many patients receive oxygen and intravenous fluids to maintain normal blood oxygen levels and blood pressure.

Depending on the patient's status, other types of treatment, such as mechanical ventilation or kidney dialysis, may be necessary. Sometimes, surgery is required to clear a local site of infection.

Many other drugs, including vasopressors and corticosteroids, may be used to treat sepsis or to revive those who have gone into septic shock. Despite years of research, scientists have not yet succeeded in developing a medicine that specifically targets the aggressive immune response that characterizes sepsis.

Are There Any Long-Term Effects of Sepsis?

Many people who survive severe sepsis recover completely and their lives return to normal. But some people, especially those who had pre-existing chronic diseases, may experience permanent organ damage. For example, in someone who already has kidney impairment, sepsis can lead to kidney failure that requires lifelong dialysis.

There is also some evidence that an episode of severe sepsis disrupts a person's immune system, making him or her more vulnerable to future infections. Studies have shown that people who have experienced sepsis have an increased risk of dying, even several years after the episode.

What Is the Economic Cost of Sepsis?

Treatment for sepsis often involves a prolonged stay in the intensive care unit and complex therapies, which incur high costs. The Agency for Healthcare Research and Quality (AHRQ) lists sepsis as the most expensive condition treated in U.S. hospitals, costing more than $20 billion in 2011.

Chapter 49

Stroke

What Happens during a Stroke

If something happens to interrupt the flow of blood, brain cells start to die within minutes because they can't get oxygen. This is called a stroke. Sudden bleeding in the brain also can cause a stroke if it damages brain cells. A stroke can cause lasting brain damage, long-term disability, or even death.

If brain cells die or are damaged because of a stroke, symptoms of that damage start to show in the parts of the body controlled by those brain cells.

Quick Treatment Is Critical for Stroke

A stroke is a serious medical condition that requires emergency care.

Types of Stroke

The main types of stroke are

- ischemic stroke

- hemorrhagic stroke

- transient ischemic attack (a warning or "mini-stroke")

This chapter includes text excerpted from "Stroke," Centers for Disease Control and Prevention (CDC), October 9, 2014.

Ischemic Stroke

Most strokes (85%) are ischemic strokes. If you have an ischemic stroke, the artery that supplies oxygen-rich blood to the brain becomes blocked.

Blood clots often cause the blockages that lead to ischemic strokes.

Hemorrhagic Stroke

A hemorrhagic stroke occurs when an artery in the brain leaks blood or ruptures (breaks open). The leaked blood puts too much pressure on brain cells, which damages them.

High blood pressure and aneurysms—balloon-like bulges in an artery that can stretch and burst—are examples of conditions that can cause a hemorrhagic stroke.

There are two types of hemorrhagic strokes:

1. **Intracerebral hemorrhage** is the most common type of hemorrhagic stroke. It occurs when an artery in the brain bursts, flooding the surrounding tissue with blood.

2. **Subarachnoid hemorrhage** is a less common type of hemorrhagic stroke. It refers to bleeding in the area between the brain and the thin tissues that cover it.

Transient Ischemic Attack (TIA)

A transient ischemic attack (TIA) is sometimes called a "mini-stroke." It is different from the major types of stroke because blood flow to the brain is blocked for only a short time—usually no more than 5 minutes.

It is important to know that

- A TIA is a warning sign of a future stroke.

- A TIA is a medical emergency, just like a major stroke.

- Strokes and TIAs require emergency care.

- There is no way to know in the beginning whether symptoms are from a TIA or from a major type of stroke.

- Like ischemic strokes, blood clots often cause TIAs.

- More than a third of people who have a TIA end up having a major stroke within 1 year if they don't receive treatment, and 10%–15% will have a major stroke within 3 months of a TIA.

Recognizing and treating TIAs can reduce the risk of a major stroke. If you have a TIA, your healthcare team can find the cause and take steps to prevent a major stroke.

Signs and Symptoms of Stroke

During a stroke, every minute counts. Fast treatment can reduce the brain damage that stroke can cause.

By knowing the signs and symptoms of stroke, you can be prepared to take quick action and perhaps save a life—maybe even your own.

Signs of Stroke in Men and Women

- Sudden **Numbness** or weakness in the face, arm, or leg, especially on one side of the body.

- Sudden **confusion**, trouble speaking, or difficulty understanding speech.

- Sudden **Trouble seeing** in one or both eyes.

- Sudden **Trouble walking**, dizziness, loss of balance, or lack of coordination.

- Sudden **Severe headache** with no known cause.

Acting F.A.S.T. Is Key for Stroke

Acting F.A.S.T. can help stroke patients get the treatments they desperately need. The most effective stroke treatments are only available if the stroke is recognized and diagnosed within 3 hours of the first symptoms. Stroke patients may not be eligible for the most effective treatments if they don't arrive at the hospital in time.

If you think someone may be having a stroke, act F.A.S.T. and do the following simple test:

F—Face: Ask the person to smile. Does one side of the face droop?

A—Arms: Ask the person to raise both arms. Does one arm drift downward?

S—Speech: Ask the person to repeat a simple phrase. Is their speech slurred or strange?

T—Time: If you observe any of these signs, call 9-1-1 immediately.

Note the time when any symptoms first appear. Some treatments for stroke only work if given in the first 3 hours after symptoms appear.

Treating a Transient Ischemic Attack

If your symptoms go away after a few minutes, you may have had a transient ischemic attack (TIA). Although brief, a TIA is a sign of a serious condition that will not go away without medical help. Tell your healthcare team about your symptoms right away.

Stroke Treatments

If you have a stroke, you may receive emergency care, treatment to prevent another stroke, rehabilitation to treat the side effects of stroke, or all three.

Emergency Treatment

Your emergency treatment starts in the ambulance. The emergency workers may take you to a specialized stroke center to ensure that you receive the quickest possible diagnosis and treatment.

If you get to the hospital within 3 hours of the first symptoms of an ischemic stroke, a healthcare provider may give you a type of medicine called a thrombolytic (a "clot-busting" drug) to break up blood clots. Tissue plasminogen activator (tPA) is a thrombolytic.

tPA improves the chances of recovering from a stroke. Studies have shown that patients with ischemic strokes who received tPA are more likely to recover fully or have less disability than patients who do not receive the drug. In addition, patients treated with tPA are less likely to need long-term care in a nursing home. Unfortunately, many stroke victims don't get to the hospital in time for tPA treatment. This is why it's so important to identify a stroke immediately.

Medicine, surgery, or other procedures may be needed to stop the bleeding and save brain tissue. For example:

- **Endovascular procedures.** Endovascular procedures may be used to treat certain hemorrhagic strokes. These procedures are less invasive and less dangerous for the patient than surgical treatments. The doctor inserts a long tube through a major artery in the leg or arm and then guides the tube to the site of the weak spot or break in a blood vessel. The tube is then used to install a device, such as a coil, to repair the damage or prevent bleeding.

- **Surgical treatment.** Hemorrhagic strokes may be treated with surgery. If the bleeding is caused by a ruptured aneurysm, a metal clip may be put in place to stop the blood loss.

Preventing Another Stroke

- 1 of 4 stroke survivors has another stroke within 5 years.

- The risk of stroke within 90 days of a TIA may be as high as 17 percent, with the greatest risk during the first week.

That's why it's important to treat the underlying causes of stroke, including heart disease, high blood pressure, atrial fibrillation (fast, irregular heartbeat), high cholesterol, and diabetes. Your doctor may give you medications or tell you to change your diet, exercise, or adopt other healthy lifestyle habits. Surgery may also be helpful in some cases.

Stroke Rehabilitation

After a stroke, you may need rehabilitation (rehab) to help you recover. Rehab can include working with speech, physical, and occupational therapists:

- Speech therapy helps people who have problems producing or understanding speech.

- Physical therapy uses exercises to help you relearn movement and coordination skills you may have lost because of the stroke.

- Occupational therapy focuses on improving daily activities, such as eating, drinking, dressing, bathing, reading, and writing.

Recovering from Stroke

Recovery time after a stroke varies—it can take weeks, months, or even years. Some people recover fully, but others have long-term or lifelong disabilities.

If you have had a stroke, you can make great progress in regaining your independence. However, some problems may continue:

- Paralysis (inability to move some parts of the body), weakness, or both on one side of the body.

- Trouble with thinking, awareness, attention, learning, judgment, and memory.

- Problems understanding or forming speech.

- Trouble controlling or expressing emotions.

- Numbness or strange sensations.

- Pain in the hands and feet that worsens with movement and temperature changes.

- Trouble with chewing and swallowing.

- Problems with bladder and bowel control.

- Depression.

Before you are discharged from the hospital, social workers can help you find care services and caregiver support to continue your long-term recovery. It is important to work with your healthcare team to find out the reasons for your stroke and take steps to prevent another stroke.

Chapter 50

Vascular Birthmarks: Hemangiomas and Vascular Malformations

Vascular Birthmarks

Vascular birthmarks, also known as vascular anomalies, affect an estimated one in ten children. Birthmarks take many forms, differing in size, shape, and location on the body. The color of birthmarks varies from shades of brown or blue to red or pink. There are two main types of vascular birthmarks: hemangiomas and vascular malformations. About half of all birthmarks are minor and require no treatment.

Hemangiomas

Hemangiomas are non-cancerous tumors that are present at birth and affect female children about three times as often as males. Due to their distinctive color, these birthmarks are also sometimes known as strawberry marks or salmon patches. They most often appear on the head or neck, but can develop anywhere on the body including internal organs. Hemangiomas may not be visible until one to four weeks after birth. These birthmarks sometimes initially appear as

---

"Vascular Birthmarks: Hemangiomas and Vascular Malformations," © 2016 Omnigraphics. Reviewed July 2016.

faint red marks. Once hemangiomas appear, they change rapidly, usually growing faster than the child grows, before reaching a peak state after about 12 months. After that, hemangiomas begin to shrink and become lighter in color. This process is known as involution or regression and can last from three to ten years. About 70 percent of hemangiomas disappear by age seven. In most cases, hemangiomas do not require treatment. Surgery may be required if the hemangioma interferes with breathing, vision, or hearing.

Vascular Malformations

Vascular malformations are non-cancerous lesions that are present at birth. These birthmarks grow with the child throughout life without involution. There are four main types of vascular malformations. Port Wine Stains can appear anywhere on the body and are typically flat and colored pink, purple, or red. Venous birthmarks are most commonly found on the jaw, cheek, tongue, and lips. These birthmarks are soft to the touch and their color disappears compressed (such as by pressing on the birthmark with a finger). Lymphatic birthmarks form as a result of excess fluid in the lymphatic vessels. Arteriovenous birthmarks appear when blood pools in capillary veins.

Causes

A tendency to develop hemangiomas and vascular malformations can be inherited, though most birthmarks of this type seem to form by chance. Hemangiomas and vascular malformations develop as a result of many different genetic syndromes with many variables affecting the chance of a child being born with a birthmark. If one parent has or had a hemangioma or vascular malformation, there is a 50 percent chance that their baby will also have such a birthmark.

Treatment

Some birthmarks can result in serious complications if the location of the birthmark impairs the body's critical functions such as breathing or blood flow. Most hemangiomas do not require treatment. Treatment is usually required for hemangiomas that interfere with vision, breathing, hearing, ability to feed, or result in other medical problems. Treatment options include surgery, laser treatment, medication, or a combination of approaches.

Treatment for vascular malformations depends upon the location and type of birthmark. Venous and lymphatic malformations are typically treated by injection therapy, in which a clotting medication is used to remove excessive blood or lymphatic fluid. Capillary malfunctions such as Port Wine Stains are usually treated with laser surgery. Arterial malformations can be treated with a process known as embolization, in which blood flow is block by injection of medication near the lesion. Treatments can also include oral medications such as steroids, radiology treatment, surgery, or a combination of approaches.

References

1. "What is a Vascular Birthmark?" University of Rochester Medical Center. 2016.

2. "Vascular Malformations and Hemangiomas," Stanford Children's Health. 2016.

Chapter 51

Vasculitis

What Is Vasculitis?

Vasculitis is a condition that involves inflammation in the blood vessels. The condition occurs if your immune system attacks your blood vessels by mistake. This may happen as the result of an infection, a medicine, or another disease or condition.

"Inflammation" refers to the body's response to injury, including injury to the blood vessels. Inflammation may involve pain, redness, warmth, swelling, and loss of function in the affected tissues.

In vasculitis, inflammation can lead to serious problems. Complications depend on which blood vessels, organs, or other body systems are affected.

Types of Vasculitis

There are many types of vasculitis. Each type involves inflamed blood vessels. However, most types differ in whom they affect and the organs that are involved.

The types of vasculitis often are grouped based on the size of the blood vessels they affect.

This chapter includes text excerpted from "Vasculitis," National Heart, Lung, and Blood Institute (NHLBI), September 23, 2014.

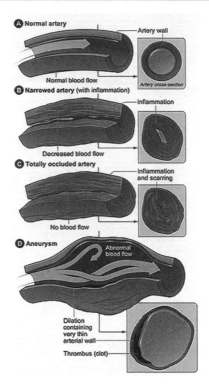

Figure 51.1. *Vasculitis*

Figure A shows a normal artery with normal blood flow. The inset image shows a cross-section of the normal artery. Figure B shows an inflamed, narrowed artery with decreased blood flow. The inset image shows a cross-section of the inflamed artery. Figure C shows an inflamed, blocked (occluded) artery and scarring on the artery wall. The inset image shows a cross-section of the blocked artery. Figure D shows an artery with an aneurysm. The inset image shows a cross-section of the artery with an aneurysm.

Mostly Large Vessel Vasculitis

These types of vasculitis usually, but not always, affect the body's larger blood vessels.

- Behçet Disease
- Cogan Syndrome
- Giant Cell Arteritis
- Polymyalgia Rheumatica
- Takayasu Arteritis

Mostly Medium Vessel Vasculitis

These types of vasculitis usually, but not always, affect the body's medium-sized blood vessels.

- Buerger Disease

- Central Nervous System Vasculitis

- Kawasaki Disease

- Polyarteritis Nodosa

Mostly Small Vessel Vasculitis

These types of vasculitis usually, but not always, affect the body's small blood vessels.

- Eosinophilic Granulomatosis with Polyangiitis

- Cryoglobulinemia Vasculitis

- IgA Vasculitis

- Hypersensitivity Vasculitis

- Microscopic Polyangiitis

Other Names for Vasculitis

- angiitis

- arteritis

What Causes Vasculitis?

Vasculitis occurs if your immune system attacks your blood vessels by mistake. What causes this to happen isn't fully known.

A recent or chronic (ongoing) infection may prompt the attack. Your body also may attack its own blood vessels in reaction to a medicine.

Sometimes an autoimmune disorder triggers vasculitis. Auto-immune disorders occur if the immune system makes antibodies (proteins) that attack and damage the body's own tissues or cells. Examples of these disorders include lupus, rheumatoid arthritis, and scleroderma. You can have these disorders for years before developing vasculitis.

Vasculitis also may be linked to certain blood cancers, such as leukemia and lymphoma.

Who Is at Risk for Vasculitis?

Vasculitis can affect people of all ages and races and both sexes. Some types of vasculitis seem to occur more often in people who:

- Have certain medical conditions, such as chronic hepatitis B or C infection
- Have certain autoimmune diseases, such a lupus, rheumatoid arthritis, and scleroderma
- Smoke

What Are the Signs and Symptoms of Vasculitis?

The signs and symptoms of vasculitis vary. They depend on the type of vasculitis you have, the organs involved, and the severity of the condition. Some people may have few signs and symptoms. Other people may become very sick.

Sometimes the signs and symptoms develop slowly, over months. Other times, the signs and symptoms develop quickly, over days or weeks.

Systemic Signs and Symptoms

Systemic signs and symptoms are those that affect you in a general or overall way. Common systemic signs and symptoms of vasculitis are:

- fever
- loss of appetite
- weight loss
- fatigue (tiredness)
- general aches and pains

Organ- or Body System-Specific Signs and Symptoms

Vasculitis can affect specific organs and body systems, causing a range of signs and symptoms.

Skin

If vasculitis affects your skin, you may notice skin changes. For example, you may have purple or red spots or bumps, clusters of small dots, splotches, bruises, or hives. Your skin also may itch.

Joints

If vasculitis affects your joints, you may ache or develop arthritis in one or more joints.

Lungs

If vasculitis affects your lungs, you may feel short of breath. You may even cough up blood. The results from a chest X-ray may show signs that suggest pneumonia, even though that may not be what you have.

Gastrointestinal Tract

If vasculitis affects your gastrointestinal tract, you may get ulcers (sores) in your mouth or have stomach pain.

In severe cases, blood flow to the intestines can be blocked. This can cause the wall of the intestines to weaken and possibly rupture (burst). A rupture can lead to serious problems or even death.

Sinuses, Nose, Throat, and Ears

If vasculitis affects your sinuses, nose, throat, and ears, you may have sinus or chronic (ongoing) middle ear infections. Other symptoms include ulcers in the nose and, in some cases, hearing loss.

Eyes

If vasculitis affects your eyes, you may develop red, itchy, burning eyes. Your eyes also may become sensitive to light, and your vision may blur. Rarely, certain types of vasculitis may cause blindness.

Brain

If vasculitis affects your brain, symptoms may include headaches, problems thinking clearly, changes in mental function, or stroke-like symptoms, such as muscle weakness and paralysis.

Nerves

If vasculitis affects your nerves, you may have numbness, tingling, and weakness in various parts of your body. You also may have a loss of feeling or strength in your hands and feet and shooting pains in your arms and legs.

How Is Vasculitis Diagnosed?

Your doctor will diagnose vasculitis based on your signs and symptoms, your medical history, a physical exam, and test results.

Diagnostic Tests and Procedures

Many tests are used to diagnose vasculitis.

- blood tests

- biopsy

- blood pressure

- urinalysis

- electrocardiogram (ekg)

- echocardiography

- chest X-Ray

- lung function tests

- abdominal ultrasound

- computed tomography scan

- magnetic resonance imaging

- other advanced imaging techniques

  - duplex ultrasonography

  - 18F-fluorodeoxyglucose positron emission tomography (FDG-PET)

  - angiography

How Is Vasculitis Treated?

Treatment for vasculitis will depend on the type of vasculitis you have, which organs are affected, and the severity of the condition.

People who have severe vasculitis are treated with prescription medicines. Rarely, surgery may be done. People who have mild vasculitis may find relief with over-the-counter pain medicines, such as acetaminophen, aspirin, ibuprofen, or naproxen.

The main goal of treating vasculitis is to reduce inflammation in the affected blood vessels. This usually is done by reducing or stopping the immune response that caused the inflammation.

Types of Treatment

Common prescription medicines used to treat vasculitis include corticosteroids and cytotoxic medicines.

Corticosteroids help reduce inflammation in your blood vessels. Examples of corticosteroids are prednisone, prednisolone, and methylprednisolone.

Doctors may prescribe cytotoxic medicines if vasculitis is severe or if corticosteroids don't work well. Cytotoxic medicines kill the cells that are causing the inflammation. Examples of these medicines are azathioprine, methotrexate, and cyclophosphamide.

Your doctor may prescribe both corticosteroids and cytotoxic medicines.

Other treatments may be used for certain types of vasculitis. For example, the standard treatment for Kawasaki disease is high-dose aspirin and immune globulin. Immune globulin is a medicine that's injected into a vein.

Certain types of vasculitis may require surgery to remove aneurysms that have formed as a result of the condition. (An aneurysm is an abnormal bulge in the wall of a blood vessel.)

How Can Vasculitis Be Prevented?

You can't prevent vasculitis. However, treatment can help prevent or delay the complications of vasculitis.

People who have severe vasculitis are treated with prescription medicines. Rarely, surgery may be done. People who have mild vasculitis may find relief with over-the-counter pain medicines, such as acetaminophen, aspirin, ibuprofen, or naproxen.

Living with Vasculitis

The outcome of vasculitis is hard to predict. It will depend on the type of vasculitis you have, which organs are affected, and the severity of the condition.

If vasculitis is diagnosed early and responds well to treatment, it may go away or go into remission. "Remission" means the condition isn't active, but it can come back, or "flare," at any time.

Flares can be hard to predict. You may have a flare when you stop treatment or change your treatment. Some types of vasculitis seem to flare more often than others. Also, some people have flares more often than others.

Sometimes vasculitis is chronic (ongoing) and never goes into remission. Long-term treatment with medicines often can control chronic vasculitis, but no cure has been found. Rarely, vasculitis doesn't respond well to treatment. This can lead to disability or even death.

Ongoing Care

The medicines used to treat vasculitis can have side effects. For example, long-term use of corticosteroids may lead to weight gain, diabetes, weakness, a decrease in muscle size, and osteoporosis (a bone-thinning condition). Long-term use of these medicines also may increase your risk of infection.

Your doctor may adjust the type or dose of medicine you take to lessen or prevent the side effects. If your vasculitis goes into remission, your doctor may carefully withdraw your medicines. However, he or she will still need to carefully watch you for flares.

While you're being treated for vasculitis, you'll need to see your doctor regularly. Talk with your doctor about any new symptoms and other changes in your health, including side effects of your medicines.

Chapter 52

Venous Disorders

Chapter Contents

Section 52.1

Arteriovenous Malformation

This section includes text excerpted from "Arteriovenous Malformations and Other Vascular Lesions of the Central Nervous System Fact Sheet," National Institute of Neurological Disorders and Stroke (NINDS), May 26, 2016.

What Are Arteriovenous Malformations?

Arteriovenous malformations (AVMs) are abnormal, snarled tangles of blood vessels that cause multiple irregular connections between the arteries and veins. These malformations most often occur in the spinal cord and in any part of the brain or on its surface, but can develop elsewhere in the body.

Normally, arteries carry oxygen-rich blood away from the heart to the body's cells, organs, and tissues; veins return blood with less oxygen to the lungs and heart. But in an AVM, the absence of capillaries—a network of small blood vessels that connect arteries to veins and deliver oxygen to cells—creates a shortcut for blood to pass directly from arteries to veins and bypass tissue, which can lead to tissue damage and the death of nerve cells and other cells. Over time, some AVMs get progressively larger as the amount of blood flow increases.

In some cases, a weakened blood vessel may burst, spilling blood into the brain (hemorrhage) that can cause stroke and brain damage. Other neurological problems include headache, weakness, seizures, pain, and problems with speech, vision, or movement. In most cases, people with neurological AVMs experience few, if any, significant symptoms.

It is unclear why AVMs form. Most often AVMs are congenital, but they can appear sporadically. In some cases the AVM may be inherited, but it is more likely that other inherited conditions increase the risk of having an AVM. The malformations tend to be discovered only incidentally, usually during treatment for an unrelated disorder or at autopsy. It is estimated that brain AVMs occur in less than one percent of the general population; each year about one percent of those with AVMs will die as a direct result of the AVM.

Treatment options depend on the type of AVM, its location, noticeable symptoms, and the general health condition of the individual.

What Are the Symptoms?

Symptoms can vary greatly in severity; in some people the severity of symptoms becomes debilitating or even life-threatening.

Seizures and headaches that may be severe are the most generalized symptoms of AVMs, but no particular type of seizure or headache pattern has been identified. Seizures can be focal (meaning they involve a small part of the brain) or generalized (widespread), involving convulsions, a loss of control over movement, or a change in a person's level of consciousness. Headaches can vary greatly in frequency, duration, and intensity, sometimes becoming as severe as migraines. Pain may be on either one side of the head or on both sides. Sometimes a headache consistently affecting one side of the head may be closely linked to the site of an AVM. Most often, the location of the pain is not specific to the malformation and may encompass most of the head.

AVMs also can cause a wide range of more specific neurological symptoms that vary from person to person, depending primarily upon the location of the AVM. Such symptoms may include:

- Muscle weakness or paralysis in one part of the body.

- A loss of coordination (*ataxia*) that can lead to such problems as gait disturbances.

- Difficulties carrying out tasks that require planning (*apraxia*).

- Back pain or weakness in the lower extremities caused by a spinal AVM.

- Dizziness.

- Visual problems such as a loss of part of the visual field, inability to control eye movement, or swelling of a part of the optic nerve.

- Difficulty speaking or understanding language (*aphasia*).

- Abnormal sensations such as numbness, tingling, or spontaneous pain.

- Memory deficits.

- Confusion, hallucinations, or dementia.

AVMs may also cause subtle learning or behavioral disorders in some people during their childhood or adolescence, long before more obvious symptoms become evident.

Symptoms caused by AVMs can appear at any age. Because the abnormalities tend to result from a slow buildup of neurological damage over time, they are most often noticed when people are in their twenties or older. If AVMs do not become symptomatic by the time people reach their late forties or early fifties, they tend to remain stable and are less likely to produce symptoms. Some pregnant women may experience a sudden onset or worsening of symptoms due to accompanying cardiovascular changes, especially increases in blood volume and blood pressure.

Although most neurological AVMs have very few, if any, significant symptoms, one particularly severe type of AVM causes symptoms to appear at, or very soon after, birth. Called a *vein of Galen defect* after the major blood vessel involved, this lesion is located deep inside the brain. It is frequently associated with *hydrocephalus* (an accumulation of fluid within certain spaces in the brain, often with visible enlargement of the head), swollen veins visible on the scalp, seizures, failure to thrive, and congestive heart failure. Children born with this condition who survive past infancy often remain developmentally impaired.

How Do AVMs Damage the Brain and Spinal Cord?

AVMs damage the brain or spinal cord through three basic mechanisms: by reducing the amount of oxygen reaching neurological tissues; by causing bleeding (hemorrhage) into surrounding tissues; and by compressing or displacing parts of the brain or spinal cord.

AVMs affect oxygen delivery to the brain or spinal cord by altering normal patterns of blood flow using the arteries, veins, and capillaries. In AVMs arteries pump blood directly into veins through a passageway called a *fistula*. Since the network of capillaries is bypassed, the rate of blood flow is uncontrolled and too rapid to allow oxygen to be dispersed to surrounding tissues. As a result, the cells that make up these tissues become oxygen-depleted and begin to deteriorate, sometimes dying off completely.

This abnormally rapid rate of blood flow frequently causes blood pressure inside the vessels located in the central portion of an AVM directly adjacent to the fistula—an area doctors refer to as the *nidus*—to rise to dangerously high levels. The arteries feeding blood into the AVM often become swollen and distorted; the veins that drain blood away from it often become abnormally constricted (a condition called *stenosis*). Also, the walls of the involved arteries and veins are often abnormally thin and weak. *Aneurysms*—balloon-like bulges in blood vessel walls that are susceptible to rupture—may develop in association with approximately half of all neurological AVMs due to this structural weakness.

- Bleeding into the brain, called intracranial hemorrhage, can result from the combination of high internal pressure and vessel wall weakness.

- Even in the absence of bleeding or significant oxygen depletion, large AVMs can damage the brain or spinal cord simply by their presence.

Where Do Neurological AVMs Tend to Form?

AVMs can form virtually anywhere in the brain or spinal cord—wherever arteries and veins exist. Some are formed from blood vessels located in the *dura mater* or in the *pia mater*, the outermost and innermost, respectively, of the three membranes surrounding the brain and spinal cord. (The third membrane, called the *arachnoid*, lacks blood vessels.) AVMs of the dura mater affect the function of the spinal cord by transmitting excess pressure to the venous system of the spinal cord. AVMs of the spinal cord affect the function of the spinal cord by hemorrhage, by reducing blood flow to the spinal cord, or by causing excess venous pressure. Spinal AVMs frequently cause attacks of sudden, severe back pain, often concentrated at the roots of nerve fibers where they exit the vertebrae, with pain that is similar to that caused by a slipped disk. These lesions also can cause sensory disturbances, muscle weakness, or paralysis in the parts of the body served by the spinal cord or the damaged nerve fibers. A spinal cord AVM can lead to degeneration of the nerve fibers within the spinal cord below the level of the lesion, causing widespread paralysis in parts of the body controlled by those nerve fibers.

AVMs on the surface of the *cerebral hemispheres*—the uppermost portions of the brain—exert pressure on the *cerebral cortex*, the brain's "gray matter." Depending on their location, these AVMs may damage portions of the cerebral cortex involved with thinking, speaking, understanding language, hearing, taste, touch, or initiating and controlling voluntary movements. AVMs located on the frontal lobe close to the optic nerve or on the occipital lobe (the rear portion of the cerebrum where images are processed) may cause a variety of visual disturbances.

AVMs also can form from blood vessels located deep inside the interior of the *cerebrum* (the main portion of the brain). These AVMs may compromise the functions of three vital structures: the *thalamus*, which transmits nerve signals between the spinal cord and upper regions of the brain; the basal ganglia surrounding the thalamus, which coordinate complex movements and plays a role in learning and memory; and the *hippocampus*, which plays a major role in memory.

AVMs can affect other parts of the brain besides the cerebrum. The *hindbrain* is formed from two major structures: the *cerebellum*, which is nestled under the rear portion of the cerebrum, and the *brain stem*, which serves as the bridge linking the upper portions of the brain with the spinal cord. These structures control finely coordinated movements, maintain balance, and regulate some functions of internal organs, including those of the heart and lungs. AVM damage to these parts of the hindbrain can result in dizziness, giddiness, vomiting, a loss of the ability to coordinate complex movements such as walking, or uncontrollable muscle tremors.

What Are the Health Consequences of AVMs?

The greatest potential danger posed by AVMs is hemorrhage. Most episodes of bleeding remain undetected at the time they occur because they are not severe enough to cause significant neurological damage. But massive, even fatal, bleeding episodes do occur. Whenever an AVM is detected, the individual should be carefully and consistently monitored for any signs of instability that may indicate an increased risk of hemorrhage.

A few physical characteristics appear to indicate a greater-than-usual likelihood of clinically significant hemorrhage:

- Smaller AVMs have a greater likelihood of bleeding than do larger ones.

- Impaired drainage by unusually narrow or deeply situated veins increases the chances of hemorrhage.

- Pregnancy appears to increase the likelihood of clinically significant hemorrhage, mainly because of increases in blood pressure and blood volume.

- AVMs that have hemorrhaged once are about nine times more likely to bleed again during the first year after the initial hemorrhage than are lesions that have never bled.

The damaging effects of a hemorrhage are related to lesion location. Bleeding from AVMs located deep inside the interior tissues, or *parenchyma*, of the brain typically causes more severe neurological damage than does hemorrhage by lesions that have formed in the dural or pial membranes or on the surface of the brain or spinal cord. (Deeply located bleeding is usually referred to as an *intracerebral* or *parenchymal* hemorrhage; bleeding within the membranes or on the surface of the brain is known as *subdural* or *subarachnoid* hemorrhage.) Therefore, location is an important factor to consider when weighing the relative risks surgery to treat AVMs.

What Other Types of Vascular Lesions Affect the Central Nervous System?

Besides AVMs, three other main types of vascular lesion can arise in the brain or spinal cord: cavernous malformations, *capillary telangiectases*, and *venous malformations*. These lesions may form virtually anywhere within the central nervous system, but unlike AVMs, they are not caused by high-velocity blood flow from arteries into veins. Instead of a combination of arteries and veins, these low-flowing lesions involve only one type of blood vessel. These lesions are less unstable than AVMs and do not pose the same relatively high risk of significant hemorrhage. In general, low-flow lesions tend to cause fewer troubling neurological symptoms and require less aggressive treatment than do AVMs.

What Causes Vascular Lesions?

The cause of vascular anomalies of the central nervous system is not yet well understood. Scientists believe the anomalies most often result from mistakes that occur during embryonic or fetal development. These mistakes may be linked to genetic mutations in some cases. A few types of vascular malformations are known to be hereditary and thus are known to have a genetic basis. Some evidence also suggests that at least some of these lesions are acquired later in life as a result of injury to the central nervous system.

During fetal development, new blood vessels continuously form and then disappear as the human body changes and grows. These changes in the body's vascular map continue after birth and are controlled by *angiogenic factors*, chemicals produced by the body that stimulate new blood vessel formation and growth. Researchers have identified changes in the chemical structures of various angiogenic factors in some people who have AVMs or other vascular abnormalities of the central nervous system. However, it is not yet clear how these chemical changes actually cause changes in blood vessel structure.

By studying patterns of occurrence in families, researchers have established that one type of cavernous malformation involving multiple lesion formation is caused by a genetic mutation in chromosome 7. This genetic mutation appears in many ethnic groups, but it is especially frequent in a large population of Hispanic Americans living in the Southwest; these individuals share a common ancestor in whom the genetic change occurred. Some other types of vascular defects of the central nervous system are part of larger medical syndromes known to be hereditary. They include *hereditary hemorrhagic telangiectasia, Sturge-Weber syndrome,* and *Klippel–Trénaunay syndrome.*

How Are AVMs and Other Vascular Lesions Detected?

One of the more distinctive signs clinicians use to diagnose an AVM is an auditory phenomenon called a *bruit*—a rhythmic, whooshing sound caused by excessively rapid blood flow through the arteries and veins of an AVM. The sound is similar to that made by a torrent of water rushing through a narrow pipe. A bruit can sometimes become a symptom when it is especially severe. When audible to individuals, the bruit may compromise hearing, disturb sleep, or cause significant psychological distress.

An array of imaging technologies can be used to uncover the presence of AVMs.

- Cerebral angiography

- CT scans (computed axial tomography)

- MRI (magnetic resonance imaging)

- Magnetic resonance angiography (MRA)

- Transcranial Doppler ultrasound

How Are AVMs and Other Vascular Lesions Treated?

There are several options for treating AVMs. Although medication can often lessen general symptoms such as headache, back pain, and seizures caused by AVMs and other vascular lesions, the definitive treatment for AVMs is either surgery or focused radiation therapy. Venous malformations and capillary telangiectases rarely require surgery. Cavernous malformations are usually well defined enough for surgical removal, but surgery on these lesions is less common than for AVMs because they do not pose the same risk of hemorrhage.

Because so many variables are involved in treating AVMs, doctors must assess the danger posed to individuals largely on a case-by-case basis. A hemorrhage from an untreated AVM can cause serious neurological deficits or death, leading many clinicians to recommend surgical intervention whenever the physical characteristics of an AVM appear to indicate a greater-than-usual likelihood of significant bleeding and subsequent neurological damage. However, surgery on any part of the central nervous system carries some risk of serious complications or death. There is no easy formula that can allow physicians and individuals to reach a decision on the best course of therapy.

An AVM grading system developed in the mid-1980s can help healthcare professionals estimate the risk of surgery based on the size of the AVM, location in the brain and surrounding tissue involvement, and any leakage.

Three surgical options are used to treat AVMs: *conventional surgery*, *endovascular embolization*, and *radiosurgery*. The choice of treatment depends largely on the size and location of an AVM. Endovascular embolization and radiosurgery are less invasive than conventional surgery and offer safer treatment options for some AVMs located deep inside the brain.

- Conventional surgery involves entering the brain or spinal cord and removing the central portion of the AVM, including the fistula, while causing as little damage as possible to surrounding neurological structures. This surgery is most appropriate when an AVM is located in a superficial portion of the brain or spinal cord and is relatively small in size. AVMs located deep inside the brain generally cannot be approached through conventional surgical techniques because there is too great a possibility that functionally important brain tissue will be damaged or destroyed.

- In endovascular embolization the surgeon guides a catheter through the arterial network until the tip reaches the site of the AVM. The surgeon then injects a substance (such as fast-drying glue-like substances, fibered titanium coils, and tiny balloons) that will travel through blood vessels and create an artificial blood clot in the center of an AVM. Since embolization usually does not permanently obliterate the AVM, it is usually used as an adjunct to surgery or to radiosurgery to reduce the blood flow through the AVM and make the surgery safer.

- Radiosurgery is an even less invasive therapeutic approach often used to treat small AVMs that haven't ruptured. A beam of highly focused radiation is aimed directly on the AVM and damages the walls of the blood vessels making up the lesion. Over the course of the next several months, the irradiated vessels gradually degenerate and eventually close, leading to the resolution of the AVM.

Embolization frequently proves incomplete or temporary, although new embolization materials have led to improved results. Radiosurgery often has incomplete results as well, particularly when an AVM is large, and it poses the additional risk of radiation damage to surrounding normal tissues. Even when successful, complete closure of an AVM takes place over the course of many months following radiosurgery. During that period, the risk of hemorrhage is still present. However, both techniques can treat deeply situated AVMs that had previously been inaccessible. And in many individuals, staged embolization followed by conventional surgical removal or by radiosurgery is now performed, resulting in further reductions in death and complication rates.

Section 52.2

Chronic Venous Insufficiency

"Chronic Venous Insufficiency," © 2016 Omnigraphics.
Reviewed July 2016.

Chronic Venous Insufficiency, also known as phlebitis, post-thrombotic syndrome, or venous leg ulcer, is a fairly common medical condition in which blood pools in the legs, resulting in increased pressure on blood vessel walls. This condition occurs most often in women, especially after multiple pregnancies, and people who are middle-aged or older. Chronic venous insufficiency affects as estimated 40 percent of people.

Symptoms

Chronic venous insufficiency can be painful, sometimes interfering with a person's ability to walk. The most common symptoms of chronic venous insufficiency mimic the symptoms of other medical conditions, sometimes making the disorder difficult to diagnose.

Symptoms of chronic venous insufficiency can include:

- pain or swelling in legs or ankles
- cramps or muscle spasms in legs
- tight feeling in calves
- itchy or restless feeling in legs
- pain when walking that stops when resting
- brown discoloration of skin on legs or ankles
- varicose veins, enlarged or twisted veins close to the skin surface
- leg ulcers

Causes

Chronic venous insufficiency can be an inherited condition. It can also develop due to certain medical conditions such as deep vein thrombosis or a blood clot in a deep vein. Factors that increase the chances of developing chronic venous insufficiency include obesity, pregnancy, traumatic leg injury, history of blood clots, high blood pressure, extended periods of sitting, lack of exercise, and smoking.

Diagnosis

Chronic venous insufficiency is diagnosed through a medical history interview, physical exam, and imaging tests that examine the structure and flow of blood in the veins in the legs.

Treatment

Treatment of chronic venous insufficiency varies according to a person's medical history, age, overall health, and the nature and prognosis of the individual case. Treatment options can include simple recommendations such as wearing compression stockings, elevating (raising) the legs, and exercise to reduce swelling and encourage increased blood flow. Medication is sometimes used to treat chronic venous insufficiency. Therapeutic procedures such as endovenous laser ablation or radiofrequency ablation introduce heat into the affected vein, to close the vein and reduce the amount of blood that pools in the leg. Sclerotherapy treatment introduces chemicals to the affected veins by injection, ending the vein's ability to carry blood. Surgical treatments include ligation, in which affected veins are tied off to end blood flow, and a process known as vein stripping, in which affected veins are removed from the body.

Chronic venous insufficiency can recur even after successful treatments. Long-term treatment plans often focus on maintaining a healthy weight, exercising regularly, wearing compression stockings, and taking prescribed medications regularly.

References

1. "Chronic Venous Insufficiency," University of Rochester Medical Center. 2016.

2. Henke, Dr. Peter K. "Chronic Venous Insufficiency," Society for Vascular Surgery.

Section 52.3

Varicose Veins

This section includes text excerpted from "Varicose Veins," National Heart, Lung, and Blood Institute (NHLBI), February 13, 2014.

What Are Varicose Veins?

Varicose veins are swollen, twisted veins that you can see just under the surface of the skin. These veins usually occur in the legs, but they also can form in other parts of the body.

Varicose veins are a common condition. They usually cause few signs and symptoms. Sometimes varicose veins cause mild to moderate pain, blood clots, skin ulcers (sores), or other problems.

Vein Problems Related to Varicose Veins

Many vein problems are related to varicose veins, such as telangiectasias, spider veins, varicoceles, and other vein problems.

Telangiectasias

Telangiectasias are small clusters of blood vessels. They're usually found on the upper body, including the face.

These blood vessels appear red. They may form during pregnancy, and often they develop in people who have certain genetic disorders, viral infections, or other conditions, such as liver disease.

Because telangiectasias can be a sign of a more serious condition, see your doctor if you think you have them.

Spider Veins

Spider veins are a smaller version of varicose veins and a less serious type of telangiectasias. Spider veins involve the capillaries, the smallest blood vessels in the body.

Spider veins often appear on the legs and face. They're red or blue and usually look like a spider web or tree branch. These veins usually aren't a medical concern.

Varicoceles

Varicoceles are varicose veins in the scrotum (the skin over the testicles). Varicoceles may be linked to male infertility. If you think you have varicoceles, see your doctor.

Other Related Vein Problems

Other types of varicose veins include venous lakes, reticular veins, and hemorrhoids. Venous lakes are varicose veins that appear on the face and neck. Reticular veins are flat blue veins often seen behind the knees. Hemorrhoids are varicose veins in and around the anus.

What Causes Varicose Veins?

Weak or damaged valves in the veins can cause varicose veins. After your arteries and capillaries deliver oxygen-rich blood to your body, your veins return the blood to your heart. The veins in your legs must work against gravity to do this.

One-way valves inside the veins open to let blood flow through, and then they shut to keep blood from flowing backward. If the valves are weak or damaged, blood can back up and pool in your veins. This causes the veins to swell.

Weak vein walls may cause weak valves. Normally, the walls of the veins are elastic (stretchy). If these walls become weak, they lose their normal elasticity. They become like an overstretched rubber band. This makes the walls of the veins longer and wider, and it causes the flaps of the valves to separate.

When the valve flaps separate, blood can flow backward through the valves. The backflow of blood fills the veins and stretches the walls even more. As a result, the veins get bigger, swell, and often twist as they try to squeeze into their normal space. These are varicose veins.

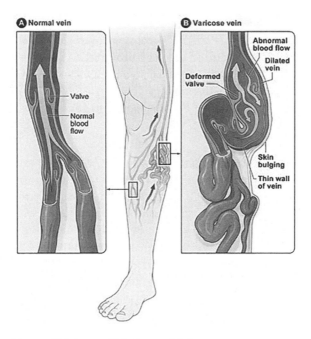

Figure 52.1. *Normal Vein and Varicose Vein*

Figure A shows a normal vein with a working valve and normal blood flow. Figure B shows a varicose vein with a deformed valve, abnormal blood flow, and thin, stretched walls. The middle image shows where varicose veins might appear in a leg.

Figure A shows a normal vein with a working valve and normal blood flow. Figure B shows a varicose vein with a deformed valve, abnormal blood flow, and thin, stretched walls. The middle image shows where varicose veins might appear in a leg.

Older age or a family history of varicose veins may raise your risk for weak vein walls. You also may be at higher risk if you have increased pressure in your veins due to overweight or obesity or pregnancy.

Who Is at Risk for Varicose Veins?

Many factors may raise your risk for varicose veins, including family history, older age, gender, pregnancy, overweight or obesity, lack of movement, and leg trauma.

Family History

Having family members who have varicose veins may raise your risk for the condition. About half of all people who have varicose veins have a family history of them.

Older Age

Getting older may raise your risk for varicose veins. The normal wear and tear of aging may cause the valves in your veins to weaken and not work well.

Gender

Women tend to get varicose veins more often than men. Hormonal changes that occur during puberty, pregnancy, and menopause (or with the use of birth control pills) may raise a woman's risk for varicose veins.

Pregnancy

During pregnancy, the growing fetus puts pressure on the veins in the mother's legs. Varicose veins that occur during pregnancy usually get better within 3 to 12 months of delivery.

Overweight or Obesity

Being overweight or obese can put extra pressure on your veins. This can lead to varicose veins.

Lack of Movement

Standing or sitting for a long time, especially with your legs bent or crossed, may raise your risk for varicose veins. This is because staying in one position for a long time may force your veins to work harder to pump blood to your heart.

Leg Trauma

Previous blood clots or traumatic damage to the valves in your veins can weaken their ability to move blood back to the heart, increasing the risk for varicose veins.

What Are the Signs and Symptoms of Varicose Veins?

The signs and symptoms of varicose veins include:

- Large veins that you can see just under the surface of your skin.
- Mild swelling of your ankles and feet.
- Painful, achy, or "heavy" legs.
- Throbbing or cramping in your legs.
- Itchy legs, especially on the lower leg and ankle. Sometimes this symptom is incorrectly diagnosed as dry skin.
- Discolored skin in the area around the varicose vein.

Signs of telangiectasias are clusters of red veins that you can see just under the surface of your skin. These clusters usually are found on the upper body, including the face. Signs of spider veins are red or blue veins in a web or tree branch pattern. Often, these veins appear on the legs and face.

See your doctor if you have these signs and symptoms. They also may be signs of other, more serious conditions.

Complications of Varicose Veins

Varicose veins can lead to dermatitis, an itchy rash. If you have varicose veins in your legs, dermatitis may affect your lower leg or ankle. Dermatitis can cause bleeding or skin ulcers (sores) if the skin is scratched or irritated.

Varicose veins also can lead to a condition called superficial thrombophlebitis. Thrombophlebitis is a blood clot in a vein. Superficial thrombophlebitis means that the blood clot occurs in a vein close to the surface of the skin. This type of blood clot may cause pain and other problems in the affected area.

How Are Varicose Veins Diagnosed?

Doctors often diagnose varicose veins based on a physical exam alone. Sometimes tests or procedures are used to find out the extent of the problem or to rule out other conditions.

Physical Exam

To check for varicose veins in your legs, your doctor will look at your legs while you're standing or sitting with your legs dangling. He or she may ask you about your signs and symptoms, including any pain you're having.

Diagnostic Tests and Procedures

- Duplex Ultrasound
- Angiogram

How Are Varicose Veins Treated?

Varicose veins are treated with lifestyle changes and medical procedures. The goals of treatment are to relieve symptoms, prevent complications, and improve appearance.

If varicose veins cause few symptoms, your doctor may simply suggest making lifestyle changes. If your symptoms are more severe, your doctor may recommend one or more medical procedures. For example, you may need a medical procedure if you have a lot of pain, blood clots, or skin disorders caused by your varicose veins.

Some people who have varicose veins choose to have procedures to improve how their veins look.

Although treatment can help existing varicose veins, it can't keep new varicose veins from forming.

Lifestyle Changes

Lifestyle changes often are the first treatment for varicose veins. These changes can prevent varicose veins from getting worse, reduce pain, and delay other varicose veins from forming. Lifestyle changes include the following:

- Avoid standing or sitting for long periods without taking a break.

- Do physical activities to get your legs moving and improve muscle tone.

- If you're overweight or obese, try to lose weight.

- Avoid wearing tight clothes, especially those that are tight around your waist, groin (upper thighs), and legs.

- Avoid wearing high heels for long periods.

Your doctor may recommend compression stockings. These stockings create gentle pressure up the leg. This pressure keeps blood from pooling and decreases swelling in the legs.

Medical Procedures

Medical procedures are done either to remove varicose veins or to close them. Removing or closing varicose veins usually doesn't cause problems with blood flow because the blood starts moving through other veins.

You may be treated with one or more of the procedures described below. Common side effects right after most of these procedures include bruising, swelling, skin discoloration, and slight pain.

The side effects are most severe with vein stripping and ligation. Rarely, this procedure can cause severe pain, infections, blood clots, and scarring.

Sclerotherapy

Sclerotherapy uses a liquid chemical to close off a varicose vein. The chemical is injected into the vein to cause irritation and scarring inside the vein. The irritation and scarring cause the vein to close off, and it fades away.

This procedure often is used to treat smaller varicose veins and spider veins. It can be done in your doctor's office, while you stand. You may need several treatments to completely close off a vein.

Treatments typically are done every 4 to 6 weeks. Following treatments, your legs will be wrapped in elastic bandaging to help with healing and decrease swelling.

Microsclerotherapy

Microsclerotherapy is used to treat spider veins and other very small varicose veins.

A small amount of liquid chemical is injected into a vein using a very fine needle. The chemical scars the inner lining of the vein, causing it to close off.

Laser Surgery

This procedure applies light energy from a laser onto a varicose vein. The laser light makes the vein fade away.

Laser surgery mostly is used to treat smaller varicose veins. No cutting or injection of chemicals is involved.

Endovenous Ablation Therapy

Endovenous ablation therapy uses lasers or radio waves to create heat to close off a varicose vein.

Your doctor makes a tiny cut in your skin near the varicose vein. He or she then inserts a small tube called a catheter into the vein. A device at the tip of the tube heats up the inside of the vein and closes it off.

You'll be awake during this procedure, but your doctor will numb the area around the vein. You usually can go home the same day as the procedure.

Endoscopic Vein Surgery

For endoscopic vein surgery, your doctor will make a small cut in your skin near a varicose vein. He or she then uses a tiny camera at the end of a thin tube to move through the vein. A surgical device at the end of the camera is used to close the vein.

Endoscopic vein surgery usually is used only in severe cases when varicose veins are causing skin ulcers (sores). After the procedure, you usually can return to your normal activities within a few weeks.

Ambulatory Phlebectomy

For ambulatory phlebectomy, your doctor will make small cuts in your skin to remove small varicose veins. This procedure usually is done to remove the varicose veins closest to the surface of your skin.

You'll be awake during the procedure, but your doctor will numb the area around the vein. Usually, you can go home the same day that the procedure is done.

Vein Stripping and Ligation

Vein stripping and ligation typically is done only for severe cases of varicose veins. The procedure involves tying shut and removing the veins through small cuts in your skin.

You'll be given medicine to temporarily put you to sleep so you don't feel any pain during the procedure.

Vein stripping and ligation usually is done as an outpatient procedure. The recovery time from the procedure is about 1 to 4 weeks.

How Can Varicose Veins Be Prevented?

You can't prevent varicose veins from forming. However, you can prevent the ones you have from getting worse. You also can take steps to delay other varicose veins from forming.

Living with Varicose Veins

Varicose veins are a common condition. They often cause few signs and symptoms. If your signs and symptoms are minor, your doctor may simply suggest making lifestyle changes.

If your condition is more severe—for example, if you have pain, blood clots, or skin ulcers (sores)—your doctor may recommend one or more medical procedures. Many treatments for varicose veins are quick and easy and don't require a long recovery.

Part Six

Additional Help and Information

Chapter 53

Glossary of Terms Related to Blood and Circulatory Disorders

acute lymphoblastic leukemia: A type of leukemia (blood cancer) that comes on quickly and is fast growing. In acute lymphoblastic leukemia, there are too many lymphoblasts (immature white blood cells) in the blood and bone marrow.

angina: A recurring pain or discomfort in the chest that happens when some part of the heart does not receive enough blood.

agranulocyte: A type of white blood cell. Monocytes and lymphocytes are agranulocytes.

albumin: A type of protein found in blood, egg white, milk, and other substances.

angiogenesis: Blood vessel formation. Tumor angiogenesis is the growth of new blood vessels that tumors need to grow.

antibody: A protein found in the blood that is produced in response to foreign substances invading the body.

This glossary contains terms excerpted from documents produced by several sources deemed reliable.

aorta: The largest artery in the body which has its origin at the heart. It gives off branches to the extremities, neck and major organs for the purpose of supplying oxygenated blood.

arteries: Blood vessels that carry oxygen and blood to the heart, brain and other parts of the body.

B cell: A small white blood cell crucial to the immune defenses.

basophil: A white blood cell that contributes to inflammatory reactions.

bilirubin: When the hemoglobin in a person's blood breaks down, causing a yellowing of the skin and whites of the eyes.

blood banking: The process that takes place in the laboratory to ensure that donated blood, or blood products, are safe before they are used in blood transfusions and other medical procedures.

blood clot: A mass of blood that forms when blood platelets, proteins, and cells stick together.

blood plasma: The fluid part of blood that contains nutrients, glucose, proteins, minerals, enzymes, and other substances.

blood pressure: Blood pressure is the force of blood against the walls of arteries.

blood test: A test done on a sample of blood to measure the amount of certain substances in the blood or to count different types of blood cells.

blood thinner: A substance that is used to prevent and treat blood clots in blood vessels and the heart.

blood transfusion: The transfer of blood or blood products from one person (donor) into another person's bloodstream (recipient).

blood vessel: An artery, vein, or capillary that carries blood to and from the heart and body tissues.

cardiovascular diseases: Disease of the heart and blood vessels.

chronic myelogenous leukemia: Chronic myelogenous leukemia is a malignant cancer of the bone marrow that causes rapid growth of the blood forming cells in the bone marrow, peripheral blood, and body tissues.

complete blood count: A blood test that measures the following components in a sample of blood: red blood cells, white blood cells, platelets, and hemoglobin.

connective tissue: The supporting or framework tissue of the body, formed of fibrous and ground substance with more or less numerous cells of various kinds.

diabetes: A disease in which blood glucose (blood sugar) levels are above normal.

diapedesis: Passage of blood cells (especially white blood cells) through intact capillary walls and into the surrounding tissue.

differential: In performing the blood count, a total of 100 cells are counted. The percent of each type found in these 100 cells is the cell "differential" for each type.

emboli: Material, usually blood clot but may be fat, bone fragment, nitrogen bubble or bullet, that travels through the circulation, eventually obstructing blood flow through a smaller calibre vessel.

erythropoietin: A glycoprotein hormone produced primarily by cells of the peritubular capillary endothelium of the kidney that is responsible for the regulation of red blood cell production.

Fanconi anemia: A rare, inherited blood disorder that leads to bone marrow failure. It causes your bone marrow to stop making enough new blood cells for your body to work normally.

gamma globulin: Component of blood serum (plasma) containing antibodies.

hematocrit: Hematocrit is the percentage of the volume of a blood sample occupied by cells, as determined by a centrifuge or device which separates the cells and other particulate elements of the blood from the plasma. The remaining fraction of the blood sample is called plasmocrit (blood plasma volume).

hemorrhage: A copious discharge of blood from the blood vessels.

heparin: A drug given directly into a vein that thins the blood when there is a danger of clotting (an anticoagulant)

immune system: The complex system in the body responsible for fighting disease.

ischemia: decrease in the blood supply to a an organ, tissue, or other part caused by the narrowing or blockage of the blood vessels.

ischemic stroke: A blockage of blood vessels supplying blood to the brain, causing a decrease in blood supply.

lymphocyte: A small white blood cell produced in the lymphoid organs and essential to immune defenses.

lymphocytopenia: An abnormally small number of lymphocytes in the circulating blood.

megakaryocyte: Very large bone marrow cells which release mature blood platelets.

myeloid: A collective term for the non-lymphocyte groups of white blood cells. It includes cells from the granulocyte, monocyte, and platelet lineages.

plasma: The fluid part of blood, lymph, or milk as distinguished from suspended material.

platelet: A cellular fragment critical for blood clotting and sealing off wounds.

pleural effusion: A collection of fluid (or blood) in the pleural space (in one side of the chest cavity around the lung).

serum: The clear liquid that separates from the blood when it is allowed to clot.

sickle cell anemia: It involves problems in the red blood cells. Normal red blood cells are round and smooth and move through blood vessels easily. Sickle cells are hard and have a curved edge. These cells cannot squeeze through small blood vessels. They block the organs from getting blood. Your body destroys sickle red cells quickly, but it can't make new red blood cells fast enough — a condition called anemia.

stem cell: An immature cell from which other cells derive.

T-cells: T-cells are thymus-derived lymphocytes. T-cells are the major component of cell-mediated immunity.

thalassemia: A group of blood diseases, that are inherited, which affect a person's hemoglobin and cause anemia. Hemoglobin is a protein in red blood cells that carries oxygen and nutrients to cells in the body.

transient ischemic attack: a mini-stroke where there is a short-term reduction in blood flow to the brain usually resulting in temporary stoke symptoms. Does not cause damage to the brain, but puts a person at higher risk of having a full stroke.

triglyceride: A type of fat in the blood stream and fat tissue. High triglyceride levels can contribute to the hardening and narrowing of arteries.

vein: A blood vessel that carries blood to the heart from the body tissues.

venous: Venous refers to the system or veins by which blood is returned to the lungs for oxygenation.

Waldenström's macroglobulinemia: Waldenström's macroglobulinemia is a cancer of white blood cells known as B lymphoctyes.

white blood cell: White blood cells are key components of the immune system and help fight infection and disease.

Chapter 54

Directory of Resources Related to Blood and Circulatory Disorders

General

American Society of Hematology
2021 L St. N.W., Ste. 900
Washington, DC 20036
Toll-Free: 866-828-1231
Phone: 202-776-0544
Fax: 202-776-0545
Website: www.hematology.org
E-mail: ash@hematology.org

Iron Disorders Institute
P.O. Box 675
Taylors, SC 29687
Toll-Free: 888-565-IRON
(888-565-4766)
Phone: 864-292-1175
Fax: 864-292-1878
Website: www.irondisorders.org
E-mail: info@irondisorders.org

National Heart, Lung, and Blood Institute (NIILBI)
P.O. Box 30105
Bethesda, MD 20824-0105
Phone: 301-592-8573
TTY: 240-629-3255
Fax: 240-629-3246
Website: www.nhlbi.nih.gov
E-mail: nhlbiinfo@nhlbi.nih.gov

Resources in this chapter were compiled from several sources deemed reliable; all contact information was verified and updated in July 2016.

National Institute of Arthritis and Musculoskeletal and Skin Diseases (NIAMS)
1 AMS Cir.
Bethesda, MD 20892-3675
Toll-Free: 877-22-NIAMS
(877-226-4267)
Phone: 301-495-4484
TTY: 301-565-2966
Fax: 301-718-6366
Website: www.niams.nih.gov
E-mail: NIAMSinfo@mail.nih.gov

National Institute of Diabetes, Digestive, and Kidney Diseases
1 Center Dr., MSC 2560
Bldg. 31, Rm. 9A063
Bethesda, MD 20892-2560
Phone: 301-496-3583
Website: www.niddk.nih.gov

National Organization for Rare Disorders (NORD)
55 Kenosia Ave.
P.O. Box 1968
Danbury, CT 06813–1968
Toll-Free: 800-999-6673
Phone: 203-744-0100
Fax: 203-798-2291
Website: www.rarediseases.org
E-mail: orphan@rarediseases.org

The Nemours Foundation / KidsHealth®
Website: kidshealth.org
E-mail: info@KidsHealth.org

Amyloidosis

Amyloidosis Foundation
7151 N. Main St.
Ste. 2
Clarkston, MI 48346
Toll-Free: 877-AMYLOID
(877-269-5643)
Webiste: www.amyloidosis.org
E-mail: info@amyloidosis.org

Anemia

American Sickle Cell Anemia Association
10900 Carnegie Ave.
Ste. DD1-201
Cleveland, OH 44106
Phone: 216-229-8600
Fax: 216-229-4500
Website: www.ascaa.org
Email: irabragg@ascaa.org

American Society of Hematology
2021 L St. N.W., Ste. 900
Washington, DC 20036
Toll-Free: 866-828-1231
Phone: 202-776-0544
Fax: 202-776-0545
Website: www.hematology.org
E-mail: ash@hematology.org

Aplastic Anemia and MDS International Foundation, Inc.
100 Park Ave., Ste. 108
Rockville, MD 20850
Toll-Free: 800-747-2820
Phone: 301-279-7202
Fax: 301-279-7205
Website: www.aamds.org
E-mail: help@aamds.org

Diamond Blackfan Anemia Foundation, Inc.
P.O. Box 1092
West Seneca, NY 14224
Phone: 716-674-2818
Website: dbafoundation.org
E-mail: dbafoundation@juno.com

Fanconi Anemia Research Fund, Inc.
1801 Willamette St.
Ste. 200
Eugene, OR 97401
Toll-Free: 888-FANCONI
(888-326-2664)
Phone: 541-687-4658
Fax: 541-687-0548
Website: www.fanconi.org
E-mail: info@fanconi.org

National Center for Chronic Disease Prevention and Health Promotion
U.S. Centers for Disease Control and Prevention
4770 Buford Hwy N.E.
MS K–40
Atlanta, GA 30341–3717
Toll-Free: 800-CDC-INFO
(800-232-4636)
TTY: 888-232-6348
Fax: 770-488-5966
Website: www.cdc.gov/nccdphp
E-mail: ccdinfo@cdc.gov

Aneurysms

American Association of Neurological Surgeons
5550 Meadowbrook Dr.
Rolling Meadows, IL 60008-3852
Toll-Free: 888-566-AANS
(888-566-2267)
Phone: 847-378-0500
Fax: 847-378-0600
Website: www.aans.org
E-mail: info@aans.org

American Stroke Association
7272 Greenville Ave.
Dallas, TX 75231-4596
Toll-Free: 888-4STROKE
(888-478-7653)
Fax: 214-706-5231
Website: www.strokeassociation.org
E-mail: strokeinfo@heart.org

The Brain Aneurysm Foundation
269 Hanover St.
Bldg. 3
Hanover, MA 02339
Toll-Free: 888-BRAIN02
(888-272-4602)
Phone: 781-826-5556
Website: www.bafound.org
E-mail: office@bafound.org

**Brain Resources and
Information Network
(BRAIN)**
National Institute of
Neurological Disorders & Stroke
P.O. Box 5801
Bethesda, MD 20824
Toll-Free: 800-352-9424
Phone: 301-496-5751
Fax: 301-402-2186
Website: www.ninds.nih.gov
E-mail: braininfo@ninds.nih.gov

Antiphospholipid Antibody Syndrome

**APS Foundation of America,
Inc.**
P.O. Box 801
LaCrosse, WI 54602-0801
Website: www.apsfa.org

Bleeding and Clotting Disorders

**Foundation for Women and
Girls with Blood Disorders**
P.O. Box 1358
Montclair, New Jersey 07042
Website: www.fwgbd.org
E-mail: ekearns@fwgbd.org

**HHT Foundation
International, Inc.**
P.O. Box 329
Monkton, MD 21111
Toll-Free: 800-448-6389
Phone: 410-357-9932
Fax: 410-357-0655
Website: curehht.org
E-mail: hhtinfo@curehht.org

**National Blood Clot Alliance
(formerly, the National
Alliance for Thrombosis and
Thrombophilia (NATT))**
8321 Old Courthouse Rd., Ste. 255
Vienna, VA 22182
Toll-Free: 877-4NO-CLOT
(877-466-2568)
Phone: 703-935-8845
Website: stoptheclot.org
E-mail: info@stoptheclot.org

Preeclampsia Foundation
6905 N. Wickham Rd., Ste. 302
Melbourne, FL 32940
Toll-Free: 800-665-9341
Phone: 321-421-6957
Fax: 321-821-0450
Website: www.preeclampsia.org
E-mail: info@preeclampsia.org

Blood Donation

**AABB (formerly, the
American Association of
Blood Banks)**
8101 Glenbrook Rd.
Bethesda, MD 20814-2749
Toll-Free: 800-793-9376
Phone: 301-907-6977
Fax: 301-907-6895
Website: www.aabb.org
E-mail: aabb@aabb.org

**American Red Cross
National Headquarters**
2025 E. St. N.W.
Washington, DC 20006
Toll-Free: 800-REDCROSS
(800-733-2767)
Phone: 202-303-4498
Website: www.redcross.org

America's Blood Centers
725 15th St. N.W., Ste. 700
Washington, DC 20005
Phone: 202-393-5725
Fax: 202-393-1282
Website: www.americasblood.org

Bone Marrow Donation and Stem Cell Transplantation

The Center for International Blood and Marrow Transplant Research
9200 W. Wisconsin Ave.
Ste. C5500
Milwaukee, WI 53226
Phone: 414-805-0700
Fax: 414-805-0714
Website: www.cibmtr.org
E-mail: contactus@cibmtr.org

International Society for Stem Cell Research
5215 Old Orchard Rd.
Ste. 270
Skokie, IL 60077
Phone: 224-592-5700
Fax: 224-365-0004
Website: www.isscr.org
E-mail: info@isscr.org

National Marrow Donor Program
500 N. 5th St.
Minneapolis, MN 55401-1206
Toll-Free: 888-999-6743
Phone: 612-627-8140
Website: www.bethematch.org
E-mail: patientinfo@nmdp.org

Circulatory Disorders

American Heart Association
7272 Greenville Ave.
Dallas, TX 75231
Toll-Free: 800-AHA-USA-1
(800-242-8721)
Website: www.americanheart.org

The Erythromelalgia Association
200 Old Castle Ln.
Wallingford, PA 19086
Phone: 610-566-0797
Website: www.erythromelalgia.org

Fibromuscular Dysplasia Association of America (FMDSA)
20325 Center Ridge Rd.
Ste. 360
Rocky River, OH 44116
Toll-Free: 888-709-7089
Phone: 216-834-2410
Website: www.fmdsa.org
E-mail: admin@fmdsa.org

UC Davis Vascular Center
Lawrence J. Ellison Ambulatory Care Center
4860 Y St., Ste. 2100
Sacramento, CA 95817
Toll-Free: 800-2-UCDAVIS
(800-282-3284)
Phone: 916-734-3800
Fax: 916-734-3801
Website: www.ucdmc.ucdavis.edu/vascular
E-mail: vascular.center@ucdmc.ucdavis.edu

Vascular Birthmarks Foundation
P.O. Box 106
Latham, NY 12110
Toll-Free: 877-VBF-4646
(877-823-4646)
Website: www.birthmark.org
E-mail: vbfpresident@gmail.com

Vascular Cures
555 Price Ave.
Ste. 180
Lakewood, CO 80226
Toll-Free: 888-VDF-4INFO
(888-833-4463)
Phone: 303-989-0500
Fax: 303-989-0200
Website: www.vdf.org

Vasculitis Foundation
P.O. Box 28660
Redwood City, CA 94063
Phone: 650-368-6022
Website: www.vascularcures.org
E-mail: info@vascularcures.org

Hemochromatosis

American Hemochromatosis Society, Inc.
P.O. Box 950871
Lake Mary, FL 32795-0871
Toll-Free: 888-655-IRON
(888-655-4766)
Phone: 407-829-4488
Fax: 407-333-1284
Website: www.americanhs.org
E-mail: mail@americanhs.org

American Liver Foundation
75 Maiden Ln.
Ste. 603
New York, NY 10038–4810
Toll-Free: 800-GO-LIVER (800-465-4837) or 888-443-7872
Phone: 212-668-1000
Fax: 212-483-8179
Website: www.liverfoundation.org
E-mail: info@liverfoundation.org

Hemophilia

Children's Cancer & Blood Foundation
333 E. 38th St.
Ste. 830
New York, NY 10016-2745
Phone: 212-297-4336
Fax: 212-297-4340
Website: www.childrenscbf.org
E-mail: info@childrenscbf.org

The Coalition for Hemophilia B
825 Third Ave.
2nd Fl.
New York, NY 10022
Phone: 212-520-8272
Fax: 212-520-8501
Website: www.hemob.org
E-mail: contact@hemob.org

Hemophilia Federation of America
820 First St. N.E., St. 720
Toll-Free: 800-230-9797
Phone: 202-675-6984
Website: www.hemophiliafed.org
E-mail: info@hemophiliafed.org

*National Hemophilia
Foundation*
116 W. 32nd St.
11th Fl.
New York, NY 10001
Toll-Free: 800-424-2634
Phone: 212-328-3700
Fax: 212-328-3799
Website: www.hemophilia.org
E-mail: handi@hemophilia.org

*World Federation of
Hemophilia*
1425 René Lévesque Blvd. W.
Ste. 1010
Montreal, Quebec
H3G 1T7
Canada
Phone: 514-875-7944
Fax: 514-875-8916
Website: www.wfh.org
E-mail: wfh@wfh.org

Leukemia

American Cancer Society
250 Williams St. N.W.
Atlanta, GA, 30303
Toll-Free: 800-ACS-2345
(800-227-2345)
TTY: 866-228-4327
Website: www.cancer.org

*Leukemia and Lymphoma
Society*
3 International Dr., Ste. 200
Rye Brook, NY 10573
Toll-Free: 800-955-4572
Phone: 914-949-5213
Fax: 914-949-6691
Website: www.lls.org
E-mail: info@lls.org

*Leukemia Research
Foundation*
191 Waukegan Rd., Ste. 105
Northfield, IL 60093
Phone: 847-424-0600
Fax: 847-424-0606
Website: www.allbloodcancers.
org

National Cancer Institute
9609 Medical Center Dr.
BG 9609 MSC 9760
Bethesda, MD 20892-9760
Toll-Free: 800-4-CANCER
(800-422-6237)
Website: www.cancer.gov

Myeloproliferative Disorders

MPN Research Foundation
180 N. Michigan Ave., Ste. 1870
Chicago, IL 60601
Toll-Free: 855-258-1943
Phone: 312-683-7249
Fax: 312-332-0840
Website: www.
mpnresearchfoundation.org

*Myelodysplastic Syndromes
Foundation*
4573 S. Broad St.
Ste. 150
Yardville, NJ 08620
Toll-Free: 800-MDS-0839
(800-637-0839)
Phone: 609-298-1035
Fax: 609-298-0590
Website: www.mds-foundation.
org
E-mail: patientliaison@mds-
foundation.org

Plasma Cell Disorders

The Amyloidosis Center
Boston University School of
Medicine
72 E. Concord St., K-503
Boston, MA 02118
Toll-Free: 800-841-4325
Phone: 617-638-4317
Fax: 617-638-4493
Website: www.bu.edu/amyloid
E-mail: amyloid@bu.edu

Amyloidosis Foundation, Inc.
7151 N. Main St., Ste. 208
Clarkston, MI 48346
Toll-Free: 877-AMYLOID
(877-269-5643)
Phone: 248-922-9610
Fax: 248-922-9620
Website: www.amyloidosis.org

International Waldenstrom's
Macroglobulinemia
Foundation (IWMF)
6144 Clark Center Ave.
Sarasota, FL 34238
Phone: 941-927-4963
Fax: 941-927-4467
Website: www.themmrf.org
E-mail: info@themmrf.org

Multiple Myeloma Research
Foundation (MMRF)
383 Main Ave.
5th Fl.
Norwalk, CT 06851
Phone: 203-229-0464
Fax: 203-972-1259
Website: www.multiplemyeloma.
org
E-mail: info@themmrf.org

Sickle Cell Disease

Sickle Cell Disease Asso-
ciation of America, Inc.
3700 Koppers St.
Ste. 570
Baltimore, MD 21227
Toll-Free: 800-421-8453
Phone: 410-528-1555
Fax: 410-528-1495
Website: www.sicklecelldisease.
org
E-mail: scdaa@sicklecelldisease.
org

Sickle Cell Information
Center
201 Dowman Dr.
Atlanta, Georgia 30322
Phone: 404-727-7857
Website: scholarblogs.emory.edu
E-mail: aplatt@emory.edu

White Blood Cell Disorders

American Partnership For
Eosinophilic Disorders
P.O. Box 29545
Atlanta, GA 30359
Phone: 713-493-7749
Fax: 713-493-7749
Website: www.apfed.org
E-mail: mail@apfed.org

Campaign Urging Research
for Eosinophilic Disease
(CURED)
P.O. Box 32
Lincolnshire, IL 60069
Website: www.curedfoundation.
org

Center for Pediatric Eosinophilic Disorders
Children's Hospital of
Philadelphia
34th St. and Civic Center Blvd.
Philadelphia, PA 19104
Toll-Free: 800-879-2467
Phone: 267-426-7003
Website: www.chop.edu/centers-programs/center-pediatric-eosinophilic-disorders

Neutropenia Support Association Inc.
971 Corydon Ave.
P.O. Box 243
Winnipeg, Manitoba
R3M 3S7
Canada
Toll-Free: 1-800-6-NEUTRO
(1-800-663-8876)
Phone: 204-489-8454
Website: www.neutropenia.ca

Index

Index